Sleep

Guest Editors

H. KLAR YAGGI, MD, MPH
TEOFILO L. LEE CHIONG Jr, MD
VAHID MOHSENIN, MD

CLINICS IN
CHEST MEDICINE

www.chestmed.theclinics.com

June 2010 • Volume 31 • Number 2

SAUNDERS an imprint of ELSEVIER, Inc.

W.B. SAUNDERS COMPANY
A Division of Elsevier Inc.

1600 John F. Kennedy Boulevard • Suite 1800 • Philadelphia, Pennsylvania 19103

http://www.theclinics.com

CLINICS IN CHEST MEDICINE Volume 31, Number 2
June 2010 ISSN 0272-5231, ISBN-13: 978-1-4377-1805-8

Editor: Sarah E. Barth
Developmental Editor: Theresa Collier

Clinics in Chest Medicine (ISSN 0272-5231) is published quarterly by Elsevier Inc., 360 Park Avenue South, New York, NY 10010-1710. Months of issue are March, June, September, and December. Periodicals postage paid at New York, NY and additional mailing offices. Subscription prices are $274.00 per year (domestic individuals), $432.00 per year (domestic institutions), $133.00 per year (domestic students/residents), $300.00 per year (Canadian individuals), $530.00 per year (Canadian institutions), $373.00 per year (international individuals), $530.00 per year (international institutions), and $186.00 per year (international and Canadian students/residents). International air speed delivery is included in all Clinics subscription prices. All prices are subject to change without notice. **POSTMASTER:** Send address changes to Clinics in Chest Medicine, Elsevier Health Sciences Division, Subscription Customer Service, 3251 Riverport Lane, Maryland Heights, MO 63043. **Customer Service: Telephone: 1-800-654-2452** (U.S. and Canada); **1-314-447-8871** (outside U.S. and Canada). **Fax: 1-314-447-8029. E-mail: journalscustomerservice-usa@elsevier.com** (for print support); **journalsonlinesupport-usa@elsevier.com** (for online support).

Reprints. For copies of 100 or more of articles in this publication, please contact the Commercial Reprints Department, Elsevier Inc., 360 Park Avenue South, New York, NY 10010-1710. Tel.: 212-633-3812; Fax: 212-462-1935; E-mail: reprints@elsevier.com.

Clinics in Chest Medicine is covered in *MEDLINE/PubMed (Index Medicus), Current Contents/Clinical Medicine, EMBASE/ Excerpta Medica, Science Citation Index,* and *ISI/BIOMED.*

Printed and bound by CPI Group (UK) Ltd, Croydon, CR0 4YY

Transferred to Digital Print 2011

Contributors

GUEST EDITORS

H. KLAR YAGGI, MD, MPH
Assistant Professor of Medicine, Division of Pulmonary and Critical Care Medicine, Yale University School of Medicine, New Haven; Director, West Haven VA Medical Center Sleep Laboratory, VA CT Health Care System, Clinical Epidemiology Research Center, West Haven, Connecticut

TEOFILO L. LEE CHIONG Jr, MD
Professor of Medicine, Division of Sleep Medicine, Department of Medicine, National Jewish Health, Denver, Colorado

VAHID MOHSENIN, MD
Professor, Department of Medicine, Yale University School of Medicine; Director, Yale Center for Sleep Medicine, New Haven, Connecticut

AUTHORS

IMRAN AHMED, MD
Assistant Professor of Neurology, Montefiore Medical Center, Albert Einstein College of Medicine; Neurology Department, Sleep-Wake Disorders Center, Bronx, New York

ALON Y. AVIDAN, MD, MPH
Associate Professor of Neurology; Neurology Residency Program Director; Director, UCLA Neurology Clinic; and Associate Director, Sleep Disorders Center, Department of Neurology, University of California Los Angeles, Los Angeles, California

LEE K. BROWN, MD
Professor of Internal Medicine and Pediatrics and Vice Chair, Clinical Program Development, Division of Pulmonary, Critical Care and Sleep Medicine, Department of Internal Medicine, University of New Mexico School of Medicine; Program in Sleep Medicine, University of New Mexico Health Sciences Center, Albuquerque, New Mexico

CAROLYN M. D'AMBROSIO, MD
Division of Pulmonary Diseases, Department of Medicine, Tufts-New England Medical Center; Division of Pulmonary Diseases, Department of Medicine, Tufts Medical School, Boston, Massachusetts

KARL DOGHRAMJI, MD
Professor of Psychiatry and Human Behavior, Professor of Medicine, Associate Professor of Neurology, Medical Director, Jefferson Sleep Disorders Center; Program Director, Fellowship in Sleep Medicine, Thomas Jefferson University, Philadelphia, Pennsylvania

NEIL FREEDMAN, MD, FCCP
Pulmonary Physicians of the North Shore, Bannockburn, Illinois; Sleep Institute Steering Committee Member of the American College of Chest Physicians, Chicago, Illinois

CHARLENE E. GAMALDO, MD
Assistant Professor of Neurology, Johns Hopkins Sleep Disorders Center at Johns Hopkins Hospital, Johns Hopkins School of Medicine, Baltimore, Maryland

JOHN HARRINGTON, MD
Assistant Professor, Division of Sleep Medicine, Department of Medicine, National Jewish Health, Denver, Colorado

MARY S.M. IP, MD
Chair Professor, Division of Respiratory Medicine, and Critical Care Medicine, Department of Medicine, Queen Mary Hospital, The University of Hong Kong, Hong Kong Special Administrative Region, Hong Kong, People's Republic of China

BEHROUZ JAFARI, MD
Senior Fellow, Section of Pulmonary,
Critical Care and Sleep Medicine,
Yale Center for Sleep Medicine,
Yale University School of Medicine,
New Haven, Connecticut

S. JAVAHERI, MD
Emeritus Professor, Department of Medicine,
University of Cincinnati College of Medicine;
Medical Director, Sleepcare Diagnostics,
Mason, Ohio

NAVEEN KANATHUR, MD
Professor, Division of Sleep Medicine,
Department of Medicine, National Jewish
Health, Denver, Colorado

NEERAJ KAPLISH, MD
Clinical Lecturer, Department of Neurology,
University of Michigan, Ann Arbor, Michigan

ELIOT S. KATZ, MD
Division of Respiratory Diseases, Department
of Medicine, Children's Hospital, Boston;
Division of Respiratory Diseases, Department
of Pediatrics, Harvard Medical School, Boston,
Massachusetts

MEIR H. KRYGER, MD
Clinical Professor of Medicine, University of
Connecticut School of Medicine, Farmington,
Connecticut; Director of Research and
Education, Gaylord Sleep Medicine,
Wallingford, Connecticut

SAMUEL T. KUNA, MD
Chief, Pulmonary, Critical Care and Sleep
Medicine Section, Department of Medicine,
Philadelphia VA Medical Center; Associate
Professor of Medicine, Division of Pulmonary,
Allergy and Critical Care Medicine, Department
of Medicine, University of Pennsylvania,
Philadelphia, Pennsylvania

TEOFILO LEE-CHIONG Jr, MD
Professor of Medicine, Division of Sleep
Medicine, Department of Medicine, National
Jewish Health, Denver, Colorado

BRANDON S. LU, MD, MS
Department of Medicine, California Pacific
Medical Center, San Francisco, California

MACY M.S. Lui, MRCP
Medical Officer, Division of Respiratory
Medicine, and Critical Care Medicine,
Department of Medicine, Queen Mary Hospital,
The University of Hong Kong, Hong Kong
Special Administrative Region, Hong Kong,
People's Republic of China

VAHID MOHSENIN, MD
Professor of Medicine and Director, Yale
Center for Sleep Medicine, Yale University
School of Medicine, New Haven, Connecticut

RUSSELL RASQUINHA, MSE
Research Coordinator, Department of
Biomedical Engineering, Johns Hopkins
University, Baltimore, Maryland

FRANCOISE J. ROUX, MD, PhD
Assistant Professor of Medicine, Section of
Pulmonary and Critical Care Medicine; Yale
Center for Sleep Medicine, Yale University
School of Medicine, New Haven, Connecticut

RACHEL E. SALAS, MD
Assistant Professor of Neurology, Division of
Pulmonary and Critical Care, Johns Hopkins
Sleep Disorders Center at Johns Hopkins
Hospital, Johns Hopkins School of Medicine,
Baltimore, Maryland

BERNARDO SELIM, MD
Post Doctoral Fellow, Division of Pulmonary
and Critical Care Medicine, Yale University
School of Medicine, New Haven, Connecticut

KINGMAN P. STROHL, MD
Professor, Department of Medicine, Case
Western Reserve School of Medicine, Director
of the Center for Sleep Education and
Research, Cleveland, Ohio

BERNIE SUNWOO, BSc(Med), MBBS
Fellow, Division of Pulmonary, Allergy and
Critical Care Medicine, Department of
Medicine, Hospital of the University of
Pennsylvania, Philadelphia, Pennsylvania

SHEILA C. TSAI, MD
Assistant Professor of Medicine, Department
of Internal Medicine, Division of Sleep
Medicine, National Jewish Health, University of
Colorado, Denver School of Medicine, Denver,
Colorado

MICHAEL THORPY, MD
Professor, Neurology, Montefiore Medical
Center, Albert Einstein College of Medicine;
Director, Neurology Department,
Sleep-Wake Disorders Center, Bronx,
New York

CHRISTINE WON, MD
Assistant Professor of Medicine, Division of
Pulmonary and Critical Care Medicine, Yale
University School of Medicine, New Haven,
Connecticut

H. KLAR YAGGI, MD, MPH
Assistant Professor of Medicine, Division of
Pulmonary and Critical Care Medicine, Yale
University School of Medicine, New Haven;
Director, West Haven VA Medical Center Sleep
Laboratory, VA CT Health Care System,
Clinical Epidemiology Research Center, West
Haven, Connecticut

PHYLLIS C. ZEE, MD, PhD
Professor, Department of Neurology,
Northwestern University, Chicago, Illinois

MICHAEL THORPY, MD
Professor, Neurology, Montefiore Medical
Center, Albert Einstein College of Medicine;
Director, Neurology Department,
Sleep-Wake Disorders Center, Bronx,
New York

CHRISTINE WON, MD
Assistant Professor of Medicine, Division of
Pulmonary and Critical Care Medicine, Yale
University School of Medicine, New Haven,
Connecticut

HKLAR YAGGI, MD, MPH
Assistant Professor of Medicine, Division of
Pulmonary and Critical Care Medicine, Yale
University School of Medicine, New Haven;
Director, West Haven VA Medical Center Sleep
Laboratory, VA CT Health Care System;
Clinical Epidemiology Research Center, West
Haven, Connecticut

PHYLLIS C. ZEE, MD, PhD
Professor, Department of Neurology,
Northwestern University, Chicago, Illinois

Contents

The objectives of this article are to (1) understand how respiratory event definitions and syndrome threshold values affect prevalence estimates of obstructive sleep apnea in adults, (2) recognize important risk factors for obstructive sleep apnea in adults, and (3) understand current theories of the underlying mechanisms for airway obstruction during sleep.

Several treatment options are available for obstructive sleep apnea syndrome (OSAS), including various types of positive airway pressure (PAP) therapy, oral appliances, surgery, and conservative approaches including weight loss and positional therapy. This article focuses on continuous positive airway pressure treatment and technological advancements in the delivery of PAP therapy for OSAS, reviews indications for treatment, treatment outcomes, and methods of improving compliance, and discusses the other non-PAP treatment options.

Cardiovascular disease has been the leading cause of death since 1900. Strategies for cardiovascular disease and prevention have helped to reduce the burden of disease, but it remains an important public health challenge. Therefore, understanding the underlying pathophysiology and developing novel therapeutic approaches for cardiovascular disease is of crucial importance. Recognizing the link between sleep and cardiovascular disease may represent one such novel approach. Obstructive sleep apnea (OSA), a common form of sleep-disordered breathing, has a high and rising prevalence in the general adult population, attributable in part to the emerging epidemic of obesity and enhanced awareness. OSA has been independently linked to specific cardiovascular outcomes such as hypertension, stroke, myocardial ischemia, arrhythmias, fatal and nonfatal cardiovascular events, and all-cause mortality. Treatment of OSA may represent a novel target to reduce cardiovascular health outcomes.

Obstructive sleep apnea syndrome (OSAS) is a common and serious cause of metabolic, cardiovascular, and neurocognitive morbidity in children. Children with OSAS have increased upper airway resistance during sleep due to a combination of soft tissue hypertrophy, craniofacial dysmorphology, neuromuscular weakness, or obesity. Consequently, children with OSAS encounter a combination of oxidative stress, inflammation, autonomic activation, and disruption of sleep homeostasis. The threshold amount of OSAS associated with adverse consequences varies widely among children, depending on genetic and environmental factors. The choice of therapy is predicated on the etiology, severity, and natural history of the increased upper airway resistance.

Central apnea is caused by temporary failure in the pontomedullary pacemaker generating breathing rhythm, which results in the loss of ventilatory effort, and if it lasts 10 seconds or more it is defined as central apnea. This article reviews current knowledge on central sleep apnea.

A wide variety of mechanisms can lead to the hypoventilation associated with various medical disorders, including derangements in central ventilatory control, mechanical impediments to breathing, and abnormalities in gas exchange leading to increased dead space ventilation. The pathogenesis of hypercapnia in obesity hypoventilation syndrome remains somewhat obscure, although in many patients comorbid obstructive sleep apnea appears to play an important role. Hypoventilation in neurologic or neuromuscular disorders is primarily explained by weakness of respiratory muscles, although some central nervous system diseases may affect control of breathing. In other chest wall disorders, obstructive airways disease, and cystic fibrosis, much of the pathogenesis is explained by mechanical impediments to breathing, but an element of increased dead space ventilation also often occurs. Central alveolar hypoventilation syndrome involves a genetically determined defect in central respiratory control. Treatment in all of these disorders involves coordinated management of the primary disorder (when possible) and, increasingly, the use of noninvasive positive pressure ventilation.

Despite proliferating literature, the exact relationship between obstructive sleep apnea (OSA) and alterations in glucose metabolism is still controversial. There is growing evidence to suggest that OSA imposes adverse effects on glucose metabolism, but the translation into clinical effect is not well delineated. Many potential mechanisms are being explored, mostly relating to peripheral tissue response to insulin and more recently regarding pancreatic β cell function of insulin secretion. The effect of OSA on glucose metabolism is likely to be influenced by many personal characteristics. Age, degree of adiposity, lifestyle, comorbidities, and even the stage of glucose disorder itself may modify the relationship between OSA and glucose metabolism. In the biologic system of the human body, all these interact to culminate in clinically relevant outcomes.

Section II: Testing

Polysomnography (PSG) is an essential tool for diagnosis of a variety of sleep disorders. The results of PSG should be interpreted in the context of a patient's history and medications and observation in the sleep laboratory. As new technologies evolve, it is expected that the field will evolve. Further work is needed to determine if computerized scoring, with or without human revision, may reliably replace visual scoring in normal and abnormal sleep. Improved techniques to measure and quantify sleep itself will allow for more meaningful assessment of sleep disruption that can lead to the recognition of new disorders and better predictions of the outcomes of these disorders.

Portable monitor testing is being increasingly used as an alternative strategy for the diagnosis and treatment of patients with obstructive sleep apnea. Portable monitors have become progressively sophisticated but lack standardization. Recent studies comparing clinical outcomes of ambulatory management pathways using portable monitor testing support their use in patients with a high pretest probability for obstructive sleep apnea. Whether ambulatory management is cost-effective and will improve patient access to diagnosis and treatment requires further investigation.

Section III: Non Pulmonary Sleep Medicine

The neurobiology of sleep is introduced in the context of interacting wake and sleep systems. Specifically, the transitions from wake to sleep and from non-rapid eye movement to rapid eye movement sleep are discussed based on the flip-flop switch hypothesis. Regulation of wake and sleep according to the opposing homeostatic and circadian systems are also presented.

Because there is insufficient cellular energy for organisms to perform their functions at the same constant rate and at the same time, all biologic processes show rhythmicity, each with its own unique frequency, amplitude, and phase. Optimal sleep and wakefulness requires proper timing and alignment of desired sleep-wake schedules and circadian rhythm-related periods of alertness. Persistent or recurrent mismatch between endogenous circadian rhythms and the conventional sleep-wake schedules of the environmental day can give rise to several circadian rhythm sleep disorders. Evaluation of suspected circadian rhythm sleep disorders requires proper monitoring of sleep diaries, often over several days to weeks. This article discusses the disorders of the circadian sleep-wake cycle and the therapeutic measures to correct the same.

Insomnia is a highly prevalent malady and adversely affects many dimensions of daily human function. Although its pathophysiology is poorly understood, it seems to arise in the context of heightened arousal in neurophysiologic and psychological systems. Because it often coexists with a wide variety of medical and psychiatric conditions, the first task in the management of this condition is to identify comorbid disorders through a comprehensive evaluation. Once identified, specific treatments can be tailored to the underlying conditions. Effective cognitive/behavioral and pharmacologic management techniques are available for primary insomnia.

providers are able to recognize these conditions to accurately diagnose, manage, and appropriately refer patients.

Medication Effects on Sleep   397

Francoise J. Roux and Meir H. Kryger

The understanding of the neuropharmacologic reciprocal interactions between the sleep and wake cycles has progressed significantly in the past decade. It was also recently appreciated that sleep disruption or deprivation can have adverse metabolic consequences. Multiple medications have a direct or indirect impact on sleep and the waking state. This article reviews how commonly prescribed medications can significantly affect the sleep-wake cycle.

Clinics in Chest Medicine

ISSUES OF RELATED INTEREST

Sleep Medicine Clinics Volume 5, Issue 1 (March 2010)
Dentistry's Role in Sleep Medicine
Edited by Dennis R. Bailey

THE CLINICS ARE NOW AVAILABLE ONLINE!

Access your subscription at:
www.theclinics.com

Preface

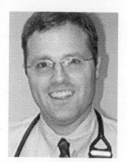
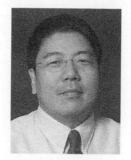
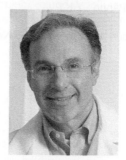

H. Klar Yaggi, MD, MPH   Teofilo L. Lee Chiong Jr, MD   Vahid Mohsenin, MD
Guest Editors

This is the fifth issue of *Clinics in Chest Medicine* dedicated to sleep disorders. Since the first issue was published 25 years ago, the care of patients with sleep-disordered breathing has become a major part of the day-to-day practice of pulmonary medicine. Competency in sleep disorders is now a required component of pulmonary training programs. We envision this issue as a primer for pulmonary/critical care physicians in training and an update for consultants in practice.

Over the past several years, there been significant advances made in sleep medicine. Prospective cohort studies and randomized trials have provided significant insight into the morbidity and mortality of sleep-disordered breathing and the benefits of treatment, respectively. There have been significant technologic advances made in the ways in which positive airway pressure is delivered for the treatment of various types of sleep-disordered breathing. There are new scoring rules for overnight polysomnography and new technologies now in use for the ambulatory monitoring of sleep in patients' homes.

With regard to content, there is appropriate emphasis on sleep-disordered breathing with state-of-the-art articles on adult and pediatric sleep apnea, treatment of sleep-disordered breathing, central sleep apnea, hypoventilation syndromes, and the cardiovascular and metabolic consequences of sleep-disordered breathing. We have also included 2 articles on monitoring, providing an update on the scoring of polysomnography and an overview of ambulatory sleep studies. Finally, we have selected several common nonpulmonary topics in sleep medicine to be reviewed: neurobiology of sleep, circadian rhythms disorders, insomnia, disorders of excessive daytime sleepiness, parasomnias, narcolepsy, movement disorders (restless legs syndrome and periodic limb movement disorder), and medication effects on sleep. The reason for this inclusion is that patients who are referred to pulmonary consultants for sleep-disordered breathing may have a nonpulmonary disorder. The knowledge gained from the reviews will help to facilitate appropriate referrals and care.

We wish to extend our sincere gratitude to the outstanding authors who have generously provided an array of excellent manuscripts. We are especially indebted to Sarah Barth and the editorial staff at Elsevier for bringing this project to fruition.

H. Klar Yaggi, MD, MPH
Division of Pulmonary and Critical Care Medicine
Yale University School of Medicine
333 Cedar Street, PO Box 208057
New Haven, CT 06520-8057, USA
West Haven VA Medical Center Sleep Laboratory
VA CT Health Care System Clinical
Epidemiology Research Center
950 Campbell Avenue
West Haven, CT 06516, USA

Teofilo L. Lee Chiong Jr, MD
Division of Sleep Medicine
Department of Medicine
National Jewish Health, 1400 Jackson Street
Denver, CO 80206, USA

Vahid Mohsenin, MD
Department of Medicine
Yale University School of Medicine
Yale Center for Sleep Medicine
New Haven, CT, USA

E-mail addresses:
henry.yaggi@yale.edu (H.K. Yaggi)
Lee-ChiongT@NJHealth.org (T.L. Lee Chiong)
vahid.mohsenin@yale.edu (V. Mohsenin)

Clin Chest Med 31 (2010) xiii–xiv
doi:10.1016/j.ccm.2010.03.003

Dedication

To Seonaid, Maddy, and Anna - HKY
To Mary Lau Ngo - TLC
To my wife Shahla and our children Amir and Neda - VM

Adult Obstructive Sleep Apnea/ Hypopnea Syndrome: Definitions, Risk Factors, and Pathogenesis

H. Klar Yaggi, MD, MPH[a,b],*, Kingman P. Strohl, MD[c]

KEYWORDS
- Epidemiology • Obstructive sleep apnea syndrome
- Pathogenesis • Risk factors

DEFINITIONS

The *International Classification of Sleep Disorders, Second Edition (ICSD-2)* classifies sleep-related breathing disorders into 3 basic categories: central sleep apnea syndrome, obstructive sleep apnea (OSA) syndrome, and sleep-related hypoventilation/hypoxic syndrome. In this classification, the term "upper airway resistance syndrome" is subsumed under the diagnosis of OSA because the pathophysiology is so similar to that of OSA. Sleep apnea is termed "obstructive" when respiratory effort is present and "central" or "nonobstructive" when this effort is absent. OSA, which is the focus of this article, is decidedly more prevalent and amenable to treatments that are directed at increasing the size of the upper airway. Clinical disease is characterized by repetitive airflow cessation (apnea) or reduction (hypopnea). The onset of an obstructive apnea occurs when forces promoting airway collapse overcome mechanisms that maintain airway patency.

An apnea is defined as the cessation of airflow for 10 seconds or longer using a valid measure of airflow; this time criteria represents approximately 2.5 cycles of normal respiration. Unlike the definition of apnea that has remained consistent over time, the definition of hypopnea has shifted over time to represent the measurable features of partial upper airway obstruction. This, in part, is a reflection of the fact that this event involves identification of a subtle reduction in airflow. A consensus conference (Chicago Criteria) provided a definition of hypopnea as including 1 of 3 features: a substantial reduction in airflow (>50%), a moderate reduction in airflow (<50%) with desaturation (>3%), or a moderate reduction in airflow (<50%) with electroencephalographic evidence of arousal.[1] Subsequently, population studies addressed various operational definitions of hypopnea. The Sleep Heart Health Study (SHHS), a large cohort study designed to relate cardiovascular disease with polysomnographic findings, defined hypopnea as a 30% decrease (from baseline) in airflow or chest wall movement for at least 10 seconds, accompanied by an oxygen desaturation of 4% or greater.[2] This definition is accompanied by a high degree of

[a] Division of Pulmonary and Critical Care Medicine, Yale University School of Medicine, 333 Cedar Street, PO Box 208057, New Haven, CT 06520-8057, USA
[b] West Haven VA Medical Center Sleep Laboratory, VA CT Health Care System, Clinical Epidemiology Research Center, 950 Campbell Avenue, West Haven, CT 06516, USA
[c] Department of Medicine, Case Western Reserve School of Medicine, Center for Sleep Education and Research, 11100 Euclid Avenue, Cleveland, OH 44106-6003, USA
* Corresponding author. Division of Pulmonary and Critical Care Medicine, Yale University School of Medicine, 333 Cedar Street, PO Box 208057, New Haven, CT 06520-8057.
E-mail address: henry.yaggi@yale.edu

Clin Chest Med 31 (2010) 179–186
doi:10.1016/j.ccm.2010.02.011
0272-5231/10/$ – see front matter © 2010 Published by Elsevier Inc.

interscorer reliability and pathophysiologic consequences.

An analysis of more than 5000 records from the SHHS underscores the effect of various hypopnea definitions. This analysis showed that the magnitude of the median apnea-hypopnea index (AHI) could vary 10 fold (ie, 29.3 when the AHI was based on events identified on the basis of flow or volume amplitude alone vs 2 for an AHI that required an associated 5% desaturation with events).[3] Varying thresholds for polysomnographic summary data also resulted in marked differences in the percentage of subjects classified as diseased. For example, using an AHI cutoff value of greater than 15 and requiring a 5% level of desaturation resulted in a prevalence estimate of 10.8. In contrast, almost the entire cohort was affected when sleep-disordered breathing (SDB) was defined using an AHI threshold value of 5 and when all hypopneas were scored regardless of associated corroborative physiologic changes. To add to the complexity of scoring clinical records, there are events called respiratory effort–related arousals (RERAs), whereby arousals are identified in the setting of heavy snoring without hypoxemia or discernible reductions in airflow; these events contribute to clinical presentations because their elimination improves symptoms.[1] Thus, there is a need for standardization across laboratories and research protocols, not necessarily to determine an individual severity but to facilitate multicenter trials and recommendations for therapy as determined by laboratory-based disease severity.

The most widely used severity criteria use "cutoffs" based on the frequency of apnea and hypopnea events. By consensus, mild sleep apnea has been defined as an AHI (number of apneas and hypopneas/hour of sleep) of 5 to 15 events per hour, moderate as greater than 15 to 30 events per hour, and severe as greater than 30 events per hour.[1] A similar measure called respiratory disturbance index (RDI) not only is based on flow, desaturations, and arousals but also uses RERAs. Most epidemiologic studies have used the AHI or RDI almost interchangeably as the single polysomnographic-derived measurement when testing the association between OSA and cardiovascular complications. However, other unidimensional indices, such as (among others) the severity of oxygen desaturation or arousal index (number of arousals per hour), are not captured by AHI. The current severity criteria based on AHI or RDI also correlate only loosely with symptom or clinical severity.[4] Furthermore, investigators have questioned whether the AHI alone is the best predictor for outcomes such as survival, cardiovascular events, or incident hypertension and metabolic dysfunction.[5,6] Available evidence supports a need to standardize these other dimensions; for example, recurrence of atrial fibrillation among OSAs may not be best predicted by the AHI but rather by the severity of nocturnal hypoxemia.[7]

PREVALENCE

According to the first major US population-based study conducted about 15 years ago, when AHI criteria based on thermistor measures of airflow are applied to a general population of middle-aged adults, 24% of men and 9% of women meet criteria for OSA.[8] These prevalence figures are based on a cutoff AHI of 5 or higher. Most of these patients (>50%) had mild sleep apnea according to current criteria. If the symptom of sleepiness is included as part of a syndromic definition (OSA syndrome), 4% of men and 2% of women meet criteria in this 1993 study. From this study and subsequent studies, more than 75% of patients with OSA are undiagnosed or untreated.[8] In view of the epidemic increase of obesity (an important determinant of OSA) in the US population since 1993, these numbers are an underestimate that the current prevalence figures. Recent results from the National Sleep Foundation *Sleep in America 2005 Poll* containing a validated instrument used to identify individuals at risk for sleep apnea, using a composite score from self-reports (the Berlin Questionnaire), indicated that as many as 1 in 4 American adults met criteria for a high pretest probability risk for OSA.[9] Not all of these individuals need definitive testing or direct therapy; however, the pool of people who could be considered at risk for OSA from a population perspective is large and perhaps more importantly at risk for its behavioral and cardiovascular consequences.

Risk Factors in Clinical Assessments

Despite the numerous advancements in the understanding and the pathogenesis and clinical consequences of OSA, great majority of patients (approximately 70%–80%) remain undiagnosed.[10] Case identification is confounded in part by the fact that patients are often unaware of the importance of associated symptoms even if they can frequently be identified by a bed partner or family member. Public knowledge of risk factors along with physician awareness needs to be addressed to inform appropriate diagnostic attention and case finding in the future.

Sex

Men are at higher risk for the development of sleep apnea; however, the effect is modest. Some of the early (largely clinic-based) studies suggested that there was a 5- to 8-fold increased risk for sleep apnea among men compared with women.[11] Subsequent population-based studies have shown this magnitude of risk to be closer to 2 to 3 fold higher among men.[8,12] These studies indicate that one does not have to be a man to have sleep apnea, but it helps. This difference between early clinic-based and population-based estimates not only relates in part to patient presentations but also may reflect differences in how women and men perceive and report symptoms of SDB. Although a prototypical male patient with sleep apnea tends to present with excessive daytime sleepiness, unrefreshing sleep, and loud snoring, community-based studies of women (which included women with significant sleep apnea) suggest that women are less likely to endorse these classic symptoms of sleep apnea and more likely to report symptoms of daytime fatigue, morning headache, and mood disturbance.[13,14] If women are less likely to report classic symptoms of sleep apnea, they are less likely to be referred to sleep clinics for evaluation and, therefore, may be underrepresented in clinic-based studies and lead down alternative diagnostic pathways.[13] Alternatively, the disease process may be different, requiring alternative case funding and assessments for risk and response to therapy.

Well-designed population-based studies confirm a clear increased expression of objectively measured SDB among men compared with women. Studies examining this difference have focused on hormonal differences. In women, a strong predictor of sleep apnea is menopausal status. Bixler and colleagues[12] found a nearly 4-fold increased risk of sleep apnea (AHI $\geq$ 5) among postmenopausal women compared with premenopausal women. Similar results were seen in the Wisconsin Sleep Cohort Study in which such an increased risk was seen even after adjusting for the confounding effects of age and body fat distribution.[15] In addition, the SHHS demonstrated a lower prevalence of sleep apnea among postmenopausal women who were taking hormone replacement therapy (HRT), compared with those who were not, implicating a potential protective effect of HRT.

In addition to the differences in event prevalence, the severity of sleep apnea and its occurrence in sleep stages may differ between men and women. There seems to be, on average, a decrease in number and shorter duration of apneic events in women compared with men.[16] Women tend to have a higher percentage of rapid eye movement (REM)–related apneas and hypopneas and are more likely to have sleep apnea that occurs entirely during REM sleep, an effect more prominent in younger populations.[17] In addition, one study suggests that women may be more symptomatic at a lower severity of sleep apnea,[18] and a proposed mechanism is the clustering of events within and hence disruption of REM sleep.

Other hypotheses for the gender differences in sleep apnea have included differences in airway caliber and compliance,[19] soft tissue structure,[20] genioglossal activity,[21] and regional fat distribution[22] (with men more likely to have upper body fat distribution and women more likely to have lower body fat deposition).

Excess weight and measures of obesity

Epidemiologic studies in the United States and Europe have consistently identified body weight as the strongest risk factor for OSA, and there seems to be little controversy regarding the causal associations seen in observational studies. In the Wisconsin Cohort Study, a 10% weight gain was associated with a 6-fold increased risk of OSA.[23] Longitudinal data from the Cleveland Family Study show that an increase in bodyweight over time increases the risk for and accelerates the progression of OSA,[24] suggesting that the incidence of sleep apnea increases as the incidence of obesity continues to increase. In the Asian population, obesity is less prevalent, but sleep apnea is not proportionately reduced, indicating an effect of craniofacial features perhaps interacting with body habitus (see later discussion).

The close link with features of obesity is a strong factor in the clinical identification of patients who have a high likelihood of sleep apnea, at least in the US population. Neck circumference (a measure of upper body obesity strongly correlated with body measures) is a strong predictor of sleep apnea.[25] Fatty tissue amounts in the neck cause narrowing of the airway, thus increasing the chances of airway closure during sleep. Imaging studies of the neck and upper airway among patients with sleep apnea show larger lateral parapharyngeal fat pads and pharyngeal walls compared with nonobese controls.[26] With weight reduction, the volume of the parapharyngeal walls and lateral paraphyngeal fat pads decreases, accompanied by an increase in airway caliber.

Weight reduction (by any means) can improve severity of sleep apnea in many patients and may be completely curative in some. Extrapolating from pooled surgical and medical weight loss studies, a 10% to 20% weight reduction is associated with an approximately 50% reduction in AHI.[27]

Age

With advancing age, sleep-related difficulties are more common, often manifested by complaints of difficulty falling asleep, increased number of and duration of night-time awakenings, and a decreased amount of night-time sleep. This age-related variability in sleep stability contributes in some way to an increasing prevalence of OSA with advancing age.

In one of the first large population-based studies of sleep apnea among older people, Ancoli-Israel and colleagues[28] examined 427 community-dwelling men and women of ages between 65 and 95 years. They found that 70% of men and 56% of women had OSA objectively defined as AHI greater than or equal to 10. This value is several folds higher than the prevalence estimates among middle-aged adults.[8] Subsequent studies from several population-based samples confirmed this higher prevalence of SDB among older individuals.[29–31] This higher prevalence with older age raises some important questions: how does aging itself have an etiologic role in the development of SDB and what is the significance of the high prevalence of OSA in the elderly?

If aging has an etiologic role in sleep apnea, then authors would expect the prevalence to continue to increase over the older-age range, but this does not seem to be the case. Most of the age-related increases in OSA occur before the age of 65 years and then plateaus subsequently.[29,31] This is not what would be expected with continued accumulation of cases and suggests several possibilities: the incidence may decrease with age older than 65 years, a cohort effect, or perhaps an increased mortality rate among older-aged patients with sleep apnea.[27]

The question arises whether OSA among older adults represents a different clinical entity compared with that seen in middle-aged adults. In particular, age-related attributable morbidity and mortality is an area of controversy. Some of the studies have shown increased risk of adverse outcomes,[32] whereas others have reported little or no association.[33] Additional samples with adequate control for confounding covariates are needed to investigate whether OSA portends excess medical risk among older people.

Ethnicity

Most population-based studies examining the prevalence of OSA have largely focused on characterizing disease prevalence in North America, Australia, and Europe. Compared with the literature on cardiac disease, there are no studies using similar methods that have examined racially, ethnically, and geographically diverse samples. In the data involving African American samples, population-based samples suggest that the prevalence of sleep apnea is as high or higher and potentially more severe among African Americans (particularly among older and younger age groups as compared with middle-aged groups). For example, Ancoli-Israel and colleagues[34] studied a random sample of persons older than 65 years of age from the community with home overnight monitoring. The overall prevalence of SDB, defined as an RDI greater than 15 per hour, was approximately the same in whites (30%) and African Americans (32%), but more African Americans had severe SDB than whites, with an RDI greater than 30 (17 vs 8%). Logistic regression showed that African American race as well as male sex, older age, and increased body mass index (BMI) were independent risk factors for an RDI greater than 30. The odds ratio for severe SDB for African Americans was 2.55 compared with whites, even after adjustment for BMI, sex, and age. A case-control study that also included family members of patients with OSA showed that African Americans with SDB tended to be younger than their white counterparts.[35] Among subjects younger than 25 years of age, African Americans had significantly higher RDIs than their white counterparts, even after adjustment for obesity, sex, familial clustering, and proband sampling. A limitation of the data that links race with an increased risk for OSA has a strong potential for confounding by pathophysiologic, cultural, and socioeconomic factors. Minority samples may have a higher prevalence of comorbid medical conditions, including obesity. These factors in conjunction with systemic factors such as economic status or access to or knowledge of health care may all contribute to a higher risk for OSA. Thus, race may, in part, be a surrogate for other predisposing factors, and this heightened risk in minority samples may disappear if confounding is adequately addressed.

In support of such ethnic and population differences, Asian samples seem to have a similar prevalence rate compared with the West (approximately 5%) despite lower levels of obesity (approximately 3%).[36] And for a given age, sex, and BMI, Asians have greater disease severity compared with whites. One explanation for such differences is in craniofacial morphology.[37]

Craniofacial morphology

The critical element in determining the onset of an obstructive apnea or hypopneas or snoring is the structure and functional control of the nasopharyngeal and pharyngeal airway. Both soft tissue and bone structure may play a role in determining the initial, passive set point of the air channel and muscle act and interact to affect airway size and wall stiffness.[38] US and European patients with obstructive sleep apnea-hypopnea syndrome (OSAHS) tend to have smaller upper airways related to a variety of structural features, including reduction in the length of the mandible, retroposition of the hyoid bone and maxilla, increased tongue volume, elongated soft palate, and increased parapharyngeal fat pads.[39] Many of these features are likely to have an inherited basis and thus play a role in the familial aggregation of OSAHS. These features could contribute to racial/population differences in sleep apnea. In one study, Asians and Caucasians with OSAHS had a more crowded posterior oropharynx (judged by Mallampati Score) and a steeper thyromental plane (line through soft tissue mentum and thyroid prominence) than the controls. Asians tended to have more severe airway narrowing by these measures and more severe OSA after accounting for BMI and neck circumference.[37] Brachycephaly, a head form associated with reduced anterior-posterior cranial dimensions, also seems to be associated with a risk for an AHI of greater than or equal to 15 in whites but not in African Americans.[40] These studies involve limited numbers of subjects, measured in a cross-sectional manner. These issues being raised begin to address predisposing and childhood risk factors for adult disease.

Thus, craniofacial abnormality may be an important risk factor for SDB independent from BMI, and its importance varies among different ethnic groups. Whether such measures are useful in individual assessments or in making decisions about therapy remains an open question. One could imagine that a comprehensive risk assessment in the future would include craniofacial profiling.

Familial/genetic factors
Familial aggregation was first recognized in the 1970s among a family with several affected members.[41] Subsequent studies indicate that first-degree relatives are at increased risk, and this increases with the number of affected family members. This effect is modest and would not drive testing for sleep apnea in unaffected members of the family of a patient. Segregation analysis models suggest that 35% of the variance of OSA severity (ie, AHI) may be attributed to genetic factors that are independent of BMI.[42] Twin studies have also demonstrated that concordance rates for snoring were significantly higher in monozygotic twins than in dizygotic twins.[43,44]

So what is the genetic substrate and what is the likelihood that studies of genetic factors might lead to therapy and individualized therapy in particular? Sleep apnea in adult disease from this perspective is similar to diabetes and hypertension in that they are "complex diseases." A complex disease is one in which no one gene or risk factor is sufficient or required to produce the disease.[45] Each of the risk factors listed earlier are also "complex" traits, and risk factors can operate either alone or in combination to result in the initiation and propagation of apneas over time not only over years but also over the course of a sleep study. In addition to the complexity of those systems affecting obesity, body fat distribution, craniofacial morphology, and self-reported sleepiness, other factors (eg, ventilatory control and sleep cycles/architecture) operating during sleep are in part the result of various genetic and environmental factors that act and interact to produce disease.

PATHOGENESIS

The upper airway in humans has a complex anatomic structure characterized by an elongated posterior pharyngeal space, a 90 degree bend in airflow, and lack of rigidity. This is in part due to its multipurpose function of phonation, swallowing, and breathing. With respect to breathing and the underlying pathogenesis of sleep apnea, the patency of the upper airway depends on a balance of forces: forces that promote airway collapse and opposing forces that maintain upper airway patency. Forces promoting airway collapse include the negative pressure of ventilation and extraluminal positive pressure imposed by factors such as adipose deposition in the soft tissues of the upper airway, fluid, obstructive lesions of the upper airway (eg, tonsillar hypertrophy), and small mandibular size. Upper airway lumen cross-sectional area also decreases somewhat during sleep because of loss of a "tracheal tug" when lung volume falls on assuming the recumbent position.[46]

With inspiration, the negative intraluminal pressure predisposes to collapse of the airway and the activity of the pharyngeal dilator muscles (eg, genioglossus) of the upper airway increases in a phasic manner to oppose these collapsing forces and maintain patency. This activity is usually maintained during sleep. The tensor pallitine dilator muscles are tonically active and help to provide some upper airway stiffness to resist collapse, however this activity falls during sleep. This, in addition to inadequate compensatory increase in phasic dilator muscle activity predisposes to collapse. Furthermore, vibratory damage to the upper airway musculature from snoring may predispose to worsen (or indeed induce) sleep apnea. Friberg and colleagues[47] studied biopsy samples of the upper airway in control subjects, snorers, and patients with OSA. Biopsy specimens were taken from other muscles (eg, anterior tibialis) as control sites. All patients had abnormalities in the upper airway biopsy findings, and 71% had morphometric signs, such as fascicular atrophy and grouped atrophy consistent with neurogenic lesions. Only 20% of control individuals had slight changes of these types. The tibialis muscle biopsies were normal in 20 of the 21 patients, indicating that no generalized muscle or neurologic abnormality was present. The degree of abnormality in the upper airway biopsy specimens was correlated with the percentage of time spent in periodic breathing on an overnight monitoring study. The authors concluded that trauma from snoring may contribute to neurogenic lesions of the upper airway, leading to increased collapsibility, and increased risk for SDB.

Recent data suggests that rostral shifts of fluid may also play an important role in the underlying pathogenesis of sleep-disordered breathing. It has previously been demonstrated that fluid displacement from the legs by inflation of anti-shock trousers increases neck circumference, narrows the pharynx, and increases collapsibility in awake healthy subjects.[48–50] The amount of fluid displaced correlates with overnight increase in neck circumference and frequency of obstructive apnea and hypopneas per hour of sleep. These findings have obvious implications for patients with conditions characterized by dependent fluid retention in the legs such as congestive heart failure and chronic renal failure. Indeed recent data suggests that nocturnal fluid shift may be directly related to the pathogenesis of sleep apnea in these conditions.[51,52]

Finally, in some patients with OSAHS, an unstable respiratory control system appears to promote cycling of respiratory effort. This produces varying levels of upper airway intraluminal negative pressure, and the inadequate compensatory increase in phasic dilator muscle activity predisposes the airway to collapse. Brief microarousals following apneas cause an increase in respiratory effort and accentuate the changes in ventilation. Resulting fluctuations in the level of Pao_2 and $Paco_2$ give feedback to neural respiratory control centers, augmenting and perpetuating respiratory cycling. Thus, upper airway patency is determined by the interaction of a number of structural and functional factors. OSAHS patients appear to have varying degrees of anatomic narrowing combined with reduced neuromuscular dilatory compensatory mechanisms during sleep. Ventilatory controller instability may also contribute to a propensity for periodic breathing and partial or complete airway closure in some patients.

REFERENCES

1. Sleep-related breathing disorders in adults: recommendations for syndrome definition and measurement techniques in clinical research. The Report of an American Academy of Sleep Medicine Task Force. Sleep 1999;22(5):667–89.
2. Meoli AL, Casey KR, Clark RW, et al. Hypopnea in sleep-disordered breathing in adults. Sleep 2001; 24(4):469–70.
3. Redline S, Kapur VK, Sanders MH, et al. Effects of varying approaches for identifying respiratory disturbances on sleep apnea assessment. Am J Respir Crit Care Med 2000;161(2 Pt 1): 369–74.
4. Gottlieb DJ, Whitney CW, Bonekat WH, et al. Relation of sleepiness to respiratory disturbance index: the Sleep Heart Health Study. Am J Respir Crit Care Med 1999;159(2):502–7.
5. Lopez-Jimenez F, Somers VK. Stress measures linking sleep apnea, hypertension and diabetes– AHI vs arousals vs hypoxemia. Sleep 2006;29(6): 743–4.
6. Veasey SC. Obstructive sleep apnea: re-evaluating our index of severity. Sleep Med 2006;7(1):5–6.
7. Gami AS, Pressman G, Caples SM, et al. Association of atrial fibrillation and obstructive sleep apnea. Circulation 2004;110(4):364–7.
8. Young T, Palta M, Dempsey J, et al. The occurrence of sleep-disordered breathing among middle-aged adults. N Engl J Med 1993;328:1230–5.
9. Hiestand DM, Britz P, Goldman M, et al. Prevalence of symptoms and risk of sleep apnea in the US population: results from the national sleep foundation sleep in America 2005 poll. Chest 2006;130(3): 780–6.
10. Punjabi NM. The epidemiology of adult obstructive sleep apnea. Proc Am Thorac Soc 2008;5(2):136–43.
11. Strohl KP, Redline S. Recognition of obstructive sleep apnea. Am J Respir Crit Care Med 1996; 154(2 Pt 1):279–89.
12. Bixler EO, Vgontzas AN, Lin HM, et al. Prevalence of sleep-disordered breathing in women: effects of gender. Am J Respir Crit Care Med 2001;163(3 Pt 1): 608–13.
13. Collop NA, Adkins D, Phillips BA. Gender differences in sleep and sleep-disordered breathing. Clin Chest Med 2004;25(2):257–68.
14. Redline S, Kump K, Tishler PV, et al. Gender differences in sleep disordered breathing in a community-based sample. Am J Respir Crit Care Med 1994;149(3 Pt 1):722–6.
15. Young T, Rabago D, Zgierska A, et al. Objective and subjective sleep quality in premenopausal, perimenopausal, and postmenopausal women in the Wisconsin Sleep Cohort Study. Sleep 2003; 26(6):667–72.

16. Ware JC, McBrayer RH, Scott JA. Influence of sex and age on duration and frequency of sleep apnea events. Sleep 2000;23(2):165–70.

17. Koo BB, Patel SR, Strohl K, et al. Rapid eye movement-related sleep-disordered breathing: influence of age and gender. Chest 2008;134(6): 1156–61.

18. Young T, Hutton R, Finn L, et al. The gender bias in sleep apnea diagnosis. Are women missed because they have different symptoms? Arch Intern Med 1996;156(21):2445–51.

19. Mohsenin V. Gender differences in the expression of sleep-disordered breathing: role of upper airway dimensions. Chest 2001;120(5):1442–7.

20. Schwab J. Sex differences and sleep apnoea. Thorax 1999;54(4):284–5.

21. Popovic RM, White DP. Influence of gender on waking genioglossal electromyogram and upper airway resistance. Am J Respir Crit Care Med 1995;152(2):725–31.

22. Millman RP, Carlisle CC, McGarvey ST, et al. Body fat distribution and sleep apnea severity in women. Chest 1995;107(2):362–6.

23. Peppard PE, Young T, Palta M, et al. Longitudinal study of moderate weight change and sleep-disordered breathing. JAMA 2000;284(23):3015–21.

24. Tishler PV, Larkin EK, Schluchter MD, et al. Incidence of sleep-disordered breathing in an urban adult population: the relative importance of risk factors in the development of sleep-disordered breathing. JAMA 2003;289(17):2230–7.

25. Flemons WW, Whitelaw WA, Brant R, et al. Likelihood ratios for a sleep apnea clinical prediction rule. Am J Respir Crit Care Med 1994;150 (5 Pt 1):1279–85.

26. Schwab RJ. Properties of tissues surrounding the upper airway. Sleep 1996;19(Suppl 10):S170–4.

27. Young T, Peppard P, Gottlieb D. Epidemiology of obstructive sleep apnea: a population health perspective. Am J Respir Crit Care Med 2002;165: 1217–39.

28. Ancoli-Israel S, Kripke DF, Klauber MR, et al. Sleep-disordered breathing in community-dwelling elderly. Sleep 1991;14(6):486–95.

29. Bixler EO, Vgontzas AN, Ten Have T, et al. Effects of age on sleep apnea in men: I. Prevalence and severity. Am J Respir Crit Care Med 1998;157(1): 144–8.

30. Duran J, Esnaola S, Rubio R, et al. Obstructive sleep apnea-hypopnea and related clinical features in a population-based sample of subjects aged 30 to 70 yr. Am J Respir Crit Care Med 2001;163(3 Pt 1): 685–9.

31. Young T, Shahar E, Nieto FJ, et al. Predictors of sleep-disordered breathing in community-dwelling adults: the Sleep Heart Health Study. Arch Intern Med 2002;162(8):893–900.

32. Yaggi H, Concato J, Kernan W, et al. Obstructive sleep apnea as a risk factor for stroke and death. N Engl J Med 2005;353:2034–41.

33. Lavie P, Lavie L, Herer P. All-cause mortality in males with sleep apnoea syndrome: declining mortality rates with age. Eur Respir J 2005;25(3):514–20.

34. Ancoli-Israel S, Klauber MR, Stepnowsky C, et al. Sleep-disordered breathing in African-American elderly. Am J Respir Crit Care Med 1995; 152(6 Pt 1):1946–9.

35. Redline S, Tishler PV, Hans MG, et al. Racial differences in sleep-disordered breathing in African-Americans and Caucasians. Am J Respir Crit Care Med 1997;155(1):186–92.

36. Ip MS, Lam B, Lauder IJ, et al. A community study of sleep-disordered breathing in middle-aged Chinese men in Hong Kong. Chest 2001;119(1):62–9.

37. Lam B, Ip MS, Tench E, et al. Craniofacial profile in Asian and white subjects with obstructive sleep apnoea. Thorax 2005;60(6):504–10.

38. Lloyd SR, Cartwright RD. Physiologic basis of therapy for sleep apnea. Am Rev Respir Dis 1987; 136(2):525–6.

39. Fogel RB, Malhotra A, White DP. Sleep. 2: pathophysiology of obstructive sleep apnoea/hypopnoea syndrome. Thorax 2004;59(2):159–63.

40. Cakirer B, Hans MG, Graham G, et al. The relationship between craniofacial morphology and obstructive sleep apnea in whites and in African-Americans. Am J Respir Crit Care Med 2001; 163(4):947–50.

41. Strohl KP, Saunders NA, Feldman NT, et al. Obstructive sleep apnea in family members. N Engl J Med 1978;299(18):969–73.

42. Palmer LJ, Redline S. Genomic approaches to understanding obstructive sleep apnea. Respir Physiolo Neurobiol 2003;135(2–3):187–205.

43. Carmelli D, Bliwise DL, Swan GE, et al. A genetic analysis of the Epworth Sleepiness Scale in 1560 World War II male veteran twins in the NAS-NRC Twin Registry. J Sleep Res 2001;10(1):53–8.

44. Carmelli D, Colrain IM, Swan GE, et al. Genetic and environmental influences in sleep-disordered breathing in older male twins. Sleep 2004;27(5): 917–22.

45. Altshuler D, Kruglyak L, Lander E. Genetic polymorphisms and disease. N Engl J Med 1998;338(22): 1626.

46. White DP. Pathogenesis of obstructive and central sleep apnea. Am J Respir Crit Care Med 2005; 172(11):1363–70.

47. Friberg D, Ansved T, Borg K, et al. Histological indications of a progressive snorers disease in an upper airway muscle. Am J Respir Crit Care Med 1998; 157:586–93.

48. Shiota S, Ryan CM, Chiu KL, et al. Alterations in upper airway cross-sectional area in response to

lower body positive pressure in healthy subjects. Thorax 2007;62:868–72.

49. Chiu KL, Ryan CM, Shiota S, et al. Fluid shift by lower body positive pressure increases pharyngeal resistance in healthy subjects. Am J Respir Crit Care Med 2006;174:1378–83.

50. Su MC, Chiu KL, Ruttanaumpawan P, et al. Lower body positive pressure increases upper airway collapsibility in healthy subjects. Respir Physiol Neurobiol 2008;161:306–12.

51. Yumino D, Redolfi S, Ruttanaumpawan P, et al. Nocturnal rostral fluid shift: a unifying concept for the pathogenesis of obstructive and central sleep apnea in men with heart failure. Circulation 2010; 121:1598–605.

52. Tang S, Lam B, Ku P, et al. Alleviation of sleep apnea in patients with chronic renal failure by nocturnal cycler-assisted peritoneal dialysis compared with conventional continuous ambulatory peritoneal dialysis. J Am Soc Nephrol 2006;17:2607–16.

Treatment of Obstructive Sleep Apnea Syndrome

Neil Freedman, MD, FCCP*

KEYWORDS

- Obstructive sleep apnea syndrome
- Continuous positive airway pressure
- Pressure-relief PAP • Auto-CPAP (APAP)
- Bilevel therapy • Oral appliances
- Upper-airway surgery • Weight loss

Several treatment options are available for obstructive sleep apnea syndrome (OSAS), including various types of positive airway pressure (PAP) therapy, oral appliances, surgery, and conservative approaches including weight loss and positional therapy. This article focuses on continuous positive airway pressure (CPAP) treatment and technological advancements in the delivery of PAP therapy for OSAS, reviews indications for treatment, treatment outcomes, and methods of improving compliance, and discusses the other non-PAP treatment options.

PAP IN THE TREATMENT OF OSAS

CPAP therapy remains the predominant therapy for the treatment of patients with OSAS, and has been shown to resolve sleep-disordered breathing events and improve several clinical outcomes. Nasal CPAP therapy was initially described as a treatment of OSAS by Sullivan and colleagues[1] in 1981. Nasal CPAP therapy has become the mainstay of treatment of patients with OSAS.[2] CPAP is conventionally delivered via a nasal mask at a fixed pressure that remains constant throughout the respiratory cycle. CPAP's proposed mechanism of action is as a pneumatic splint that maintains the patency of the upper airway in a dose-dependent fashion. It does not exert its effects by increasing upper-airway muscle activity,[3] and acts only as a treatment, and not a cure, for the syndrome.

CPAP therapy is currently indicated for the treatment of moderate to severe OSAS and for patients with mild OSAS and associated symptoms, and/or underlying cardiovascular disease.[2,4,5] In 2008, the Centers for Medicare and Medicaid Services (CMS), based on recommendations from the Practice Parameters Committee from the American Academy of Sleep Medicine (AASM)[5] and other professional societies, updated and modified its position on the requirements for CPAP therapy in patients with OSAS.[6] Given the modifications in the CMS requirements for CPAP therapy and their constant state of change, the authors encourage interested persons to review the National Coverage Determinant at http://www.cms.gov and Local Coverage Determinants polices, which may be specific to given coverage areas.

DETERMINING THE OPTIMAL CPAP SETTING

The optimal CPAP settings for home use may be defined as the minimal pressure required to resolve all apneas, hypopneas, snoring, and arousals related to these events in all stages of sleep and in all positions.[2,5,7,8] The optimal CPAP setting should resolve all sleep-disordered breathing in supine rapid eye movement (REM) sleep, to account for the effects of gravity and changes in muscle tone that may occur in different

---

Financial disclosures: American College of Chest Physicians – Sleep Institute Steering Committee.
Pulmonary Physicians of the North Shore, Bannockburn, IL 60015, USA
* 33944 Wooded Glen Drive, Grayslake, IL 60030.
E-mail address: neilfreedman@comcast.net

Clin Chest Med 31 (2010) 187–201
doi:10.1016/j.ccm.2010.02.012

sleep stages and positions.[9–11] The most current AASM Practice Parameters Committee recommends a full night of CPAP titration based on the criteria outlined previously.[5,8] A repeat CPAP titration need only be performed if symptoms of OSAS reappear despite compliance with CPAP therapy, if a patient sustains a significant weight loss through diet or bariatric surgery, or if CPAP compliance and benefits remain suboptimal by CMS standards. Although there are current recommendations for how to manually titrate CPAP therapy in a laboratory-based setting, these recommendations largely serve as guidelines, as they are principally based on the consensus of expert opinion and not on randomized trials showing their superiority compared with other methods of manual titration.[7] The use of home sleep testing (HST) is currently not recommended for the titration of CPAP or other PAP therapies because there are insufficient data evaluating the reliability of HST for this indication. Given the absence of data regarding HST for CPAP titration, CMS will not reimburse providers who use HST for this indication.

A split-night sleep study, in which the initial portion of the study is used to objectively document an individual's sleep-disordered breathing, followed by a CPAP titration during the second portion of the night, may be indicated in certain situations.[5,7,8] A split-night sleep study may be indicated when the following criteria have been met: (1) an apnea hypopnea index (AHI) of 40 or more events per hour is recorded during the initial 2 hours of polysomnography (PSG); and (2) at least 3 hours remain during the PSG to conduct an adequate CPAP titration. A second full night of CPAP titration should be performed if an optimal CPAP pressure setting cannot be achieved during the second portion of the split-night study. Split-night studies can also be considered for individuals who have less severe OSA with an AHI of 20 to 40 events/h during the initial 2 hours of a sleep study, although data suggest that CPAP titrations in this subgroup of patients may be less accurate when performed in the split-night protocol setting. Although split-night studies potentially reduce waiting times to initiate home CPAP therapy, especially in areas with long sleep-laboratory waiting times, a significant portion of patients with OSAS may undergo suboptimal CPAP titrations using this format.[12]

Although current recommendations warrant that CPAP titrations occur during a full, overnight, in-laboratory PSG, some data suggest that conventional fixed-pressure CPAP can be successfully initiated in an unattended home setting.[13–20] Specifically, these studies confirm that CPAP

therapy initiated in an unattended home setting can be successful in most patients with uncomplicated OSAS when CPAP settings are determined by a clinical prediction formula,[19] by CPAP self-adjusted to resolve snoring,[16,17] or by auto-CPAP (APAP) therapy.[13–15,20] All of these methods typically offer only a starting pressure for initiating CPAP therapy. Many patients required pressure adjustments based on symptoms and problems with therapy during most of these study protocols. If results such as these continue to be reproduced in future studies, positive-pressure therapy may potentially be initiated in the home for many patients with uncomplicated OSAS. It is also possible that in-laboratory CPAP titrations may be reserved for patients with OSAS and concomitant cardiac or respiratory disease, those with obesity hypoventilation syndrome, and those who are having difficulty with CPAP initiated in an unattended setting. If this mode of CPAP treatment comes to fruition, patients with OSAS may benefit by realizing shorter waiting times to CPAP therapy and health care dollars could be saved by reducing the need for unnecessary polysomnograms.[14,15,17,18,21]

BENEFITS OF CPAP THERAPY

It is the perception of many non–sleep practitioners and the lay public that CPAP treatment consistently resolves or improves several important outcomes including sleep architecture, daytime sleepiness, neurocognitive function, mood, quality of life, and cardiovascular disease.

When titrated appropriately, CPAP therapy has been shown to resolve all sleep-disordered breathing across the spectrum of disease severity, and has been shown to be superior to placebo, conservative management, and positional therapy regarding this outcome.[4,5] Randomized controlled trials have also shown CPAP therapy to be superior to placebo at improving stages 3, 4, and REM sleep. The effects of CPAP on other sleep parameters, including stages 1 and 2 sleep, total sleep time, and the arousal index, have been inconsistent.[4,5]

CPAP Treatment and Daytime Sleepiness

Several randomized controlled studies have repeatedly shown that CPAP therapy significantly improves or resolves subjective symptoms of daytime sleepiness in patients with OSAS who suffer from this complaint, predominantly in those who suffer from severe disease (AHI>30 events/h).[17,20,22–28] The minimal and optimal amounts of nocturnal use necessary to improve symptoms of daytime sleepiness are not well defined, as even partial nocturnal use (as little as 2 hours per night) has been associated with significant improvements in daytime symptoms.[29] Although the minimal amount of time required on a nightly basis to improve symptoms of daytime sleepiness is not well established, it is clear that CPAP therapy is required for a least a portion of each night because symptoms of daytime sleepiness reappear when CPAP therapy is discontinued for as little as 1 night.[30,31] A specific threshold for nightly use of CPAP in terms of improvements in symptoms of daytime sleepiness does not exist.[29] In general, more CPAP use on a nightly basis has been associated with greater improvements in symptoms of daytime sleepiness.

The data regarding the effects of CPAP on more objective measures of daytime sleepiness are more inconclusive across the spectrum of disease severity.[4,22] In randomized controlled trials comparing CPAP therapy with placebo or conservative management, a large meta-analysis found only a small, but statistically significant, improvement in the mean sleep latency as measured on the multiple sleep latency or maintenance of wakefulness tests. Across all studies, the mean sleep latency improved by 0.93 minutes ($P = .04$). Whether this small improvement in objective sleepiness is clinically significant is unclear.

Although most patients with daytime sleepiness related to OSAS will achieve significant improvements in symptoms after CPAP therapy has been instituted, this is not the case for all patients. A subgroup of patients with OSAS continues to suffer from symptoms of residual daytime sleepiness despite adequate compliance with CPAP therapy.[29,32,33] The prevalence of residual daytime sleepiness in CPAP-compliant patients remains undefined. Prospective observational data have shown that as many as 30% of those patients who are compliant with their CPAP therapy for greater than or equal to 7 hours per night may still complain of subjective sleepiness (Epworth sleepiness scale score >10) after 3 months of treatment.[29] The mechanisms responsible for this syndrome of residual daytime sleepiness also remain unclear, but may be related to the oxidative-injury effects of long-term intermittent hypoxemia on the sleep-wake–promoting regions in the brain.[34]

Effects of CPAP Treatment on Neurocognitive Function, Mood, and Quality of Life

Many studies have assessed the effects of sleep-disordered breathing on neurocognitive functioning, mood, and quality of life.[5,28,35–46] Most randomized controlled studies find inconsistent,

if any, improvements in several neurobehavioral performance parameters.[4,28,31,35–37] The data regarding the therapeutic effects of CPAP treatment on mood and quality of life are also variable and inconsistent, with most randomized trials finding no clear benefits of CPAP therapy compared with placebo or conservative treatments.[4] One possible explanation for the inconsistent effect of CPAP at improving these outcomes is the use of multiple different measures of function to assess similar parameters. For example, there is near-universal use of the Epworth Sleepiness Scale for assessing improvements in subjective sleepiness, but there are multiple different tests that are used across several studies to assess for improvements in mood, neurocognitive function, and quality of life. Further research is required to evaluate the role of CPAP therapy in alleviating these symptoms and deficits in susceptible patients.

CPAP Treatment and Cardiovascular Disease

The literature on the beneficial effects of CPAP on cardiovascular disease has also been inconsistent and variable.[4,5] Although CPAP treatment seems to augment the adverse effects of untreated sleep apnea on nocturnal blood pressure, most randomized controlled studies show little or no beneficial effects on daytime blood pressure control.[47–51] Two recent meta-analyses that reviewed the randomized controlled data on CPAP and blood pressure showed that overall CPAP therapy may lead to a small (-1.33 to -2.22 mm Hg), but statistically significant ($P = .001$), reduction in 24-hour mean blood pressure.[52,53] Improvements in blood pressure were associated with greater severity of disease and greater duration of CPAP use.

The Haentjens data showed that, although the overall results confirmed an improvement in 24-hour mean blood pressure, these data were inconsistent.[52] Specifically, only 4 of the 12 studies that they reviewed found statistically significant improvements in blood pressure. Of these 4 studies, 2 had a total of 64 patients, with 1 of these studies having a 50% dropout rate by the end of the study.

The inconsistent outcomes related to the effect of CPAP on blood pressure may in part be related to limitations of the data. In the Haentjens data,[52] of the 12 studies that used 24-hour mean blood pressure as an outcome measure, most of the studies enrolled patients without hypertension at baseline. Specifically, 9 of the studies enrolled 31% or less of their patients with hypertension at baseline, and 3 studies had no patients with hypertension. In addition, most of the patients with hypertension at enrollment were on antihypertensive medications during the studies. Most of the studies were of short duration (≤ 12 weeks), which may not be enough treatment time to improve long-standing hypertension. It is therefore possible that CPAP treatment may have a more robust effect on blood pressure, but our current literature has been limited in terms of the patient populations studied and the duration of treatment.

Two small, randomized, controlled trials have shown a beneficial effect on left ventricular ejection fraction (LVEF) in patients with concomitant obstructive sleep apnea and congestive heart failure.[54,55] Compared with optimal medical management alone, heart-failure patients with moderate to severe obstructive sleep apnea showed LVEF improvements of 5% to 9% in 1 to 3 months, respectively.[54,55]

There are currently no long-term randomized controlled data evaluating CPAP and any cardiovascular outcomes, including mortality. The most convincing long-term data regarding the potential beneficial effects of CPAP therapy on cardiovascular outcomes come from Marin and colleagues.[49] They followed a large group of male patients with OSAS with the spectrum of disease severity in a prospective observational study for a period of 10 years.[49] Their results showed 2 important findings: (1) compared with normal controls, patients with untreated severe sleep apnea (AHI >30 events/h) had a significant increase in fatal and nonfatal cardiovascular events; and (2) CPAP treatment (>4 h/night) in patients with severe disease reduced their cardiovascular risks to levels similar to normal nonsnoring controls. A more recent observational study has also found improvements in cardiovascular mortality across the spectrum of disease severity, although the data are limited by the absence of a control group.[56] Given the inconclusive nature of CPAP therapy on cardiovascular outcomes in general, this option has been recommended only as an adjunctive therapy to lower blood pressure in hypertensive patients with OSAS.[5]

PROBLEMS AND COMPLIANCE WITH CPAP THERAPY

Patients with OSAS should ideally use their CPAP therapy all night every night. However, as with therapies for other chronic diseases, compliance with CPAP therapy for OSAS is imperfect. Although there are no formal definitions of what constitutes compliance with CPAP therapy, most studies have defined compliance as use greater than 4 hours per night for 70% of the observed nights.[57] Patients who are asked about their CPAP use

indicate that subjective compliance ranges between 65% and 90%. Objective measures of CPAP compliance have shown that new and long-term patients usually overestimate their CPAP usage.[57,58] Short-term follow-up of patients with OSAS shows that there are 2 patterns of CPAP usage: (1) patients who use their CPAP for more than 90% of nights, with an average usage time of greater than 6 hours per night; and (2) patients who use their CPAP intermittently, with an average usage of less than 3.5 hours per night.[59] Long-term objective follow-up has shown that approximately 68% of patients with OSAS continue to use their CPAP therapy after 5 years.[58]

A pattern of CPAP compliance can usually be determined within the first few days, and certainly by 3 months, of therapy.[58-61] Some studies have suggested certain parameters that may predict short- and long-term usage, although reliable predictors of compliance currently do not exist. Suggested predictors of long-term CPAP compliance have included symptoms of subjective sleepiness (Epworth Sleepiness Scale >10), severity of OSAS (AHI >30), and average nightly use within the first 3 months of therapy.[58] Patients reporting problems during their initial night with CPAP therapy are typically less likely to use CPAP on a regular basis.[60] The level of CPAP pressure has not been shown to be a predictor of CPAP use. As noted earlier, most studies have not been able to establish factors that consistently predict compliance with CPAP therapy.[24,57,62-64]

Typical problems that may lead to reduced compliance with CPAP therapy include claustrophobia, nasal congestion, and poor mask fit leading to leaks and skin irritation. Several interventions have been proposed and instituted in an attempt to improve CPAP compliance. Several studies have found that the addition of heated humidification improves symptoms of nasal congestion and increases objective CPAP use,[65-67] although this finding has not been consistent. Patient education has also been shown to improve CPAP compliance in many, but not all, studies.[57,68,69] Simple interventions such as weekly phone calls and mailings may improve compliance, especially if performed in the initial weeks of therapy.[69] In general, increased intensity of patient education or the frequency of health-provider contact improve CPAP adherence.[4,5]

Although proper initial mask fit may be a key to CPAP acceptance, the optimum form of CPAP delivery interface remains unclear.[70] Changing masks once a problem has developed has not been shown to improve long-term compliance. Although a ramp feature that slowly increases pressure to a therapeutic level is common on most of the current CPAP devices, there is no peer-reviewed literature evaluating the effect of ramp on compliance with CPAP therapy. The use of prescription hypnotics has not been consistently shown to improve compliance when used during the first month of CPAP therapy.

Given the studies mentioned earlier, the addition of heated humidification and a systematic educational program are recommended as standards to improve adherence to CPAP therapy.[4,5] There are few, if any, data to guide providers as to when or how often patients on CPAP should have follow-up. Current recommendations, based predominantly on expert opinion, suggest that patients should have initial follow-up in the first few weeks after CPAP therapy has been initiated. Thereafter, CPAP patients should be followed on an annual basis and as needed to troubleshoot problems as they arise.[4,5] CMS, as described earlier, has defined its own rules regulating how and when patients on CPAP should have office follow-up.

CPAP SUMMARY

CPAP therapy remains the mainstay of treatment of patient with moderate to severe OSAS. The literature clearly shows that CPAP therapy resolves sleep-disordered breathing events and improves symptoms of daytime sleepiness in patients with more severe disease. There are inconsistent data concerning the benefits of CPAP therapy in regard to neurocognitive function, mood, quality of life, and cardiovascular outcomes. The data regarding the benefits of CPAP therapy in patients with more mild disease are even more controversial, predominantly related to a paucity of well-performed studies in this patient population. There are few data on which to base recommendations in patients with OSAS without associated symptoms across the spectrum of disease severity. Despite its potential to improve several clinical outcomes, long-term compliance remains suboptimal. The data clearly show that the addition of heated humidification and a systematic education program improve CPAP compliance. Although CPAP remains the mainstay of therapy, it is clear that future research is required to better define the role of CPAP therapy in regard to several clinical outcomes and across the spectrum of disease severity.

TECHNOLOGICAL ADVANCEMENTS IN THE DELIVERY OF PAP THERAPY FOR OSAS: APAP AND BEYOND

Although CPAP remains the mainstay of therapy for OSAS, there are several other methods of delivering PAP therapy. Clinicians, patients, and industry are continually evaluating better methods to make PAP treatment a more acceptable therapy for OSAS. This article focuses on newer technological advancements in the delivery of positive pressure therapy, including bilevel therapy, expiratory-pressure relief devices, and APAP.

BILEVEL POSITIVE PRESSURE THERAPY

The potential benefits of bilevel therapy in treating patients with OSAS were first described in 1990.[71] As opposed to CPAP therapy, which allows a fixed pressure throughout the respiratory cycle, bilevel therapy allows the independent adjustment of the expiratory positive airway pressure (EPAP) and the inspiratory positive airway pressure (IPAP). In its initial description, bilevel therapy showed that obstructive events could be eliminated at a lower EPAP compared with conventional CPAP pressures.[71] Although, intuitively, bilevel ought to increase compliance by reducing unwanted pressure-related side effects, there are no convincing data that bilevel therapy improves compliance or efficacy compared with CPAP therapy for patients with uncomplicated OSAS.[4,5,72]

Newer bilevel systems have been introduced by several companies. Respironics (Respironics, Inc; Murrysville, PA) introduced a novel bilevel device (BiFlex) that differs from conventional bilevel systems in 2 major respects. First, the inspiratory pressure is reduced slightly near the end of inspiration, and the expiratory pressure is slightly reduced near the beginning of expiration. Second, the magnitude of change of the IPAP and EPAP is proportional to patient effort. In a randomized study of 27 newly diagnosed patients with OSAS over a 1-month period, this bilevel system was as effective as conventional nasal CPAP. There were no differences in compliance or measures of subjective sleepiness and quality of life.[73] This report confirms the findings of previous studies that the role of bilevel-type devices in otherwise uncomplicated OSA remains unclear.

Although the data regarding the use of traditional bilevel and BiFlex therapies do not show any advantages compared with CPAP therapy in patients with newly diagnosed OSAS, a study by Ballard and colleagues[74] has shown a potential role for BiFlex therapy in patients who are noncompliant with CPAP therapy. Ballard and colleagues[74] studied a large group of OSAS patient who were noncompliant with CPAP therapy despite significant education, attention to proper mask fitting, and the addition of heated humidification. After 3 months of therapy, those patients randomized to BiFlex therapy showed significantly better nightly compliance ($P = .03$) compared with those who were retitrated on standard CPAP therapy. As BiFlex technology provides PAP via is own unique algorithm, these findings cannot be generalized to other bilevel therapies. Although these data are intriguing, further studies will be required to confirm these findings.

Overall, bilevel therapy remains a viable option for CPAP-intolerant patients with OSAS, OSAS with concurrent respiratory disease, or obesity hypoventilation syndrome.[2,4,5] The role of bilevel therapy, and its variants, in otherwise uncomplicated OSA remains unclear.[75]

EXPIRATORY-PRESSURE RELIEF SYSTEMS

A common complaint in many patients with OSAS is the uncomfortable feeling of exhaling against positive pressure. This consequence is a potential barrier to the long-term acceptance of CPAP therapy. Expiratory-pressure relief (EPR) systems have been developed in an attempt to remedy this potential problem. EPR technologies allow pressure relief during exhalation in an attempt to make CPAP therapy more comfortable. In simple terms, EPR technologies briefly reduce the CPAP pressure during exhalation before returning the pressure to its baseline CPAP setting before the initiation of inspiration. Certain EPR technologies monitor the patient's airflow during exhalation and reduce the expiratory pressure in response to the airflow and patient effort. The amount of pressure relief varies on a breath-by-breath basis, depending on the patient's airflow, and is also dictated by patient preference. This technology is comparable with a modified bilevel device with a narrower range of difference between the inspiratory and expiratory pressures (maximum difference is 3 cm H_2O).

Although Respironics (Respironics, Inc; Murrysville, PA) and Resmed (Resmed; North Ryde, Australia) have developed EPR devices for the marketplace, only the Respironics technology (CFLEX) has been evaluated in the peer-reviewed literature.[76,77] There are only 2 peer-reviewed studies of EPR devices, both comparing CFLEX (Respironics, Inc; Murrysville, PA) with conventional CPAP therapy.[76,77] The only randomized controlled study evaluating the CFLEX technology evaluated 52 newly diagnosed CPAP-naive patients with OSAS and allocated them to fixed CPAP or CFLEX therapy.[77] After 7 weeks of treatment, CPAP and CFLEX groups showed equal objective compliance (5.2 hours vs 5.3 hours, respectively). Both treatments also showed equal improvements in subjective daytime sleepiness

and reductions in the AHI. CFLEX therapy offered no significant benefits in that subgroup of patients that required pressures of more than 9 cm H_2O. Based on limited data from 1 randomized controlled trial, CFLEX technology offers no significant benefits compared with fixed CPAP therapy regarding compliance and other typical outcomes.

Although EPR technologies offer an alternative method for delivering PAP for the treatment of OSAS, further randomized controlled trials will be necessary to determine whether this technology offers any objective advantages compared with fixed CPAP therapy. Based on the paucity of peer-reviewed data currently available on EPR technology, no recommendations can be made regarding its use in clinical practice.[75]

APAP

APAP (also known as auto-, automated, autoadjusting, or autotitrating positive airway pressure) further advances PAP therapy with the ability to detect and respond to changes in upper-airway flow and resistance in real time.[78] This review focuses on the literature related to APAP in the treatment of patients already diagnosed with OSAS, as there is currently little evidence to support the use of APAP technology in the diagnosis of OSAS.[79]

Before reviewing the APAP outcomes data and comparisons with conventional fixed CPAP, this article first reviews APAP as a technology. Unlike conventional CPAP, in which the technology is standardized across all manufacturers, APAP represents several different technologies from several different companies. As mentioned earlier, most currently available APAP devices noninvasively detect and respond to variations in patterns of upper-airway inspiratory flow or resistance. Sensors used to detect the spectrum of these upper-airway changes, as well as the algorithms responsible for responding to them, vary among the different APAP machines and companies.

Most APAP machines with which the reader would be familiar are flow-based devices. These devices monitor a combination of changes in inspiratory flow patterns, including inspiratory flow limitation, snoring (indirectly measured via mask pressure vibration), and absence of flow (which is interpreted by these devices as apneas). Changes in airflow are detected via a pneumotachograph, nasal pressure monitor, or alterations in compressor speed. Most units detect flow limitation via an algorithm using a flow-versus-time profile. The other less commonly used technology uses the forced oscillation technique (FOT) method, which is an alternative method that detects changes in upper-airway resistance or impedance.[80–82] Because the FOT method measures changes in upper-airway resistance that are independent of patient activity and ventilatory effort, this technology has the potential advantage of better differentiating central from obstructive apneas or mask leak.

Once upper-airway flow or impedance changes have been detected, the APAP devices automatically increase the pressure until the flow or resistance has been normalized. Once a therapeutic pressure has been achieved, the APAP devices reduce pressure until flow limitation or increases in airway resistance resume. Each APAP device follows different proprietary algorithms to increase and decrease pressure in response to changes in airway flow or resistance over a set period of time. Most devices have a therapeutic pressure range between 4 and 20 cm H_2O, with the ability to adjust the upper and lower pressure limits based on the clinical conditions. Because pressures changes occur throughout the sleep period, it has been postulated that APAP devices may increase sleep fragmentation.[83] This concern has not been substantiated in studies evaluating changes in sleep structure or in clinical trials that have measured subjective sleepiness as a main outcome. Specifically, the frequency of microarousals and sleep fragmentation induced by APAP devices seems to be small,[84] and clinical outcomes related to subjective sleepiness also show no significant differences compared with conventional CPAP therapy.[17,85–87]

Currently available APAP machines have several potential limitations. Most flow-based APAP devices are limited in their ability to distinguish between central and obstructive apneas as well as large mask leaks.[88–91] These flow patterns are interpreted by these devices as an absence of flow, which, in the cases of central apneas and leaks, may erroneously lead to increases in pressure and worsening of the central events or leaks. In addition, the ability of the APAP devices to respond to sustained hypoventilation in the absence of upper-airway obstruction is unclear, as most APAP studies have excluded patients at high risk, including those patients with obesity hypoventilation syndrome or chronic respiratory diseases. Given these limitations, the current AASM Practice Parameters regarding the use of APAP recommends that APAP devices only be used for patients with uncomplicated moderate to severe obstructive sleep apnea.[79,92,93] The committee recommended that APAP devices not be used in the following groups of patients: (1) congestive heart failure; (2) lung diseases such as chronic obstructive pulmonary disease (COPD); and (3) patients expected to have nocturnal arterial oxyhemoglobin desaturation caused by conditions other than OSAS (eg, obesity hypoventilation syndrome). Patients who do not snore (as a result of palatal surgery or naturally) should not be titrated with an APAP device that relies on vibration or sound in the device's algorithm.[79,92,93] APAP devices are not recommended for split-night titrations because of the lack of data to support such a practice.

Comparisons of APAP with Conventional CPAP for the Treatment of OSAS

Several randomized controlled trials have compared APAP technology with conventionally titrated CPAP therapy.[17,18,75,82,85–87,94–103] These studies have concluded that, compared with standard CPAP, APAP are almost always associated with a reduction in mean pressure. Aside from this difference, APAP and standard CPAP are similar in several outcomes, including objective compliance, ability to eliminate respiratory events, and ability to improve subjective daytime sleepiness as measured by the Epworth Sleepiness Scale.

Most of the literature concerning APAP technology has evaluated patients with uncomplicated predominantly severe OSAS (AHI >30 events/h), and therefore the results and recommendations that have been reviewed predominantly apply to this group of patients. There is currently only 1 study comparing the efficacy of APAP versus conventionally titrated CPAP in patients with more mild disease.[103] This study found similar efficacy and outcomes between APAP and CPAP. Aside from this lone study evaluating APAP in patients with less severe disease, it is difficult to make reliable recommendations for this subgroup of patients.

Although most studies have found equal efficacy between APAP technologies as a group and conventionally titrated CPAP, several questions still need to be addressed. Specifically: (1) are all APAPs the same? (2) Can APAP be used to predict conventional CPAP pressure. (3) Can APAP be used in an unattended setting without in-laboratory confirmation of efficacy?

Are all APAPs the Same?

Although there have been few studies comparing different APAP devices in a head to head manner, it seems clear from clinical[102,104,105] and bench studies[88–91] that all APAP devices are not the same. As a group, APAPs are different technologies with different proprietary algorithms for the detection of, and response to, sleep-disordered breathing events. It is not clear from the current literature which, if any, algorithm for event detection or response to respiratory events is superior. Because of these inherent differences, unlike CPAP, results from an individual clinical trial using a particular APAP device are specific to that machine and cannot be generalized across the entire technology of APAP devices.[79]

Can APAP Titrations be Used to Determine a Therapeutic Pressure Setting for Conventional Fixed CPAP Devices?

The literature has clearly demonstrated the efficacy of various APAP devices used in an attended setting to determine a fixed CPAP pressure for home use.[79,92,93] Based on the available literature, the current AASM Practice Parameters have recommended that certain APAP devices may be used during attended PSG titration studies to identify a single, effective, conventional CPAP pressure.[79]

The use of unattended APAP to determine a therapeutic setting for fixed CPAP therapy remains controversial. There are several potential methods that can be used in an attempt to determine a fixed CPAP pressure from APAP devices used in an unattended setting. The 2 most common methods are (1) visual inspection of the downloaded raw data from 1 or several nights of home APAP and using the highest pressure; and (2) using the P90 or P95 from the downloaded data. The P90 and P95 are the maximum pressures at which the device operates for 90% or 95% of the treatment time, respectively. These methods have problems that may lead the evaluator to make erroneous conclusions about a fixed CPAP setting.

Several laboratory-based clinical studies have shown that using the P95 data from various APAP devices gives inconsistent estimates of effective CPAP pressures.[94,106,107] Several randomized clinical trials that have looked at the usefulness of using an APAP determined P95 to ascertain a fixed CPAP pressure setting for home therapy.[13–15,20] In general, these studies have shown similar outcomes to CPAP titrated conventionally in a laboratory-based setting. Although these studies show similar outcomes using the unattended home APAP P95 (primarily using Resmed APAP technology) as a starting point to determine home fixed CPAP pressures, the data remain limited. Given these limitations and the potential controversies regarding these results, unattended APAP titrations to determine optimal treatment pressures for conventional CPAP use

should be used cautiously.[79] Patients being treated with fixed CPAP on the basis of an unattended APAP titration must be followed closely to determine treatment efficacy and safety. A reevaluation and, if necessary, a standard CPAP titration should be performed if symptoms do not resolve or if CPAP treatment seems to lack efficacy.

Can Unattended Home APAP be Used as the Sole Treatment of Patients with OSAS Without the use of PSG?

Until recently, there were minimal data to support unattended APAP use as the sole treatment of OSAS without objectively confirming treatment efficacy via PSG. Since 2003, there have been several studies evaluating the use of APAP in CPAP-naive and current CPAP users in unattended settings.[14,17,18,86,87] All of these studies have found that, in an unattended setting, various APAPs and conventional CPAP therapy result in similar treatment outcomes. Specifically, these studies found no significant differences in objective compliance, and similar improvements in daytime sleepiness and quality of life. Despite these studies finding similar efficacy between unattended APAP treatment and conventional CPAP treatment, the AASM Practice Parameters committee has recommended unattended APAP use only as an option for patients with moderate to severe uncomplicated OSAS.[79]

APAP technology seems to be as effective as conventional fixed CPAP therapy when used in attended and unattended settings in patients with moderate to severe uncomplicated OSAS.[79] Although APAP technologies reduce the mean treatment pressure across the night, they seem to result in similar objective compliance rates and improvements in other important clinical outcomes. Although APAP therapy has been shown to have some shortcomings in the peer-reviewed literature, the technology is rapidly advancing. It is possible that APAP therapy may take the place of the standard in-laboratory CPAP titration in the near future. The main benefits of APAP technology will likely be the ability to provide faster treatment to patients with uncomplicated OSAS, and possibly the saving of health care dollars by eliminating unnecessary sleep studies.[17,18,86]

ORAL APPLIANCE THERAPY

Oral appliance therapy offers a reasonable treatment option for many patients with mild to moderate disease, as well as for those patients with more severe disease who are unable to tolerate CPAP therapy. The proposed mechanisms of action for oral appliances for improving sleep-disordered breathing include an increase in upper-airway patency and improvements in upper-airway muscle tone. There are many forms of oral appliance, with most studies evaluating the efficacy of mandibular advancement devices. Tongue-retaining devices have been studied to a lesser extent. The best form of oral appliance therapy is not known.

In randomized controlled studies, oral appliances are less efficacious at reducing the AHI compared with CPAP therapy, with only 42% of oral-appliance patients achieving an optimal titration as defined by a residual AHI of less than 5 events per hour.[108,109] Oral appliances also seem to be inferior to CPAP in improving oxygenation, especially in patients with more severe disease.[110] Most studies show that oral appliances result in similar improvements in daytime sleepiness, as defined by the Epworth Sleepiness Scale, compared with CPAP in patients with mild to moderate disease.[111] The explanation for this discordance between improvements in AHI and subjective sleepiness is unclear. Better adherence to oral appliance therapy versus CPAP treatment has been proposed as one explanation for this inconsistency, although it is difficult to support based on the current literature. There are limited data comparing oral-appliance therapy with upper-airway surgery. Compared with uvulopalatopharyngoplasty (UPPP) in patients with less severe OSA, oral appliances were more likely to result in maintenance of an AHI less than 5 at 1 year.[109,110,112] Overall, there are few data regarding the effect of oral appliances on other important outcomes such as cardiovascular disease; the data in patients with mild to moderate OSA are mixed.[113,114]

Predicting treatment success may be difficult. The success rate of a given study is based on the type of device used as well as a given study's definition of success. In addition to the type of device used, several other variables may affect the efficacy of treatment: (1) severity of OSA, (2) degree of protrusion, and (3) body mass index (calculated as weight in kilograms divided by the square of height in meters). In general, oral appliance therapy is less likely to be successful, by any definition, in those patients with more severe disease (AHI >30 events per hour) and in those with a higher body mass index. Given the inability to accurately predict treatment success before initiating therapy, objective testing to document the efficacy of oral appliance therapy is recommended. This testing may be done through in-laboratory full PSG or via unattended HST devices.[109]

Oral appliances are currently recommended for patients with mild to moderate OSA who: (1) prefer oral appliances to CPAP, (2) do not respond to CPAP, (3) are not appropriate candidates for CPAP, or (4) fail CPAP therapy.[108,110] Because CPAP is more effective than oral appliances in patients with severe disease, patients with severe OSA should be offered a trial of CPAP before initiating oral-appliance therapy. Adequate follow-up with objective documentation of efficacy is currently recommended.

UPPER-AIRWAY SURGERY

The role of upper-airway surgery in the management of adult obstructive sleep apnea remains unclear. There are several upper-airway surgical procedures that are currently being performed with the goal of increasing upper-airway patency. Types of procedures include, but are not limited to, UPPP, genioglossus advancement, tongue radiofrequency, midline glossectomy, hyoid suspension, maxillomandibular advancement (MMA), and combinations of the various procedures. It is unclear which procedure, if any, will benefit a given patient or group of patients. Although tracheostomy is the ultimate corrective surgery for the treatment of OSA, its use in clinical practice has been limited to those with life-threatening disease who have been unable to tolerate other treatments.

There are several reasons why the use of surgery for the treatment of OSA remains controversial. First and foremost, there are few well-designed studies comparing the various surgeries with placebo or other types of controls. Most of the evidence-based data are primarily case series (level 4 evidence), with only a few level 1 and 2 studies.[115,116] Although surgical reviews of this literature have concluded that hypopharyngeal surgery for obstructive sleep apnea results in improved outcomes,[115] the most recent Cochrane Database Systematic Review concluded that, based on a limited number of trials assessing diverse surgical techniques, the available evidence does not support the use of surgery for patients with OSA.[116]

Second, it is difficult to determine success rates from the surgical literature, because the definition of success varies widely from study to study. Using a traditional surgical definition of success (a 50% reduction of the AHI, AHI <20, or both), success rates vary between 55% for limited (phase 1) procedures and 86% for the more complicated (phase 2) MMA procedure. If a more stringent definition of success (having a residual AHI <5 events per hour) is applied to the same group of studies, the success rates drop dramatically to 13% and 43% for the limited and MMA procedures, respectively.[117,118] Another reason for controversy is a significant heterogeneity throughout the literature, with most phase 1 studies evaluating combinations of various procedures. Many studies are limited by the lack of adequate or uniform follow-up. It is difficult to draw any reliable conclusions about upper-airway surgical procedures for the treatment of OSA based on the current lack of robust, well-designed studies. Future research should focus on well-designed, randomized, controlled trials with clearly defined outcomes and uniform follow-up. When this type of information is available, it may help us better determine which surgical procedures are efficacious, which clinically significant outcomes are improved, and which patient groups may benefit from the various types of procedures.

CONSERVATIVE TREATMENTS AND MEDICAL THERAPIES

Although obesity is an independent risk factor for OSAS in adults up to 60 years of age, the role of weight loss as a primary treatment remains unclear because there has been little robust evidence specifically concerning OSA as a primary outcome of various weight-loss therapies. The amount of weight loss required to significantly reduce a given patient's sleep-disordered breathing also remains unknown, with some patients showing significant residual sleep-disordered breathing despite considerable weight loss. Currently, medical weight loss through diet, counseling, and exercise is recommended only as an adjunct to primary treatments such as PAP and oral appliance therapies.[33,119]

Although the risks related to various types of bariatric surgeries have improved,[120] the role of bariatric surgery as a treatment of OSA remains unclear. A recent meta-analysis, which included 12 studies (n = 342 patients) that required patients to be tested with PSG before and at least 3 months after bariatric surgery, found that bariatric surgery can result in significant reductions in the severity of OSA as defined by the AHI. As is the case with medical weight-loss therapy, residual OSA was evident in many patients after surgical weight loss, with a mean residual AHI of 15.8 events per hour (baseline AHI 54.7 events per hour).[121] Other studies of surgical weight loss have found that some patients may have increases in their AHI over time after initial improvement, with and without associated weight gain.[122] Given that the

amount of weight loss necessary to significantly improve OSA remains unclear, and that many patients who lose weight by any means regain some or most of the weight that they initially lost over time, repeat PSG is recommended to objectively document a given patient's improvement before decisions to stop primary treatments such as CPAP or oral-appliance therapy are considered.

In addition to weight loss, no other medical therapies are recommended as primary treatments for OSA of any severity. Positional therapy is an effective secondary therapy or adjunct to a primary treatment in patients with predominantly supine-dependent disease. Nasal steroids may be useful as an adjunctive treatment in patients with OSA and concurrent rhinitis.[33,119] Modafinil and armodafinil are approved for use in patients with OSA who have residual daytime sleepiness despite adequate CPAP use. Randomized placebo-controlled trials with both of these stimulant agents show that the improvements in subjective daytime sleepiness and objective alertness, although statistically significant, are small, with most patients sustaining abnormal residual daytime sleepiness.[32,119] Other pharmacologic agents, including various classes of antidepressants, methylxanthine derivatives, and estrogen replacement, have shown no significant benefits and are currently not recommended as primary or adjunctive therapies for the treatment of OSA.[33,119]

SUMMARY

CPAP therapy remains the mainstay of treatment of patient with moderate to severe OSAS. Despite its potential to improve several clinical outcomes, long-term compliance remains suboptimal. Newer technologies, specifically APAP, have the potential to improve treatment of OSAS. Although these technologies differ, many have been shown to be as effective as in-laboratory titrated CPAP in patients with uncomplicated, moderate to severe OSAS. Although the role of APAP in the treatment of OSAS is still poorly defined, it has the potential to improve the delivery of PAP therapy by reducing the current sleep laboratory waiting times, replacing laboratory-based PAP titrations in uncomplicated OSAS patients and thus potentially reducing health care spending. Other technological advancements, such as EPR and bilevel devices, are supported by limited data and seem to offer no advantages compared with conventionally titrated CPAP therapy in most patients with OSAS. Oral appliances may be used in patients with mild to moderate OSAS and in those with more severe disease who are unable to tolerate CPAP therapy. It is possible that oral appliances may become more widely used in the future as the technology advances. The role of upper-airway surgery in the treatment of OSAS remains unclear at this time. Limited data assessing the role of bariatric surgery in the treatment of OSAS show significant improvements in the AHI, although many patients have moderate residual disease as assessed by the AHI. There are no other medical therapies that are recommended as primary treatments for OSA of any severity.

REFERENCES

1. Sullivan C, Issa F, Berthon-Jones M, et al. Reversal of obstructive sleep apnea by continuous positive airway pressure applied through the nares. Lancet 1981;1:862–5.
2. Loube D, Gay P, Strohl K, et al. Indications for positive airway pressure treatment of adult obstructive sleep apnea patients: a consensus statement. Chest 1999;115(3):863–6.
3. Strohl K, Redline S. Nasal CPAP therapy, upper airway muscle activation and obstructive sleep apnea. Am Rev Respir Dis 1986;134:555–8.
4. Gay P, Weaver T, Loube D, et al. Evaluation of positive airway pressure treatment for sleep related breathing disorders in adults. Sleep 2006;29(3):381–401.
5. Kushida C, Littner M, Hirshkowitz M, et al. Practice parameters for the use of continuous and bilevel positive airway pressure devices to treat adult patients with sleep-related breathing disorders. Sleep 2006;29(3):375–80.
6. Centers for Medicare and Medicaid Services. Continuous positive airway pressure (CPAP) therapy for obstructive sleep apnea (OSA). Updated August 28, 2008. Available at: www.cms. gov. Accessed February 12, 2010.
7. Kushida C, Chediak A, Berry R, et al. Clinical guidelines for the manual titration of positive airway pressure in patients with obstructive sleep apnea. J Clin Sleep Med 2008;4(2):157–71.
8. Kushida C, Littner M, Morgenthaler T, et al. Practice parameters for the indications for polysomnography and related procedures: an update for 2005. Sleep 2005;28(4):499–521.
9. Pevernagie D, Shepard J. Relations between sleep stage, posture and effective nasal CPAP levels in OSA. Sleep 1992;15(2):162–7.
10. Series F, Marc I. Importance of sleep stage and body position-dependence of sleep apnoea determining benefits of auto-CPAP therapy. Eur Respir J 2001;18(1):170–5.
11. Oksenberg A, Silverberg D, Arons E, et al. The sleep supine position has a major effect on optimal nasal continuous positive airway pressure. Chest 1999;116:1000–6.
12. Sanders M, Kern N, Costatino J, et al. Adequacy of prescribing positive airway pressure therapy by mask for sleep apnea on the basis of a partial night trial. Am Rev Respir Dis 1993;147:1169–74.
13. Mulgrew A, Fox N, Ayas N, et al. Diagnosis and initial management of obstructive sleep apnea without polysomnography: a randomized validation study. Ann Intern Med 2007;146(3):157–66.
14. West S, Jones D, Stradling J. Comparison of three ways to determine and deliver pressure during nasal CPAP therapy for obstructive sleep apnoea. Thorax 2006;61(3):226–31.
15. Cross M, Vennelle M, Engleman H, et al. Comparison of CPAP titration at home or the sleep laboratory in the sleep apnea hypopnea syndrome. Sleep 2006;29(11):1451–5.
16. Fitzpatrick M, Alloway C, Wakeford T, et al. Can patients with obstructive sleep apnea titrate their own continuous positive airway pressure? Am J Respir Crit Care Med 2003;167(5):716–22.
17. Masa J, Jimenez A, Duran J, et al. Alternative methods of titrating continuous positive airway pressure: a large multicenter study. Am J Respir Crit Care Med 2004;170(11):1218–24.
18. Planes C, d'Ortho M, Foucher A, et al. Efficacy and cost of home-initiated Auto-nCPAP versus conventional nCPAP. Sleep 2003;26(2):156–60.
19. Oliver Z, Hoffstein V. Predicting effective continuous positive airway pressure. Chest 2000;117:1061–4.
20. Berry R, Hill G, Thompson L, et al. Portable monitoring and autotitration versus polysomnography for the diagnosis and treatment of sleep apnea. Sleep 2008;31(10):1423–31.
21. Hukins C. Arbitrary-pressure continuous positive airway pressure for obstructive sleep apnea syndrome. Am J Respir Crit Care Med 2005;171(5):500–5.
22. Patel S, White D, Malhotra A, et al. Continuous positive airway pressure therapy for treating sleepiness in a diverse population with obstructive sleep apnea: results of a meta-analysis. Arch Intern Med 2003;163(5):565–71.
23. Engleman H, Douglas N. Sleep 4: sleepiness, cognitive function, and quality of life in obstructive sleep apnoea/hypopnoea syndrome. Thorax 2004;59(7):618–22.
24. Douglas N, Engleman H. CPAP therapy: outcomes and patient use. Thorax 1998;53(90003):47S–48.
25. Douglas N. Systematic review of the efficacy of nasal CPAP. Thorax 1998;53(5):414–5.
26. Jenkinson C, Davies R, Mullins R, et al. Comparison of therapeutic and sub-therapeutic nasal continuous airway pressure for obstructive sleep

apnea: a randomized prospective parallel trial. Lancet 1999;353:2100–5.

27. Ballester E, Badia J, Hernandez L, et al. Evidence of the effectiveness of continuous positive airway pressure in the treatment of sleep apnea/hypopnea syndrome. Am J Respir Crit Care Med 1999;159(2):495–501.

28. Engleman H, Martin S, Kingshott R, et al. Randomised, placebo-controlled trial of daytime function after continuous positive airway pressure therapy for the sleep apnoea/hypopnoea syndrome. Thorax 1998;53:341–5.

29. Weaver T, Maislin G, Dinges D, et al. Relationship between hours of CPAP use and achieving normal levels of sleepiness and daily functioning. Sleep 2007;30:711–9.

30. Kribbs N, Pack A, Kline L, et al. Effects of one night without nasal CPAP treatment on sleep and sleepiness in patients with obstructive sleep apnea. Am J Respir Crit Care Med 1993;147(5):1162–8.

31. Zimmerman ME, Arnedt JT, Stanchina M, et al. Normalization of memory performance and positive airway pressure adherence in memory-impaired patients with obstructive sleep apnea. Chest 2006;130(6):1772–8.

32. Black J, Hirshkowitz M. Modafinil for the treatment of residual excessive sleepiness in nasal continuous positive airway pressure-treated obstructive sleep apnea/hypopnea syndrome. Sleep 2005;28(4):464–71.

33. Morgenthaler T, Kapen S, Lee-Chiong T, et al. Practice parameters for the medical therapy of obstructive sleep apnea. Sleep 2006;29(8):1031–5.

34. Veasey S, Davis C, Fenik P, et al. Long-term intermittent hypoxia in mice: protracted hypersomnolence with oxidative injury to sleep-wake brain regions. Sleep 2004;27(2):194–201.

35. Engleman H, Martin S, Deary I, et al. The effect of continuous positive airway pressure therapy on daytime function in the sleep apnoea/hyponoea syndrome. Lancet 1994;343:572–5.

36. Engleman H, Martin S, Deary I, et al. Effect of CPAP therapy on daytime function in patients with mild sleep apnoea/hypopnoea syndrome. Thorax 1997;52:114–9.

37. Engleman H, Kingshott R, Wraith P, et al. Randomized placebo-controlled crossover trial of CPAP for mild sleep apnea/hypopnea syndrome. Am J Respir Crit Care Med 1999;159:461–7.

38. Engleman H, Kingshott R, Martin S, et al. Cognitive function in the sleep apnea/hypopnea syndrome (SAHS). Sleep 2000;23(Suppl 4):S102–8.

39. Greenberg G, Watson R, Deptula D. Neuropsychological dysfunction in sleep apnea. Sleep 1987;10:254–62.

40. Redline S, Strauss M, Adams N, et al. Neuropsychological function in mild sleep-disordered breathing. Sleep 1997;20:160–7.

41. Kim H, Young T, Matthews C, et al. Sleep-disordered breathing and neuropsychological deficits: a population based study. Am J Respir Crit Care Med 1997;156:1813–9.

42. Bedard M, Montplaisir J, Richer F, et al. Obstructive sleep apnea syndrome: pathogenesis of neuropsychological deficits. J Clin Exp Neuropsychol 1991;13:950–64.

43. Borak J, Cieslicki J, Koziej M, et al. Effects of CPAP treatment on psychological status in patients with severe obstructive sleep apnea. J Sleep Res 1996;5(2):123–7.

44. Naegele B, Thouvard V, Pepin J, et al. Deficits of cognitive executive functions in patients with sleep apnea syndrome. Sleep 1995;18:43–52.

45. Ramos Platon M, Espinar, Sierra J. Changes in psychopathological symptoms in sleep apnea patients after treatment with nasal continuous airway pressure. Int J Neurosci 1992;62(3-4):173–95.

46. Munoz A, Mayoralas L, Barbe F, et al. Long-term effects of CPAP on daytime functioning in patients with sleep apnoea syndrome. Eur Respir J 2000;15(4):676–81.

47. Doherty LS, Kiely JL, Swan V, et al. Long-term effects of nasal continuous positive airway pressure therapy on cardiovascular outcomes in sleep apnea syndrome. Chest 2005;127(6):2076–84.

48. Barnes M, McEvoy RD, Banks S, et al. Efficacy of positive airway pressure and oral appliance in mild to moderate obstructive sleep apnea. Am J Respir Crit Care Med 2004;170(6):656–64.

49. Marin J, Carrizo S, Vincente E, et al. Long-term cardiovascular outcomes in men with obstructive sleep apnoea-hypopnea with or without treatment with continuous positive airway pressure: an observational study. Lancet 2005;365(9464):1046–53.

50. Campos-Rodriguez F, Grilo-Reina A, Perez-Ronchel J, et al. Effect of continuous positive airway pressure on ambulatory BP in patients with sleep apnea and hypertension: a placebo-controlled trial. Chest 2006;129(6):1459–67.

51. Arzt M, Bradley TD. Treatment of sleep apnea in heart failure. Am J Respir Crit Care Med 2006;173(12):1300–8.

52. Haentjens P, Van Meerhaeghe A, Moscariello A, et al. The impact of continuous positive airway pressure on blood pressure in patients with obstructive sleep apnea syndrome: evidence from a meta-analysis of placebo-controlled randomized trials. Arch Intern Med 2007;167(8):757–64.

53. Bazzano L, Khan Z, Reynolds K, et al. Effect of nocturnal nasal continuous positive airway

pressure on blood pressure in obstructive sleep apnea. Hypertension 2007;50(2):417–23.

54. Mansfield D, Gollogly N, Kaye D, et al. Controlled trial of continuous positive airway pressure in obstructive sleep apnea and heart failure. Am J Respir Crit Care Med 2004;169(3):361–6.

55. Kaneko Y, Floras J, Usui K, et al. Cardiovascular effects of continuous positive airway pressure in patients with heart failure and obstructive sleep apnea. N Engl J Med 2003;348(13):1233–41.

56. Buchner NJ, Sanner BM, Borgel J, et al. Continuous positive airway pressure treatment of mild to moderate obstructive sleep apnea reduces cardiovascular risk. Am J Respir Crit Care Med 2007; 176(12):1274–80.

57. Kribbs N, Pack A, Kline L, et al. Objective measurement of patterns of nasal CPAP use by patients with obstructive sleep apnea. Am Rev Respir Dis 1993; 147:887–95.

58. Mcardle N, Devereux G, Heidarnejad H, et al. Long-term use of CPAP therapy for sleep apnea/hypopnea syndrome. Am J Respir Crit Care Med 1999;159(4):1108–14.

59. Weaver T, Kribbs N, Pack A, et al. Night to night variability in CPAP use over the first three months of treatment. Sleep 1997;20(4):278–83.

60. Lewis K, Seale L, Bartle I, et al. Early predictors of CPAP use for the treatment of obstructive sleep apnea. Sleep 2004;27(1):134–8.

61. Budhiraja R, Parthasarathy S, Drake C, et al. Early CPAP use identifies subsequent adherence to CPAP therapy. Sleep 2007;30:320–4.

62. Reeves-Hoche M, Meck R, Zwillich C, et al. An objective evaluation of patient compliance. Am J Respir Crit Care Med 1994;149(1):149–54.

63. Rauscher H, Formanek D, Popp W, et al. Self-reported vs measured compliance with nasal CPAP for obstructive sleep apnea. Chest 1993;103(6):1675–80.

64. Engleman H, Martin S, Douglas N. Compliance with CPAP therapy in patients with the sleep apnoea/hypopnoea syndrome. Thorax 1994;49(3):263–6.

65. Massie C, Hart R, Peralez K, et al. Effects of humidification on nasal symptoms and compliance in sleep apnea patients using continuous positive airway pressure. Chest 1999;116(2):403–8.

66. Martins de Araujo M, Vieira S, Vasquez E, et al. Heated humidification or face mask to prevent upper airway dryness during continuous positive airway pressure therapy. Chest 2000;117(1):142–7.

67. Rakotonanahary D, Pelletier-Fleury N, Gagnadoux F, et al. Predictive factors for the need for additional humidification during nasal continuous positive airway pressure therapy. Chest 2001;119(2):460–5.

68. Wiese H, Boethel C, Phillips B, et al. CPAP compliance: video education may help. Sleep Med 2005; 6:171–4.

69. Chervin R, Theut S, Bassetti C, et al. Compliance with nasal CPAP can be improved by simple interventions. Sleep 1997;20(4):284–9.

70. Giles T, Lasserson T, Smith B, et-al. Continuous positive airways pressure for obstructive sleep apnoea in adults. Cochrane Database Syst Rev 2006 (2). CD001106. DOI:10.1002/14651858.CD001106.pub3.

71. Sanders M, Kern N. Obstructive sleep apnea treated by independently adjusted inspiratory and expiratory positive airway pressures via nasal mask. Physiologic and clinical implications. Chest 1990;98(2):317–24.

72. Reeves-Hoche M, Hudgel D, Meck R, et al. Continuous versus bilevel positive airway pressure for obstructive sleep apnea. Am J Respir Crit Care Med 1995;151(2):443–9.

73. Gay P, Herold D, Olson E. A randomized, double-blind clinical trial comparing continuous airway pressure with a novel bilevel pressure system for the treatment of obstructive sleep apnea. Sleep 2003;26(7):864–9.

74. Ballard R, Gay P, Strollo P. Interventions to improve compliance in sleep apnea patients previously non-compliant with continuous positive airway pressure. J Clin Sleep Med 2007;3:706–12.

75. Smith I, Lasserson T. Pressure modification for improving usage of continuous positive airway pressure machines in adults with obstructive sleep apnoea. Cochrane Database Syst Rev 2009;(4):CD003531.

76. Aloia M, Stanchina M, Arnedt J, et al. Treatment adherence and outcomes in flexible vs standard continuous positive airway pressure therapy. Chest 2005;127(6):2085–93.

77. Nilius G, Happel A, Domanski U, et al. Pressure-relief continuous positive airway pressure vs constant continuous positive airway pressure: a comparison of efficacy and compliance. Chest 2006;130(4):1018–24.

78. Roux F, Hilbert J. Continuous positive airway pressure: new generations. In: Lee-Chiong T, Mohsenin V, editors, In: Clinics in Chest Medicine, vol. 24. Philadelphia: W.B. Saunders Company; 2003. p. 315–42.

79. Morgenthaler T, Aurora R, Brown T, et al. Practice parameters for the use of autotitrating continuous positive airway pressure devices for titrating pressures and treating adult patients with obstructive sleep apnea syndrome: an update for 2007. An American Academy of Sleep Medicine Report. Sleep 2008;31:141–7.

80. Randerath W, Parys K, Feldmeyer F, et al. Self-adjusting nasal continuous positive airway pressure therapy based on measurement of

impedance: a comparison of two different maximum pressure levels. Chest 1999;116(4):991–9.

81. Randerath W, Schraeder O, Galetke W, et al. Autoadjusting CPAP therapy based on impedance efficacy, compliance and acceptance. Am J Respir Crit Care Med 2001;163(3):652–7.

82. Randerath W, Galetke W, David M, et al. Prospective randomized comparison of impedance-controlled auto-continuous positive airway pressure (APAPfot) with constant CPAP. Sleep Med 2001;2:115–24.

83. Marrone O, Insalaco G, Bonsignore MR, et al. Sleep structure correlates of continuous positive airway pressure variations during application of an autotitrating continuous positive airway pressure machine in patients with obstructive sleep apnea syndrome. Chest 2002;121(3):759–67.

84. Fuchs F, Wiest G, Frank M, et al. Auto-CPAP for obstructive sleep apnea: induction of microarousals by automatic variations of CPAP pressure? Sleep 2002;25(2):514–8.

85. Ayas N, Patel S, Malhotra A, et al. Auto-titrating vs standard continuous positive airway pressure for the treatment of obstructive sleep apnea: results of a meta-analysis. Sleep 2004;27(2):249–53.

86. Hukins CA. Comparative study of autotitrating and fixed-pressure CPAP in the home: a randomized, single-blind crossover trial. Sleep 2004;27(8):1512–7.

87. Nussbaumer Y, Bloch KE, Genser T, et al. Equivalence of autoadjusted and constant continuous positive airway pressure in home treatment of sleep apnea. Chest 2006;129(3):638–43.

88. Abdenbi F, Chambille B, Escourrou P. Bench testing of auto-adjusting positive airway pressure devices. Eur Respir J 2004;24(4):649–58.

89. Rigau J, Montserrat JM, Wohrle H, et al. Bench model to simulate upper airway obstruction for analyzing automatic continuous positive airway pressure devices. Chest 2006;130(2):350–61.

90. Farre R, Montserrat J, Rigau J, et al. Response of automatic continuous positive airway pressure devices to different sleep breathing patterns: a bench study. Am J Respir Crit Care Med 2002;166(4):469–73.

91. Lofaso F, Desmarais G, Leroux K, et al. Bench evaluation of flow limitation detection by automated continuous positive airway pressure devices. Chest 2006;130(2):343–9.

92. Berry R, Parish J, Hartse K. The use of auto-titrating continuous positive airway pressure for the treatment of adult obstructive sleep apnea. Sleep 2002;25(2):148–73.

93. Littner M, Hirshkowitz M, Davilla D, et al. Practice parameters for the use of autotitrating continuous positive airway pressure devices for titrating pressures and treating adult patients with obstructive sleep apnea syndrome. Sleep 2002; 25(2):143–7.

94. Massie CA, McArdle N, Hart RW, et al. Comparison between automatic and fixed positive airway pressure therapy in the home. Am J Respir Crit Care Med 2003;167(1):20–3.

95. Teschler H, Wessendorf T, Farhat A, et al. Two months auto-adjusting versus conventional nCPAP for obstructive sleep apnoea syndrome. Eur Respir J 2000;15(6):990–5.

96. Meurice J, Marc I, Series F. Efficacy of auto-CPAP in the treatment of obstructive sleep apnea/hypopnea syndrome. Am J Respir Crit Care Med 1996;153(2):794–8.

97. Series F, Marc I. Efficacy of automatic continuous positive airway pressure therapy that uses an estimated required pressure in the treatment of the obstructive sleep apnea syndrome. Ann Intern Med 1997;127(8_Part_1):588–95.

98. Hudgel D, Fung C. A long-term randomized crossover comparison of auto-titrating and standard nasal continuous positive airway pressure. Sleep 2000;23:1–4.

99. d'Ortho MP, Grillier-Lanoir V, Levy P, et al. Constant vs automatic continuous positive airway pressure therapy: home evaluation. Chest 2000;118(4):1010–7.

100. Konermann M, Sanner B, Vyleta M, et al. Use of conventional and self-adjusting nasal continuous positive airway pressure for treatment of severe obstructive sleep apnea syndrome: a comparative study. Chest 1998;113(3):714–8.

101. Noseda A, Kempenaers C, Kerkhofs M, et al. Constant vs auto-continuous positive airway pressure in patients with sleep apnea hypopnea syndrome and a high variability in pressure requirement. Chest 2004;126(1):31–7.

102. Pevernagie D, Proot P, Hertegonne K, et al. Efficacy of flow- vs impedance-guided autoadjustable continuous positive airway pressure: a randomized cross-over trial. Chest 2004;126(1):25–30.

103. Nolan G, Doherty L, McNicholas W. Auto-adjusting versus fixed positive pressure therapy in mild to moderate obstructive sleep apnoea. Sleep 2007; 30(2):189–94.

104. Senn O, Brack T, Matthews F, et al. Randomized short-term trial of two AutoCPAP devices versus fixed continuous positive airway pressure for the treatment of sleep apnea. Am J Respir Crit Care Med 2003;168(12):1506–11.

105. Stammnitz A, Jerrentrup A, Penzel T, et al. Automatic CPAP titration with different self-setting devices in patients with obstructive sleep apnoea. Eur Respir J 2004;24(2):273–8.

106. Kessler R, Weitzenblum E, Chaouat A, et al. Evaluation of unattended automated titration to determine therapeutic continuous positive airway

pressure in patients with obstructive sleep apnea. Chest 2003;123(3):704–10.

107. Lloberes P, Marti S, Sampol G, et al. Predictive factors of quality-of-life improvement and continuous positive airway pressure use in patients with sleep apnea-hypopnea syndrome: study at 1 year. Chest 2004;126(4):1241–7.

108. Kushida C, Morgenthaler T, Littner M, et al. Practice parameters for the treatment of snoring and obstructive sleep apnea with oral appliances: an update for 2005. Sleep 2006;29(2):240–3.

109. Ferguson K, Cartwright RR, Rogers R, et al. Oral appliances for snoring and obstructive sleep apnea: a review. Sleep 2006;29(2):244–62.

110. Lim J, Lasserson T, Fleetham JA, et al. Oral appliances for obstructive sleep apnoea. Cochrane Database Syst Rev 2008;(1):CD004435.

111. Hoffstein V. Review of oral appliances for the treatment of sleep disordered breathing. Sleep Breath 2007;11:1–22.

112. Wilhelmsson B, Tegelberg A, Walker-Engstron M, et al. A prospective randomized study of a dental appliance compared with uvulopalatopharyngoplasty in the treatment of obstructive sleep apnoea. Acta Otolaryngol 1999;119:503–9.

113. Gotsolpoulos H, Kelly J, Cistulli P. Oral appliance therapy reduces blood pressure in obstructive sleep apnea: a randomized controlled trial. Sleep 2004;27(5):934–41.

114. Lam B, Sam K, Mok W, et al. Randomised study of three non-surgical treatments in mild to moderate obstructive sleep apnoea. Thorax 2007;62:354–9.

115. Kezirian E, Goldberg A. Hypopharyngeal surgery in obstructive sleep apnea: an evidence-based review. Arch Otolaryngol Head Neck Surg 2006; 132:206–13.

116. Sundaram S, Lim J, Lasserson T. Surgery for obstructive sleep apnoea in adults. Cochrane Database Syst Rev 2008;(4):CD001004.

117. Elshaug A, Moss J, Southcott A, et al. An analysis of the evidence-practice continuum: is surgery for obstructive sleep apnoea contraindicated? J Eval Clin Pract 2007;13:3–9.

118. Elshaug A, Moss J, Southcott A, et al. Redefining success in airway surgery for obstructive sleep apnea: a meta-analysis and synthesis of the evidence. Sleep 2007;30(4):461–7.

119. Veasey S, Guilleminault C, Strohl K, et al. Medical therapy for obstructive sleep apnea: a review by the medical therapy for obstructive sleep apnea task force of the standards of practice committee of the American Academy of Sleep Medicine. Sleep 2006;29(8):1036–44.

120. The Longitudinal Assessment of Bariatric Surgery Consortium. Perioperative safety in the longitudinal assessment of bariatric surgery. N Engl J Med 2009;361:445–54.

121. Greenburg D, Lettieri C, Eliasson A. Effects of surgical weight loss on measures of obstructive sleep apnea: a meta-analysis. Am J Med 2009; 122(6):535–42.

122. Pillar G, Peled R, Lavie P. Recurrence of sleep apnea without concomitant weight increase 7.5 years after weight reduction surgery. Chest 1994; 106:1702–4.

Cardiovascular Consequences of Sleep Apnea

Bernardo Selim, MD[a], Christine Won, MD[a],
H. Klar Yaggi, MD, MPH[a,b],*

KEYWORDS

- Sleep-disordered breathing • Obstructive sleep apnea
- Stroke • Myocardial infarction • Hypertension
- Pulmonary hypertension • Congestive heart failure
- Arrhythmia

Sleeping is no mean art: for its sake one must stay awake all day.

Friedrich Nietzsche

Cardiovascular disease has been the leading cause of death since 1900 every year except 1918 (influenza epidemic), and approximately one-third of all deaths from cardiovascular disease occurs prematurely (before average life expectancy). Strategies for cardiovascular disease and prevention have helped to reduce the burden of disease, but it remains an important public health challenge. Therefore, understanding the underlying pathophysiology and developing novel therapeutic approaches for cardiovascular disease is of crucial importance.

Recognizing the link between sleep and cardiovascular disease may represent one such novel approach. A recent Institute of Medicine report, entitled *Sleep Disorders and Sleep Deprivation: An Unmet Public Health Challenge*, estimated that 50 to 70 million Americans suffer from a chronic sleep disorder. A major aspect of this "unmet public health challenge" is the cardiovascular health consequences of sleep-disordered breathing. Obstructive sleep apnea (OSA), a common form of sleep-disordered breathing, has a high and rising prevalence in the general adult population, attributable in part to the emerging epidemic of obesity and enhanced awareness. The prevalence of OSA in adults is estimated to be 6%, 75% of whom remain undiagnosed.[1] Population-based longitudinal studies, such as the Wisconsin Sleep Cohort and the Busselton Health Study, have shown that severe OSA had a threefold greater risk of all-cause mortality and a higher cardiovascular mortality at 18-year follow-up, respectively.[2,3] OSA has been independently linked to specific cardiovascular outcomes such as hypertension,[4] stroke,[5,6] myocardial ischemia,[7,8] arrhythmias,[9] fatal and nonfatal cardiovascular events,[10,11] and all-cause mortality.[2,3] Treatment of OSA may represent a novel target to reduce cardiovascular health outcomes.

CARDIOVASCULAR MODULATION IN NORMAL SLEEP AND IN OBSTRUCTIVE SLEEP APNEA

Studies in healthy humans using microneurography (which allows for direct recording of peripheral sympathetic nerve traffic) suggest that the cardiovascular influence of sleep is more complex than a generalized inhibition of the sympathetic nervous system.[12] In non–rapid eye movement (NREM)

[a] Division of Pulmonary and Critical Care Medicine, Yale University School of Medicine, 333 Cedar Street, PO Box 208057, New Haven, CT 06520-8057, USA
[b] West Haven VA Medical Center Sleep Laboratory, VA CT Health Care System, Clinical Epidemiology Research Center, 950 Campbell Avenue, West Haven, CT 06516, USA
* Corresponding author. Division of Pulmonary and Critical Care Medicine, Yale University School of Medicine, 333 Cedar Street, PO Box 208057, New Haven, CT 06520-8057.
E-mail address: henry.yaggi@yale.edu

Clin Chest Med 31 (2010) 203–220
doi:10.1016/j.ccm.2010.02.010
0272-5231/10/$ – see front matter © 2010 Published by Elsevier Inc.

sleep, parasympathetic tone increases and sympathetic tone decreases resulting in a decrease of heart rate, blood pressure, systemic vascular resistance, and cardiac output. This sleep phase, which represents 75% to 85% of sleep time, is a period of increased cardiac stability. Opposite to NREM sleep, the rapid eye movement (REM) stage is characterized by a decrease in parasympathetic and an increase in sympathetic tone, resulting in an elevation of blood pressure and heart rate to levels similar to those registered during wakefulness. This cardiovascular modulation is well documented in 24-hour ambulatory pressure monitoring of normotensive patients.[13] Blood pressure falls to its lowest level during the first few hours of sleep, followed by a marked surge in the morning hours coinciding with the transition from sleep to wakefulness. The average difference between waking and sleeping systolic and diastolic pressure is 10% to 20% (normal dipping pattern). These observations might explain why myocardial ischemia, infarction, and stroke are less common during the night than during daytime periods of similar duration, particularly the morning hours.[14] In contrast, this observed morning circadian pattern of adverse cardiovascular events appears to be inverted among patients with OSA, in whom the peak circadian time for sudden cardiac death occurs during the sleeping hours between midnight and 6 AM.[11]

PATHOPHYSIOLOGIC INFLUENCE OF OBSTRUCTIVE SLEEP APNEA IN CARDIOVASCULAR DISEASE

Patients with sleep apnea have recurrent "cycles" of sleep, airway obstruction, arousal, and

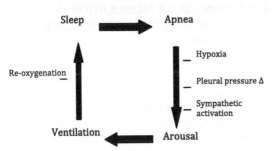

Fig. 1. The sleep apnea cycle. Patients with obstructive sleep apnea have recurrent "cycles" of sleep, airway obstruction, arousal, and resumption of ventilation. Multiple physiologic stresses occur with intermittent upper airway occlusion including: intermittent hypoxemia of varying frequency, duration, and severity; strenuous respiratory efforts that result in the generation of severely negative intrathoracic pressures; frequent arousals with significant increases in sympathetic nerve activity; and sleep deprivation.

resumption of ventilation (**Fig. 1**). Several physiologic stresses arise from this intermittent airway occlusion during sleep including cyclical hypoxemia of varying duration and severity, strenuous respiratory efforts against an occluded airway resulting in the generation of severely negative intrathoracic pressures, sympathetic activation, parasympathetic withdrawal, and reduced total sleep time. These stresses, specific to sleep apnea, serve as potential mechanisms for the independent increased risk of adverse cardiovascular events such as stroke, hypertension, myocardial ischemia, arrhythmias, congestive heart failure (HF), and pulmonary hypertension.

Inflammation and Intermittent Hypoxia

Cardiovascular/cerebrovascular events

Systemic inflammation plays an important role in the development of atherosclerosis. The pathogenesis of inflammation and atherosclerosis in sleep apnea has not been entirely elucidated; however, intermittent hypoxia followed by reoxygenation (common to sleep apnea) appears to play a key role. Repetitive episodes of hypoxia may selectively activate vascular inflammatory pathways[15,16] A higher frequency of repetitive oxygen desaturations has been correlated with increasing severity of atherosclerosis.[17] It is suggested that intermittent hypoxia promotes the formation of reactive oxygen species (ROS), particularly during the reoxygenation period, which can be deleterious to cell endothelial cells, leukocytes, and platelets. These cells, in turn, express adhesion molecules and proinflammatory cytokines that may lead to endothelial injury and dysfunction, and consequently, to atherosclerosis.[18–23]

Pulmonary hypertension

Hypoxemia-induced pulmonary vasoconstriction leading to vascular remodeling contributes to the development of chronic pulmonary hypertension (PH) in some OSA patients. Cyclical oscillations in both pulmonary and systemic arterial pressures during sleep are well described in OSA patients.[24] Pulmonary arterial pressures increase during an apneic episode, often reaching maximum at the termination of an apnea, and decrease when ventilation is restored. The degree of pulmonary arterial pressure fluctuations coincides with oxyhemoglobin saturation (Sao_2) and arterial oxygen tension (Pao_2) nadir, and tends to be less severe during oxygen administration.[25] Repetitive apneas may result in an increase in mean pulmonary artery pressure as the night progresses if the pulmonary vasculature fails to recover before subsequent Sao_2 changes.[26] Chronic or daytime pulmonary hypertension results when the pulmonary vasculature undergoes remodeling following chronic hypoxemic vasoconstriction and reperfusion injury.[27]

Nocturnal Sympathetic Activation

Cardiovascular/cerebrovascular events

Sympathetic overactivity in the pathogenesis of cardiovascular/cerebrovascular complications in OSA has been suggested for several years, and evidence continues to accumulate. Early reports found increased plasma and urinary catecholamine levels in patients with sleep apnea and a decrease in these levels after treatment with tracheostomy.[28] Others employed more direct measures of sympathetic nerve activity through the use of a tungsten microelectrode in the peroneal nerve. This methodology demonstrated increased muscle sympathetic nerve activity following acute apneic events.[29] Superimposed on these bursts of sympathetic activation are "surges" of blood pressure of up to 240 mm Hg at apnea termination. These acute blood pressure elevations during apnea appear to be driven by changes in baroreceptor sensitivity during sleep and chemoreceptor responses to progressive hypoxia.[30] Considering that humans typically spend one-third of their lives sleeping, these nocturnal increases in blood pressure might in themselves contribute to hypertensive cardiovascular and cerebrovascular consequences. In addition, patients with sleep apnea commonly do not have the normal nocturnal fall or "dipping" in blood pressure.[31–33] Among patients with hypertension, those who exhibit a diminished nocturnal decline in blood pressure, "nondippers,"[34] have been reported to have more cardiovascular target-organ damage than dippers,[35,36] including silent cerebrovascular damage.[37] Three longitudinal studies conducted in patients with hypertension have confirmed that a diminished nocturnal decline in blood pressure predicted cardiovascular events,[38,39] including worse stroke prognosis.[40] Moreover, diminished nocturnal decline of blood pressure is a risk factor for cardiovascular mortality independent of overall blood pressure load during a 24-hour period, with 5% decrease in nocturnal dipping being associated with a 20% increase in cardiovascular mortality.[41]

Heart failure

Increased sympathetic nervous system activity (SNSA) is not only a characteristic compensatory mechanism of HF but also a shared pathophysiologic effect of OSA and central sleep apnea (CSA) independently of HF. The combined hyperadrenergic drive of OSA and HF causes a greater SNSA response than either disease alone. This increased SNSA, regardless of its trigger, is associated with adverse outcomes in patients with HF.[13,42] Long-term exposure to recurrent elevated SNSA can cause cardiac myocyte apoptosis, β-adrenoceptor down-regulation, decreased heart rate variability (HRV), arrhythmias, and an increase in mortality rate.[42,43]

Pulmonary hypertension

Sympathetic activity modulates endogenous vasoconstrictors and vasodilators, and plays a role in pulmonary vascular remodeling. Norepinephrine and angiotensin II, both released by increased peripheral sympathetic tone, act as growth-promoting or trophic factors on the heart and vasculature. These 2 hormones can contribute to long-term changes in vessel wall and ventricular compliance through hypertrophy of smooth muscle and myocardium. As mentioned earlier, studies have consistently shown that nocturnal and 24-hour norepinephrine levels increase with the number of respiratory disturbances.[44,45] Moreover, when catecholamine levels were examined in 38 patients with OSA who were prospectively treated with therapeutic continuous positive airway pressure (CPAP) or sham CPAP, both plasma and urinary catecholamine levels fell by nearly 50% in the treated patients while remaining unchanged in the untreated group.[46]

Mechanical Load

Heart failure

Recurrent high negative intrathoracic pressures are generated by Mueller maneuvers (up to −65 mm Hg) during OSA events, while attempting to inspire against an obstructed upper airway. The transmural pressure across the heart and great thoracic vessels (afterload) translates into an increment of myocardial wall stress, atrial size,[47] and impairment of ventricular function,[48] more specifically diastolic function.[49,50] Venous return (preload) is also enhanced during these pressure swings, producing a right ventricular distension and left shift of interventricular septum with concomitant compromise of left ventricular filling. This increase in right- and left-side cardiac load mediated by increase of myocardial demand and increase of adrenergic tone plays an important role in myocardial dilation and ventricular dysfunction.[51]

Pulmonary hypertension

Nocturnal oscillations in pulmonary artery pressure also occur in synchrony with intrathoracic pressure changes. Large negative intrathoracic pressures generated during obstructive apneas may increase left ventricular transmural pressure causing greater myocardial oxygen demand, reduced cardiac output, and increased pulmonary capillary wedge pressure. Large negative intrathoracic pressures may also increase wall stiffness of large vessels and increase their impedance, resulting in increased right ventricular load by up to 30% to 40%. The pulmonary conductance vessels are unable to store and deliver the entire stroke volume of the right ventricle, which ultimately results in loss of pulmonary flow during diastole. Pulsatile flow is required by distal pulmonary artery endothelial cells for optimal nitric oxide (NO) production for normal pulmonary vasodilation.[52] Down-regulation of NO, the body's most potent vasodilator, through generation of superoxide anions or NO synthase alterations occurs in OSA, and rapidly reverses with CPAP therapy.[53] In contrast, endothelin-1, a powerful endogenous vasoconstrictor, is notably elevated in subjects with OSA.[54] The end result of this imbalance in vasodilator and vasoconstriction factors is an increase in resting vascular tone.[55] This increase has been demonstrated in OSA patients by blunted vasodilator and vasoconstrictor dose-response curves. Another potential pathway for pulmonary hypertension in OSA is by alteration in the apelin signaling pathway. The peptide apelin is localized in the vascular endothelium and highly expressed in pulmonary tissue. During normoxemic conditions, apelin has a modulating effect on vasoconstriction, which is lost in chronic hypoxemia. Untreated OSA has recently been associated with elevated plasma apelin levels and altered apelin secretory dynamics, both of which were restored following CPAP therapy.[56]

Arrhythmias

Mechanical-electric stress also plays an arrhythmogenic role in OSA patients. The cardiac stretch secondary to negative intrathoracic pressures may also predispose to arrhythmias by distortion of cardiac mechanoreceptors[57] and changes in atrial transmural pressures.[58,59]

Heart Rate Variability and Cardiac Arrhythmias

Heart failure/arrhythmias

HRV refers to the rhythmic R-R (beat to beat) alterations in heart rate during the breathing cycle. In inspiration, there is a cardio-acceleration followed by a cardio-deceleration during expiration. These changes correlate with increased vagal efferent tone to the cardiac sinus node during expiration followed by an attenuated vagal tone (increased sympathetic activity) during inspiration. Thus, reduced HRV has been used as a marker of reduced vagal activity. In cardiac patients, alteration of autonomic regulation manifested by a decrease in HRV is an independent predictor of cardiovascular events. For example, after myocardial infarction a decreased HRV is a prognostic indicator of both arrhythmic complications and cardiac death,[60,61] and it is also a predictor of morbidity and mortality in patients with HF.[62] But even in the absence of cardiovascular disease such as hypertension or HF, cardiovascular variability is also reduced in patients with OSA. The severity of HRV is predominant in patients with moderate to severe OSA,[63] with possible implications in the subsequent development or exacerbation of cardiovascular disease and arrhythmias.

Arrhythmias

Sleep-disordered breathing (SDB) may specifically establish proarrhythmogenic pathways through abnormal spontaneous cardiac impulse formation (pacemaker activity) and reentrant mechanism[64] secondary to nightly exposure to recurrent hypoxia, acidosis, arousals, intrathoracic pressure swings, and increase in adrenergic drive.[65] The following abnormal electrophysiological mechanisms in SDB are proposed: (1) spontaneous cardiac impulse formation (abnormal automaticity) possible secondary to apneic-related hypoxemia and respiratory acidosis[64]; (2) abnormal pacemaker activity (triggered automaticity) related to hyperadrenergic drive in a background of respiratory-related recurrent hypoxemia and arousals[66]; and (3) increased vagal tone related to inspiration against a closed glottis (Mueller maneuver), with subsequent increased dispersion of atrial repolarization and intra-atrial entry (reentry mechanism).[67]

Abnormal Coagulation

Cardiovascular/cerebrovascular events

Sleep apnea may act through multiple mechanisms to predispose to acute thrombosis and thus cardiovascular and cerebrovascular events. Platelets play a key role in ischemic cerebrovascular disease, and increases in platelet aggregability and activation have been demonstrated in patients with sleep apnea,[68–73] which improves with CPAP.[68,73] The mechanism for increased platelet reactivity in patients with sleep apnea is possibly the cyclic hypoxemia, hypercapnia, and catecholamine surges that are part of sleep apnea and have also been reported to cause platelet activation.[28,45,74] In one study,[73] the arousal index was the independent factor best associated with baseline platelet activation, supporting a pathophysiologic paradigm of sleep arousal precipitating increased neural activation and leading to increased platelet activation.[75] The observation that CPAP reduces platelet activation supports this same paradigm, and suggests that treatment intervention for sleep apnea may be protective against cardiovascular disease and stroke. Whether such a benefit of CPAP would be additive to the effects of antiplatelet therapy is not known.

Metabolic Dysregulation

There is significant overlap between sleep apnea and the cluster of cardiovascular risk factors that constitutes the "metabolic syndrome." In fact there is accumulating evidence to suggest that sleep restriction may worsen these metabolic abnormalities. Sleep curtailment has been linked to impaired carbohydrate tolerance and insulin resistance,[76] and even the development of type 2 diabetes.[77] Several studies have also demonstrated that SDB increases the risk for glucose intolerance,[78] insulin resistance,[79,80] and overt clinical diabetes.[81] A recent published observational cohort study by Botros and colleagues[82] has shown not only that sleep apnea is an independent risk factor for the development of diabetes but also that there is a direct correlation between increasing severity of sleep apnea and increasing risk for the development of diabetes. Furthermore, among patients with moderate to severe sleep apnea, regular use of positive airway pressure is associated with an attenuated risk for the development of incident diabetes. Several potential mechanistic pathways might explain how sleep apnea and its physiologic sequelae (intermittent hypoxemia and recurrent arousals) ultimately lead to metabolic abnormalities. In fact, there are firm data to support the association between severity of hypoxemia and the degree of glucose intolerance and insulin resistance.[78,83]

SLEEP APNEA AND SELECTED CARDIOVASCULAR DISEASES
Hypertension, Stroke, and Myocardial Infarction

Epidemiologic observations

In addition to acute blood pressure swings at night, evidence supports that sustained *diurnal* hypertension can arise from obstructive apnea. This hypertension appears to be in part related to a "carryover" phenomenon of heightened sympathetic activity[29] Two large observational longitudinal-based studies have measured the relation of baseline OSA severity and the risk of development of hypertension in a community-based cohort free of hypertension over a 2- to 5-year follow-up period. In the Sleep Heart Health Study,[84] sleep apnea had a modest, not statistically significant association with the development of hypertension. Subjects with an apnea/hypopnea index (AHI; number of apneas and hypopneas per hour of sleep) of 30 events/h or more had an adjusted 1.5-fold increased odds of developing hypertension compared with subjects without OSA as baseline. From the prospective results of the Wisconsin Sleep Cohort, the presence of sleep apnea at baseline was accompanied by a statistically significant increased risk for future hypertension at 4-year follow-up.[4] Even after adjusting for baseline age, gender, body mass index (BMI; weight in kilograms divided by height in meters squared), waist and neck circumference, and weekly alcohol and cigarette use, the risk for hypertension remained elevated. Subjects with an AHI of 15 events/h or more had a 3.2-fold increased odds of developing hypertension relative to subjects without OSA at baseline. Despite these apparent discrepant results, possibly related to difference in study populations and study designs, there is a strong clinical implication of a modest causal association between OSA and blood pressure. Considering the growing prevalence of OSA, the population-level impact of a modest causal OSA-blood pressure association on cardiovascular outcomes may be significant. In fact, the Seventh Report of the Joint Committee on Prevention, Detection, Evaluation, and Treatment of High Blood Pressure (JCN 7) recognizes the etiologic role of sleep apnea as an identifiable cause of hypertension.[85]

When considered separately from cardiovascular disease, stroke is the third leading cause of death and ranks as the leading cause of long-term disability.[86] Recent prospective observational cohort studies have clarified this temporal relationship and have demonstrated that sleep apnea increases the risk for stroke,[5,6] stroke and all-cause mortality,[87] and fatal and nonfatal cardiovascular events.[88] In one study, after excluding prevalent stroke and adjusting for traditional cerebrovascular risk factors (including hypertension, which itself may be on the causal pathway between sleep apnea and stroke), sleep apnea was associated with a twofold increased risk for transient ischemic attack (TIA), stroke, or all-cause-mortality.[87] In a trend analysis, increasing severity of sleep apnea at baseline was associated with an increased risk for the development of the composite end point ($P = .005$).[87] Those patients in the highest severity quartile of the cohort (AHI>36) had a greater than threefold increased risk for the development of stroke or death. A similar magnitude of risk has recently been described in other population population-based cohort studies.[5,6]

Coronary artery disease is not only highly prevalent in the United States but continues to be the leading cause of death in this country. Among patients with coronary artery disease, OSA is particularly common, with a prevalence as high as 37% among men and 30% among women. From mouse models demonstrating that chronic intermittent hypoxia induces atherosclerosis to human studies showing early signs of atherosclerosis in patients with OSA who are free of cardiovascular comorbidities, an independent association between OSA and atherosclerosis is suggested.[16,89] In fact, a recent published observational cohort study has shown among men and women with a wide range of OSA severity an increased risk for development of myocardial infarction, coronary revascularization events, or cardiovascular death, independent of other cardiovascular risk factors. Proportional to the severity of OSA, there is up to a twofold increase in coronary events and cardiovascular death in patients with severe OSA (AHI > 30 events/h).[90] Furthermore, current evidence supports that the harmful effect of OSA on the cardiovascular system may be even multiplied in the presence of a second cardiovascular risk factor such as dyslipidemia and hypertension.[91]

Treatment studies

To date no published *long-term* prospective, randomized controlled trials have demonstrated that the treatment of sleep apnea decreases the risk of cardiovascular events in terms of either primary or secondary prevention. However, *long-term* longitudinal observational cohort studies have evaluated the impact of CPAP therapy on cardiovascular outcomes, and *short-term* randomized controlled trials have evaluated the impact of CPAP on hypertension and intermediate cardiac end points in patients with sleep apnea.

Short-term randomized controlled trials with CPAP and the end point of blood pressure and selected intermediate cardiovascular end points

With respect to cardiovascular outcomes, short-term (up to 3 months) randomized controlled trials have been published looking at arterial blood pressure as the outcome. Although the studies vary with respect to the magnitude of blood pressure reduction, overall there appears to be a clinically important blood pressure reduction in both 24-hour systolic and diastolic pressures. The characteristics of the patients selected for these trials give clues to those most likely to gain any blood pressure lowering benefits. In general, those more likely to experience benefit have more severe

and symptomatic sleep apnea, are hypertensive or on hypertensive therapy at baseline, receive more effective therapy for sleep apnea (longer use), and have more frequent oxygen desaturations.[92–94] Those less likely to experience benefit are normotensive at baseline, asymptomatic, and have milder sleep apnea.[95,96] A recent systematic literature review conducted by the Cochrane Collaboration[97] found that mean 24-hour systolic and diastolic pressures were significantly lower on CPAP (−7.24 mm Hg systolic, −3.07 mm Hg diastolic). Other meta-analyses have indicated a lower *overall* blood pressure reduction on the order of 2 mm Hg[98,99]; however, the magnitude of the blood pressure reduction increases significantly with more severe sleep apnea and longer effective nighttime use of CPAP.[99] When extrapolated to antihypertensive epidemiologic data, such blood pressure lowering effects would be predicted to significantly reduce stroke and coronary heart disease event risk.[93,100]

Positive airway pressure treatment effects on atherosclerotic intermediate mediators, such as systemic inflammation, sympathetic activation, production of ROS, and endothelial dysfunction has also been examined. A recent 4-month follow-up randomized CPAP study of severe OSA patients with no other cardiovascular comorbidities (hypertension, diabetes, coronary artery disease, and so forth) showed an improvement in markers of early signs of atherosclerosis (intima-media thickness, arterial stiffness, C-reactive protein, and catecholamines) in patients treated with CPAP in comparison with those with no CPAP treatment.[101] Even though the effect of CPAP in chronic atherosclerotic lesions is still unknown, a recent observational study published by Bayram and colleagues[102] confirmed a reversal of endothelium-dependent flow-mediated dysfunction measured by ultrasound after 6 months of CPAP therapy.

Long-term observational studies and the influence of CPAP use in cardiovascular end points

Prospective observational cohorts designed to examine the impact of treatment on long-term cardiovascular outcomes in patients with sleep apnea have demonstrated that CPAP therapy may reduce mortality in severe sleep apnea[103] and protect against death from cardiovascular disease.[104] In a study conducted by Marin and colleagues[88] the incidence of fatal and nonfatal cardiovascular events was highest in patients with severe untreated sleep apnea. Patients who received and complied with CPAP (who largely had severe sleep apnea) had a significantly reduced cardiovascular risk, suggesting that long-term therapy with CPAP may reduce the risk of fatal and nonfatal cardiovascular events. For example, a recently published 5-year prospective observational follow-up study regarding ischemic stroke and CPAP treatment showed that CPAP treatment provides a reduction of excess risk of cardiovascular mortality. In fact, the mortality reduction of patients tolerating the CPAP was similar to that of the group without OSA or with mild disease.[105] Regarding CPAP impact in cardiovascular outcomes, benefits have been inferred mostly from available observational data. However, all of the aforementioned studies were observational cohorts and not randomized controlled trials, and the observed risk reductions may also be that those patients who used CPAP were also complying with other medical therapy and otherwise leading healthier lifestyles. Prospective randomized studies are needed to demonstrate the efficacy of treating sleep apnea in reducing cardiovascular outcome events.

Obstructive Sleep Apnea/Central Sleep Apnea and Heart Failure

Prevalence of sleep-disordered breathing in the general population and in the heart failure population

There is a high prevalence of SDB in patients with left ventricular dysfunction regardless of the etiology (ischemic vs idiopathic), type (systolic vs diastolic), and New York Heart Association (NYHA) class. In the HF population, previous case series studies have reported that approximately 41% to 75% of patients with stable, optimally treated HF (β-blockers, angiotensin-converting enzyme inhibitors, angiotensin II receptor antagonists, and aldosterone antagonists) will have SDB, either obstructive (31%) or central (30%) in origin.[106–109] Population-based studies such as the Sleep Heart Health Study have also shown that the presence of OSA conferred a 2.38 relative increase in the likelihood of having HF independent of other traditional cardiovascular risk factors.[10] Furthermore, the presence of OSA in HF patients is strongly associated with arrhythmias such as atrial fibrillation[110] and poorer NYHA functional class in comparison with patients with HF without SDB.[108]

Risk factors associated with obstructive sleep apnea and central sleep apnea in heart failure patients

In clinical practice, it is usually difficult to distinguish risk factors for OSA from that for HF. Several risk factors such as obesity, male gender, and age are shared by SDB and cardiovascular diseases alike. Based on recent studies, among the most common independent risk factors identified for developing OSA in patients with congestive HF are increased BMI (>35 kg/m^2) in males and increased age (>60 years) in females. Independent risk factors identified for CSA in the HF population are male gender, increasing age (>60 years), presence of atrial fibrillation, and decreasing awake Pco_2 in male and female patients alike.[107]

Hypertension and Diastolic Ventricular Dysfunction

Community-based studies have shown that 55% of individuals with HF have preserved left ventricular ejection fraction (LVEF) and 44% have isolated diastolic dysfunction.[111] Of the diastolic dysfunction population, it is estimated that 55% suffer from SDB, mainly obstructive apneas.[112] A strong physiopathological association between SDB, hypertension, and diastolic dysfunction exists. Taking into account that the most common cause of diastolic dysfunction is hypertension and that 40% to 60% of all patients with OSA are hypertensive,[113] the high prevalence of SDB in patients with diastolic dysfunction comes as no surprise. However, elevated blood pressure alone is unlikely to explain the complex physiopathology of diastolic failure in OSA.[114] Other mechanisms, such as increased negative intrathoracic pressures, hyperadrenergic drive, and recurrent hypoxemic events may promote disease progression and confer increase in morbidity independently of underlying cardiac dysfunction and blood pressure control.

Right Heart Failure and Left Heart Failure

Moderated-severe OSA (AHI ≥ 15) has been shown to have a deleterious effect over right[115,116] and left ventricular contractility[117] independently of other risk factors such as obesity, and pulmonary and arterial systolic pressure respectively.[47] Of importance is that global and diastolic myocardial function of the left ventricle is impaired in OSA, even when systolic function is not. Concomitant atrial enlargement has also been reported in this population.[118] The increase in atrial volume index could explain the predisposition of these patients to develop atrial fibrillation[119] with concomitant complications and/or perpetuation of HF. OSA is associated with increased right ventricular wall thickening but, contrary to left ventricular hypertrophy, right ventricular hypertrophy has not been confirmed as an independent predictor of adverse cardiovascular outcomes.[120,121]

Association of Heart Failure and Central Sleep Apnea: Cheyne-Stokes Respiration

CSA, although rare in the general population,[122] is highly prevalent (30%–55%) even in patients with asymptomatic, well-compensated left ventricular dysfunction (LVEF $\leq$ 40%).[123] In contrast to OSA, CSA manifested as Cheyne-Stokes respiration (CSR) likely arises as a consequence of HF.[124] CSR is the most common nonhypercapnic CSA in patients with HF. CSR is characterized by a crescendo-decrescendo ventilatory pattern during NREM sleep followed by central apneas. In patients with heart failure, CSR is considered to be the result of a high ventilatory loop gain (increase chemosensitivity stimulating hyperventilation) combined with a prolonged circulation time, pushing the Pco_2 concentration below the apnea threshold and thus triggering central apneas.[125] Although controversial, CSA-CSR may simply be a compensatory or protective mechanism for patients with HF by increasing pulmonary oxygen store due to increase in end-expiratory lung volume (crescendo ventilation) concomitant with an increase in cardiac muscle contractility secondary to alkalosis. Even though CSA severity does not parallel cardiac hemodynamic impairment (LVEF, Vo_2, and so forth) there is a clear influence of CSA in cardiac autonomic control (reflected by decreased HRV) and in increased cardiac arrhythmias.[123] These pathophysiological influences shared with OSA could propose CSA as an independent risk for mortality in patients with HF.[126]

Treatment of Sleep-Disordered Breathing Heart Failure Patients

CPAP treatment of sleep-disordered breathing patients with heart failure

Several randomized trials have shown that CPAP treatment for OSA in patients with HF decreases sympathetic nervous system activity,[29,127] blood pressure,[97,98] heart rate, and nocturnal ventricular ectopies.[128–130] Such treatment also increases vagal modulation of heart rate with consequent increase of HRV[131] and LVEF.[129] It is known that HF patients with moderate to severe OSA have an increased risk of death independently of confounding factors.[132,133] However, whether CPAP treatment of OSA patients with HF improves morbidity and mortality has not yet been proven.

There are controversial data regarding the benefit of CPAP use in patients with CSA-CSV and HF. Although CSA-CSV is not the cause of HF but an effect, treatment of CSA may have a beneficial effect. Early studies have shown that the use of CPAP in HF patients with CSA may improve LVEF and mortality.[134] In 2000, a randomized controlled study demonstrated that CPAP improves cardiac function in HF patients with CSR-CSA but not in those without it. This small study also suggests that CPAP may reduce the composite outcome of mortality-cardiac transplantation rate in compliant CSR-CSA patients on CPAP.[135,136] However, data from a larger randomized controlled Canadian trial (CanPAP trial) did not demonstrate benefits. In this study, it was shown that CPAP improved intermediate cardiovascular end points such as nocturnal oxygenation, and increased the ejection fraction and distance walk in 6 minutes, but it did not affect the main primary outcome of survival.[139] In recent years, adaptive servoventilation (ASV) has emerged as an alternative treatment tool for patients with CSA and CHF. ASV provides an expiratory positive airway pressure with an inspiratory pressure support, guaranteeing a minute ventilation in these patients. ASV has been shown not only to reduce CSA events and AHI severity but also to increase LVEF and quality of life at 6 months' follow-up.[137,138] However, further longitudinal studies are needed to clarify the role of ASV in morbidity and mortality of patients with CSA-HF.

OBSTRUCTIVE SLEEP APNEA AND ARRHYTHMIAS
Prevalence of Cardiac Arrhythmias in Obstructive Sleep Apnea

In healthy subjects, physiologic nocturnal changes in autonomic activity result in various types of benign, stable cardiac rhythms such as sinus bradycardia, sinus pause, first-degree atrioventricular (AV) block, and Mobitz type I second-degree AV block.

In patients with OSA, typical nocturnal cardiac rhythm disturbances, such as bradycardia with or without alternating tachycardia, have been well described.[139,140] However, the extension of the association between OSA and pathologic cardiac rhythm disturbances in the general population has only been recently addressed by 2 landmark studies. The Sleep Heart Study (SHHS), a multicenter longitudinal community-based study, has shown that there is a clear cross-sectional association between SDB and nocturnal cardiac arrhythmias. There is 4-times the odds of atrial fibrillation (odds ratio [OR] 4.02; 95% confidence interval [CI] 1.03–15.74), 3-times the odds of nonsustained ventricular tachycardias (OR 3.40; 95% CI 1.03–11.20), and almost twice the odds of complex ventricular ectopies (CVE) such as bigeminy, trigeminy, quadrigeminy, and nonstained ventricular tachycardias (OR 1.74; 95%

CI 1.11–2.74) in patients with severe SDB (respiratory disturbance index [RDI] $\geq$ 30 events/h) in comparison with patients with no SDB.[9] This strong association carried on even after adjustment for cardiovascular risk factors such as age, sex, BMI, and prevalence of coronary heart disease. However, the arrhythmias mentioned above are not only limited to severe cases of SDB. Recent published data from the Outcomes of Sleep Disorders in Older Men Study (MrOS Sleep Study) confirms the dose-response relationships between indices of SDB severity and arrhythmia occurrence. In addition, CVE has a stronger association with OSA and hypoxemia, and atrial fibrillation (AF) has a stronger association with CSA, Cheyne-Stokes respirations/CSA, and underlying CVD.[141]

Types of Arrhythmias in Obstructive Sleep Apnea

Sinus arrhythmias
Sinus arrhythmias, such as bradycardia with or without alternating tachycardia, have been regarded as the most distinct cardiac rhythm abnormalities seen in OSA. Sinus arrhythmias are characterized by bradycardia during the apneic phase of OSA followed by tachycardia on arousal with resumption of the respiration. The bradyarrhythmia linked to the apneic event is produced by a reflex vagal activation ("diving reflex"), which occurs mainly during REM sleep in the absence of any conduction system disease. The tachyarrhythmia is produced by hyperadrenergic drive during arousal, the result of vagal withdrawal in the postapneic phase. The calculated occurrence of bradyarrhythmias in severe OSA is around 18%.[142] The risk is directly correlated with the severity of the OSA (AHI>30) and the degree of obesity.[143] Of importance is that CPA therapy has been shown to abolish the majority of bradyarrhythmias in OSA patients.[144,145]

Supraventricular tachycardias: atrial fibrillation
In the United States, paroxysmal or persistent AF prevalence is estimated in 2.2 million people. During the past 20 years, there has been an unexplained increase in AF cases.[146] Increasing SDB prevalence from the obesity epidemic[147,148] may contribute to this increase. The parallel epidemics of AF and obesity might be related to a comorbid state such as OSA. However, obesity and severe OSA can independently predict the incidence of AF in patients younger than 65 years over 5 years of follow-up.[119,149] Patients with a history of AF have a higher prevalence of OSA (49%) in comparison with those without AF (32%), with an adjusted OR of 2.19 (95% CI 1.40–3.42).[150] AF patients with SDB have a higher rate of recurrence after cardioversion in comparison with patients without a known SDB diagnosis.[151] Furthermore, the SHHS has shown that patients in the community with severe OSA (RDI >30 events/h) have a fourfold increase in the prevalence of atrial fibrillation.[9]

Ventricular arrhythmias
There is a strong association between SDB and ventricular arrhythmias in patients with left ventricular failure (HF).[130] Data collected from overnight polysomnography (PSG), 24-hour Holter,[142,152] and implantable cardioverter defibrillator[153] in HF patients support not only that SDB is more prevalent in this population but also that SDB is an independent predictor of life-threatening nocturnal ventricular arrhythmias. It is thought that left ventricular dysfunction contributes to ventricular arrhythmias[154] in OSA patients by increasing autonomic nervous system imbalance against a background of intermittent apnea-induced hypoxia and increase in left ventricular afterload elicited by repeated cycles of apnea-Mueller maneuvers. However, recent results show that up to 60% patients with ventricular arrhythmias and normal ventricular function had SDB.[155] Regarding the prevalence of ventricular arrhythmias in OSA patients, the SHHS has shown almost twice the odds of CVEs such as bigeminy, trigeminy, quadrigeminy, and nonstained ventricular tachycardias (OR 1.74; 95% CI 1.11–2.74) in patients with severe SDB (RDI $\geq$ 30 events/h) in comparison with patients with no SDB.[9]

Sudden cardiac death
The relative risk (RR) of sudden cardiac death doubles from midnight to 6 AM (RR 2.57; 95% CI 1.87–3.52) for patients with OSA.[11] Untreated severe OSA has a higher incidence of fatal and nonfatal cardiovascular events in comparison with patients with no SDB.[88] These findings may in fact be explained by the increased rate of serious nocturnal arrhythmias occurring in individuals with severe OSA.[141] It is possible that recurrent myocardial ischemia secondary to hypoxemia, and increased afterload and sympathetic activity could predispose these patients to fatal ventricular arrhythmias.

Treatment

Atrial arrhythmias and CPAP treatment
Regarding CPAP use in arrhythmias, first-line treatment of bradyarrhythmias in the setting of OSA and normal conduction system would consist of treatment of OSA. Improvement has also been shown in ventricular ectopy and sympathetic activation after CPAP treatment in HF patients with

sleep apnea.[130] In fact, among patients with OSA who underwent electrical cardioversion for AF, in those treated with CPAP a 50% reduction in the recurrence rate for AF throughout a 1-year follow-up was reported, in comparison with those with untreated OSA.[151]

Atrial overdrive

Based on recent published data, in patients with sleep apnea syndrome and permanent atrial-synchronous ventricular pacemaker for symptomatic sinus bradycardia, atrial overdrive pacing significantly reduced (50%) the number of episodes of CSA or OSA, and increased oxyhemoglobin saturation without reducing the total sleep time.[156] The indications for atrial overdrive pacing in these patients had the goal of reducing the incidence of atrial tachyarrhythmias.[156,157] Based on these results, comparison studies of overdrive pacing versus CPAP were performed in patients with arrhythmias and OSA. Data comparing atrial overdrive with CPAP confirm that despite a mild effect of atrial overdrive pacing on respiratory events in some HF patients with OSA, it is not therapeutically effective in improving SDB, unlike CPAP.[158,159]

OBSTRUCTIVE SLEEP APNEA AND PULMONARY HYPERTENSION
Prevalence of Pulmonary Hypertension in Obstructive Sleep Apnea

PH is common in patients with OSA, with reported estimates ranging between 16% and 42%.[160,161] Discrepancies in prevalence estimates result from differences in study methodology. For example, most studies include only a small number of patients often unselected for comorbidities, and use varying definitions of pulmonary hypertension as well as modalities to measure pulmonary arterial pressure (**Table 1**). Most experts, however, estimate the prevalence of PH in uncomplicated OSA patients to be about 20%. The occurrence of PH in OSA patients is associated with obesity, poor lung function, degree and duration of hypoxemia, and hypercapnia, and does not appear to be associated with age, gender, or OSA severity as measured by the AHI.[162–164] When pulmonary hypertension does occur with OSA, mean pulmonary artery pressure is generally only mildly elevated (20–52 mm Hg), unless there is underlying lung or heart disease, or chronic daytime hypoxemia or hypercapnia, in which case pulmonary hypertension may be severe.[165]

CPAP Therapy

CPAP is highly efficacious therapy for OSA, and has been shown to improve serum markers of cardiac and vascular injury. Serum and urinary norepinephrine levels are dramatically reduced both acutely and chronically in treated OSA patients. Similarly, one night of CPAP therapy for OSA patients was able to significantly raise plasma levels of nitric oxide derivatives in OSA patients to comparable levels of healthy volunteers.[166,167]

Few studies, however, explore the effect of CPAP directly on pulmonary artery hemodynamics. In a prospective uncontrolled study, Sajkov and colleagues[168] treated 22 subjects with OSA with CPAP for 4 months, and found the mean pulmonary artery pressures (mPAP)

Table 1
Prevalence of daytime PH in obstructive sleep apnea

Study	N	M/F	Patient Selection	PH	Measurement
Podszus et al, 1986[160]	65	61/4	Unknown	20%	RHC
Fletcher et al, 1987[176]	24	24/0	Associated with lung disease	73%	RHC
Weitzenblum et al, 1988[164]	46	42/4	Unselected	20%	RHC
Krieger et al, 1989[177]	114	108/6	Unselected	19%	RHC
Sajkov et al, 1994[178]	27	26/1	No lung or heart disease	41%	Echo
Shinozaki et al, 1995[179]	25	Unknown	Unselected	32%	RHC
Laks et al, 1995[180]	100	Unknown	Unselected	42%	RHC
Chaouat et al, 1996[162]	220	207/13	Unselected	17%	RHC
Sanner et al, 1997[181]	92	81/11	No lung disease	20%	RHC
Bady et al, 2000[182]	44	37/7	No lung or heart disease	27%	RHC
Hawrylkiewicz et al, 2004[161]	67	Unknown	No lung disease	16%	RHC

Abbreviation: RHC, right heart catheterization.

decreased from 16.8 ± 1.2 mm Hg to 13.9 ± 0.6 mm Hg ($P<.05$) and pulmonary vascular resistance decreased from 231 ± 88 to 186 ± 55 dyne/s·cm^5 ($P<.05$). These investigators also tested the hypoxemic response by having subjects inspire 0.11, 0.21, and 0.50 fractions of oxygen, and found significant decreases in mPAP and pulmonary vascular resistance at all fractions of inspired oxygen levels after 4 months of CPAP therapy. The greatest treatment effect occurred in the only 2 subjects with elevated pulmonary artery pressures (mPAP>25 mm Hg). In another prospective study, Alchanatis and colleagues[134] found that 6 months of CPAP therapy in 29 OSA subjects reduced the mPAP from 17.2 ± 5.2 to 13.2 ± 3.8 mm Hg ($P<.001$). Of the 29 subjects, however, only 6 had PH with very mildly elevated pressures ranging from 20 to 30 mm Hg. Again, CPAP demonstrated greatest efficacy in those with higher baseline mPAP. Arias and colleagues[169] conducted the only randomized, controlled CPAP study in pulmonary hypertension to date, and found similar improvements in mPAP after 3 months of therapeutic CPAP. The 23 subjects with OSA in this study also had mild pulmonary hypertension with an average mPAP of 29.8 ± 8.8 mm Hg. Consistent with previous studies, the greatest treatment effect was found in those with higher baseline mPAP.

These studies suggest that CPAP therapy for OSA may be effective therapy for concomitant pulmonary hypertension. Because the effect appears to be greater in more severe disease, the true benefit of identifying and treating OSA may apply to those with significant pulmonary hypertension. Unfortunately, no study specifically addresses OSA treatment in this particularly vulnerable group of moderate to severe pulmonary hypertensives.

Most studies use mPAP as their primary outcome; however, mPAP is not a survival correlate in PH. As PH progresses, the right ventricle fails and may cause mPAP to actually decrease over time. Hence changes in mPAP do not reliably reflect pulmonary hemodynamic changes. Further studies are required to evaluate important clinical outcomes, such as cardiovascular morbidity and mortality as well as functional outcomes in patients with OSA and pulmonary hypertension, and evaluate the effect of CPAP therapy in this population.

Obstructive Sleep Apnea and Pulmonary Hypertension in Obesity-Hypoventilation Syndrome and Overlap Syndrome

Obesity-hypoventilation syndrome
Obesity-hypoventilation syndrome (OHS) is defined as a combination of obesity (ie, BMI $\geq$ 30 kg/m^2) and daytime or chronic hypercapnia (ie, Paco$_2$ $\geq$ 45 mm Hg) accompanied by SDB. In approximately 90% of patients with OHS, the SDB consists of OSA.[170] The remaining 10% of patients with OHS have an AHI of less than 5, and their sleep-disordered breathing consists of nocturnal hypoventilation defined as a greater than 10 mm Hg increase in Paco$_2$ during sleep compared with wakefulness.

OHS patients tend to be extremely obese and report similar symptoms of OSA, such as sleepiness, snoring, nocturnal gasping, and morning headaches. A restrictive ventilatory defect is seen on pulmonary function tests. In contrast to patients with uncomplicated OSA, OHS patients have a greater prevalence of low Sao$_2$ during wakefulness, peripheral edema, and pulmonary hypertension. Pulmonary hypertension is more common (>50% vs 20%, respectively) and more severe in patients with OHS than in those with uncomplicated OSA, presumably due to more chronic hypoxemia and hypercapnia as well as metabolic derangements associated with obesity contributing to cardiac and endothelial dysfunction.[88]

In patients with OSA, minute ventilation during sleep does not decrease due to the large increase in the minute ventilation between the obstructive respiratory events. Obstructive respiratory events can, however, lead to acute hypercapnia if the duration of the hyperventilation is inadequate to eliminate the accumulated CO$_2$. This acute hypercapnia causes a small increase in serum bicarbonate level that is not corrected before the next apneic episode.[171] The elevated bicarbonate level blunts the ventilatory response to CO$_2$ and ultimately results in a higher daytime CO$_2$ level. In the subgroup of patients with OHS without OSA, tidal volume and hence minute ventilation decreases by 25% during NREM sleep and by 40% during REM sleep.[172] Hypercapnia triggers metabolic compensation that ultimately results in chronic hypoventilation, hypercapnia, and hypoxemia, and puts the patient at greater likelihood of developing pulmonary hypertension.

Overlap syndrome
Overlap syndrome is the term used to describe the association of chronic obstructive pulmonary disease (COPD) and OSA. The prevalence of overlap syndrome among patients with OSA is between 10% and 15%,[165] similar to the prevalence of the general population.[173] Patients with overlap syndrome have an obstructive pattern on spirometry and, in comparison with patients with uncomplicated OSA, are more likely to have hypoxemia, hypercapnia, and PH.[174] Hypercapnia develops in patients with overlap syndrome at

a lower BMI and AHI than that of patients with OHS, and at a higher FEV_1 (forced expiratory volume in 1 second) than hypercapnic patients with pure COPD.

Most studies have emphasized the role of an associated COPD in the pathogenesis of hypoxemia, hypercapnia, and PH in OSA patients.[163,165,175] Overlap patients tend to have lower Pao_2, higher $Paco_2$, and greater resting and exercise pulmonary arterial pressures compared with uncomplicated OSA patients. In OSA patients with daytime PH, bronchial obstruction is generally not severe and the level of hypoxemia and hypercapnia is modest[162] compared with COPD patients with pulmonary hypertension and/or cor pulmonale, whose values are significantly worse.[162,164,175] For a given FEV_1, Pao_2 is generally lower in OSA patients, likely due to obesity and diminished chemosensitivity. Similarly, for a given daytime Pao_2, pulmonary artery pressure is generally better in OSA patients.

SUMMARY/PUBLIC HEALTH IMPLICATIONS

Multiple prospective observational cohort studies have demonstrated that OSA significantly increases the risk of cardiovascular disease independent of potential confounding risk factors. This finding implies that there are mechanisms mediated by sleep apnea that confer vascular risk. The current literature suggests that such mechanisms include: intermittent hypoxia, systemic inflammation, and atherosclerosis; nocturnal sympathetic activation; diurnal hypertension; metabolic dysregulation; cardiac arrhythmia (including AF); mechanical load; and abnormal coagulation.

The increasing prevalence of SDB in the population suggests that the population attributable risk percent (the percentage of the total risk of cardiovascular disease and stroke due to sleep apnea) is high, making this an important public health issue; this is particularly true given that sleep apnea is a potentially modifiable risk factor.

Short-term randomized controlled trials of CPAP in cardiovascular end points and long-term observational cohort studies with follow-up of cardiovascular outcomes suggest a clinically significant cardiovascular risk reduction associated with the use of CPAP. However, there are currently no prospective randomized studies demonstrating the efficacy of treating sleep apnea in reducing cardiovascular outcome events. Such studies are critical before large-scale sleep apnea screening guidelines are instituted. In the meantime, clinicians should have a low threshold for evaluating symptoms in their patients consistent with SDB.

REFERENCES

1. Punjabi NM. The epidemiology of adult obstructive sleep apnea. Proc Am Thorac Soc 2008; 5(2):136–43.
2. Young T, Finn L, Peppard PE, et al. Sleep disordered breathing and mortality: eighteen-year follow-up of the Wisconsin sleep cohort. Sleep 2008;31(8):1071–8.
3. Marshall NS, Wong KK, Liu PY, et al. Sleep apnea as an independent risk factor for all-cause mortality: the Busselton Health Study. Sleep 2008; 31(8):1079–85.
4. Peppard P, Young T, Palta M, et al. Prospective study of the association between sleep-disordered breathing and hypertension. N Engl J Med 2000; 342:1378–84.
5. Arzt M, Young T, Finn L, et al. Association of sleep-disordered breathing and the occurrence of stroke. Am J Respir Crit Care Med 2005;172(11):1447–51.
6. Munoz R, Duran-Cantolla J, Martinez-Vila E, et al. Severe sleep apnea and risk of ischemic stroke in the elderly. Stroke 2006;37(9):2317–21.
7. Mooe T, Rabben T, Wiklund U, et al. Sleep-disordered breathing in women: occurrence and association with coronary artery disease. Am J Med 1996; 101(3):251–6.
8. Peled N, Abinader EG, Pillar G, et al. Nocturnal ischemic events in patients with obstructive sleep apnea syndrome and ischemic heart disease: effects of continuous positive air pressure treatment. J Am Coll Cardiol 1999;34(6):1744–9.
9. Mehra R, Benjamin EJ, Shahar E, et al. Association of nocturnal arrhythmias with sleep-disordered breathing: the Sleep Heart Health Study. Am J Respir Crit Care Med 2006;173(8):910–6.
10. Shahar E, Whitney C, Redline S, et al. Sleep-disordered breathing and cardiovascular disease: cross-sectional results of the Sleep Heart Health Study. Am J Respir Crit Care Med 2001;163:19–25.
11. Gami AS, Howard DE, Olson EJ, et al. Day-night pattern of sudden death in obstructive sleep apnea. N Engl J Med 2005;352(12):1206–14.
12. Somers VK, Dyken ME, Mark AL, et al. Sympathetic-nerve activity during sleep in normal subjects. N Engl J Med 1993;328(5):303–7.
13. Pickering TG, Harshfield GA, Kleinert HD, et al. Blood pressure during normal daily activities, sleep, and exercise. Comparison of values in normal and hypertensive subjects. JAMA 1982; 247(7):992–6.
14. Marler JR, Price TR, Clark GL, et al. Morning increase in onset of ischemic stroke. Stroke 1989; 20(4):473–6.
15. Ryan S, Taylor CT, McNicholas WT. Selective activation of inflammatory pathways by intermittent

hypoxia in obstructive sleep apnea syndrome. Circulation 2005;112(17):2660–7.

16. Savransky V, Nanayakkara A, Li J, et al. Chronic intermittent hypoxia induces atherosclerosis. Am J Respir Crit Care Med 2007;175(12):1290–7.

17. Hayashi M, Fujimoto K, Urushibata K, et al. Nocturnal oxygen desaturation correlates with the severity of coronary atherosclerosis in coronary artery disease. Chest 2003;124:936–41.

18. Dyugovskaya L, Lavie P, Lavie L. Increased adhesion molecule expression and production of reactive oxygen species in leukocytes of sleep apnea patients. Am J Respir Crit Care Med 2002;165:934–9.

19. El-Solh A, Mador M, Sikka P, et al. Adhesion molecules in patients with coronary artery disease and moderate-to-severe obstructive sleep apnea. Chest 2002;121:1541–7.

20. Ohga E, Nagase T, Tomita T, et al. Increased levels of circulating I-CAM-1, VCAM-1, and L-selectin in obstructive sleep apnea syndrome. J Appl Physiol 1999;87:10–4.

21. Lavie L. Obstructive sleep apnoea syndrome—an oxidative stress disorder. Sleep Med Rev 2003;7: 35–51.

22. Lavie L, Dyugovskaya L, Lavie P. Sleep-apnea-related intermittent hypoxia and atherogenesis: adhesion molecules and monocytes/endothelial cells interactions. Atherosclerosis 2005;183(1): 183–4.

23. Lavie L. Sleep-disordered breathing and cerebrovascular disease: a mechanistic approach. Neurol Clin 2005;23(4):1059–75.

24. Tilkian AG, Guilleminault C, Schroeder JS, et al. Hemodynamics in sleep-induced apnea. Studies during wakefulness and sleep. Ann Intern Med 1976;85(6):714–9.

25. Marrone O, Bellia V, Pieri D, et al. Acute effects of oxygen administration on transmural pulmonary artery pressure in obstructive sleep apnea. Chest 1992;101(4):1023–7.

26. Marrone O, Bonsignore MR, Romano S, et al. Slow and fast changes in transmural pulmonary artery pressure in obstructive sleep apnoea. Eur Respir J 1994;7(12):2192–8.

27. Carlson JT, Rangemark C, Hedner JA. Attenuated endothelium-dependent vascular relaxation in patients with sleep apnoea. J Hypertens 1996; 14(5):577–84.

28. Fletcher E, Miller J, Schaaf J. Urinary catecholamines before and after tracheostomy in patients with obstructive sleep apnea and hypertension. Sleep 1987;10:35–44.

29. Somers V, Dyken M, Clary M, et al. Sympathetic neural mechanisms in obstructive sleep apnea. J Clin Invest 1995;96:1897–904.

30. O'Donnell C, King E, Schwartz A, et al. Relationship between blood pressure and airway obstruction during sleep in the dog. J Appl Physiol 1994;77: 1819–28.

31. Hla KM, Young T, Finn L, et al. Longitudinal association of sleep-disordered breathing and nondipping of nocturnal blood pressure in the Wisconsin Sleep Cohort Study. Sleep 2008;31(6):795–800.

32. Akashiba T, Minemura H, Yamamoto H, et al. Nasal continuous positive airway pressure changes blood pressure "nondippers" to "dippers" in patients with obstructive sleep apnea. Sleep 1999;22(7):849–53.

33. Ancoli-Israel S, Stepnowsky C, Dimsdale J, et al. The effect of race and sleep-disordered breathing on nocturnal BP "dipping": analysis in an older population. Chest 2002;122(4):1148–55.

34. O'Brien E, Sheridan J, O'Malley K. Dippers and non-dippers. Lancet 1988;2(8607):397.

35. Bianchi S, Bigazzi R, Baldari G, et al. Diurnal variations of blood pressure and microalbuminuria in essential hypertension. Am J Hypertens 1994; 7(1):23–9.

36. Verdecchia P, Schillaci G, Guerrieri M. Circadian blood pressure changes and left ventricular hypertrophy. Circulation 1990;81:528–36.

37. Shimada K, Kawamoto A, Matsubayashi K, et al. Silent cerebrovascular disease in the elderly. Correlation with ambulatory pressure. Hypertension 1990;16(6):692–9.

38. Verdecchia P, Porcellati C, Schillaci G, et al. Ambulatory blood pressure. An independent predictor of prognosis in essential hypertension. Hypertension 1994;24(6):793–801.

39. Staessen JA, Thijs L, Fagard R, et al. Predicting cardiovascular risk using conventional vs ambulatory blood pressure in older patients with systolic hypertension. Systolic Hypertension in Europe Trial Investigators. JAMA 1999;282(6):539–46.

40. Kario K, Pickering TG, Matsuo T, et al. Stroke prognosis and abnormal nocturnal blood pressure falls in older hypertensives. Hypertension 2001;38(4): 852–7.

41. Ohkubo T, Hozawa A, Yamaguchi J, et al. Prognostic significance of the nocturnal decline in blood pressure in individuals with and without high 24-h blood pressure: the Ohasama study. J Hypertens 2002;20(11):2183–9.

42. Cohn JN, Levine TB, Olivari MT, et al. Plasma norepinephrine as a guide to prognosis in patients with chronic congestive heart failure. N Engl J Med 1984;311(13):819–23.

43. Floras JS. Clinical aspects of sympathetic activation and parasympathetic withdrawal in heart failure. J Am Coll Cardiol 1993;22(4 Suppl A): 72A–84A.

44. Fletcher EC. Sympathetic over activity in the etiology of hypertension of obstructive sleep apnea. Sleep 2003;26(1):15–9.

45. Dimsdale JE, Coy T, Ziegler MG, et al. The effect of sleep apnea on plasma and urinary catecholamines. Sleep 1995;18(5):377–81.

46. Ziegler MG, Mills PJ, Loredo JS, et al. Effect of continuous positive airway pressure and placebo treatment on sympathetic nervous activity in patients with obstructive sleep apnea. Chest 2001;120(3):887–93.

47. Romero-Corral A, Somers VK, Pellikka PA, et al. Decreased right and left ventricular myocardial performance in obstructive sleep apnea. Chest 2007;132(6):1863–70.

48. Buda AJ, Pinsky MR, Ingels NB, et al. Effect of intrathoracic pressure on left ventricular performance. N Engl J Med 1979;301(9):453–9.

49. Arias MA, Garcia-Rio F, Alonso-Fernandez A, et al. Obstructive sleep apnea syndrome affects left ventricular diastolic function: effects of nasal continuous positive airway pressure in men. Circulation 2005;112(3):375–83.

50. Bradley TD, Hall MJ, Ando S, et al. Hemodynamic effects of simulated obstructive apneas in humans with and without heart failure. Chest 2001;119(6): 1827–35.

51. Cohn JN, Ferrari R, Sharpe N. Cardiac remodeling—concepts and clinical implications: a consensus paper from an international forum on cardiac remodeling. Behalf of an International Forum on Cardiac Remodeling. J Am Coll Cardiol 2000;35(3):569–82.

52. Black S, Fineman J, Johengen M, et al. Increased pulmonary blood flow alters the molecular regulation of vascular reactivity in the lamb. Chest 1998; 114(Suppl 1):39S.

53. Alonso-Fernandez A, Garcia-Rio F, Arias MA, et al. Effects of CPAP on oxidative stress and nitrate efficiency in sleep apnoea: a randomised trial. Thorax 2009;64(7):581–6.

54. Belaidi E, Joyeux-Faure M, Ribuot C, et al. Major role for hypoxia inducible factor-1 and the endothelin system in promoting myocardial infarction and hypertension in an animal model of obstructive sleep apnea. J Am Coll Cardiol 2009;53(15):1309–17.

55. Tahawi Z, Orolinova N, Joshua IG, et al. Altered vascular reactivity in arterioles of chronic intermittent hypoxic rats. J Appl Physiol 2001;90(5): 2007–13 [discussion: 2000].

56. Henley DE, Buchanan F, Gibson R, et al. Plasma apelin levels in obstructive sleep apnea and the effect of continuous positive airway pressure therapy. J Endocrinol 2009;203(1):181–8.

57. Abboud FM. Ventricular syncope: is the heart a sensory organ? N Engl J Med 1989;320(6): 390–2.

58. Franz MR. Mechano-electrical feedback in ventricular myocardium. Cardiovasc Res 1996;32(1): 15–24.

59. Somers VK, Dyken ME, Skinner JL. Autonomic and hemodynamic responses and interactions during the Mueller maneuver in humans. J Auton Nerv Syst 1993;44(2–3):253–9.

60. Kleiger RE, Miller JP, Bigger JT Jr, et al. Decreased heart rate variability and its association with increased mortality after acute myocardial infarction. Am J Cardiol 1987;59(4):256–62.

61. Fei L, Copie X, Malik M, et al. Short- and long-term assessment of heart rate variability for risk stratification after acute myocardial infarction. Am J Cardiol 1996;77(9):681–4.

62. Ponikowski P, Anker SD, Chua TP, et al. Depressed heart rate variability as an independent predictor of death in chronic congestive heart failure secondary to ischemic or idiopathic dilated cardiomyopathy. Am J Cardiol 1997;79(12):1645–50.

63. Narkiewicz K, Montano N, Cogliati C, et al. Altered cardiovascular variability in obstructive sleep apnea. Circulation 1998;98(11):1071–7.

64. Zipes D. Autonomic modulation of cardiac arrhythmias. Cardiac electrophysiology: from cell to bedside. 2nd edition. Philadelphia: Sauders; 1995.

65. Narkiewicz K, van de Borne PJ, Cooley RL, et al. Sympathetic activity in obese subjects with and without obstructive sleep apnea. Circulation 1998; 98(8):772–6.

66. Wit AL, Rosen MR. After depolarization and triggered activity. The heart and the cardiovascular system. New York: Raven Press; 1886.

67. Conti JB. Cardiac arrhythmias. J Am Coll Cardiol 2005;45(11 Suppl B):30B–2B.

68. Bokinsky G, Miller M, Ault K, et al. Spontaneous platelet activation and aggregation during obstructive sleep apnea and its response to therapy with nasal continuous positive airway pressure: a preliminary investigation. Chest 1995;108:625–30.

69. Eisensehr I, Ehrenberg BL, Noachtar S, et al. Platelet activation, epinephrine, and blood pressure in obstructive sleep apnea syndrome. Neurology 1998;51(1):188–95.

70. Sanner BM, Konermann M, Tepel M, et al. Platelet function in patients with obstructive sleep apnoea syndrome. Eur Respir J 2000;16(4):648–52.

71. Geiser T, Buck F, Meyer BJ, et al. In vivo platelet activation is increased during sleep in patients with obstructive sleep apnea syndrome. Respiration 2002;69(3):229–34.

72. von Kanel R, Dimsdale JE. Hemostatic alterations in patients with obstructive sleep apnea and the implications for cardiovascular disease. Chest 2003;124(5):1956–67.

73. Hui DS, Ko FW, Fok JP, et al. The effects of nasal continuous positive airway pressure on platelet activation in obstructive sleep apnea syndrome. Chest 2004;125(5):1768–75.

74. Wedzicha J, Syndercombe-Court D, Tan K. Increased platelet aggregate formation in patients with chronic airflow obstruction and hypoxemia. Thorax 1991;46:504–7.

75. Olson LJ, Olson EJ, Somers VK. Obstructive sleep apnea and platelet activation: another potential link between sleep-disordered breathing and cardiovascular disease. Chest 2004;126(2): 339–41.

76. Spiegel K, Leproult R, Van Cauter E. Impact of sleep debt on metabolic and endocrine function. Lancet 1999;354(9188):1435–9.

77. Yaggi HK, Araujo AB, McKinlay JB. Sleep duration as a risk factor for the development of type 2 diabetes. Diabetes Care 2006;29(3):657–61.

78. Sulit L, Storfer-Isser A, Kirchner HL, et al. Differences in polysomnography predictors for hypertension and impaired glucose tolerance. Sleep 2006;29(6):777–83.

79. Ip MS, Lam B, Ng MM, et al. Obstructive sleep apnea is independently associated with insulin resistance. Am J Respir Crit Care Med 2002; 165(5):670–6.

80. Punjabi N, Sorkin J, Katzel L, et al. Sleep-disordered breathing and insulin resistance in middle-aged and overweight men. Am J Respir Crit Care Med 2002;165:677–82.

81. Reichmuth KJ, Austin D, Skatrud JB, et al. Association of sleep apnea and type II diabetes: a population-based study. Am J Respir Crit Care Med 2005; 172(12):1590–5.

82. Botros N, Concato J, Mohsenin V, et al. Obstructive sleep apnea as a risk factor for type 2 diabetes. Am J Med 2009;122(12):1122–7.

83. Punjabi NM, Polotsky VY. Disorders of glucose metabolism in sleep apnea. J Appl Physiol 2005; 99(5):1998–2007.

84. Neito F, Young T, Lind B, et al. Association of sleep-disordered breathing, sleep apnea, and hypertension in a large community based study. JAMA 2000;283:1829–36.

85. Chobanian AV, Bakris GL, Black HR, et al. The Seventh Report of the Joint National Committee on prevention, detection, evaluation, and treatment of high blood pressure: the JNC 7 report. JAMA 2003;289(19):2560–72.

86. AHA. 2005 Heart and stroke statistical update. Dallas (TX): American Heart Association; 2005.

87. Yaggi H, Concato J, Kernan W, et al. Obstructive sleep apnea as a risk factor for stroke and death. N Engl J Med 2005;353:2034–41.

88. Marin JM, Carrizo SJ, Vicente E, et al. Long-term cardiovascular outcomes in men with obstructive sleep apnoea-hypopnoea with or without treatment with continuous positive airway pressure: an observational study. Lancet 2005;365(9464): 1046–53.

89. Drager LF, Bortolotto LA, Lorenzi MC, et al. Early signs of atherosclerosis in obstructive sleep apnea. Am J Respir Crit Care Med 2005;172(5): 613–8.

90. Shah NA, Yaggi HK, Concato J, et al. Obstructive sleep apnea as a risk factor for coronary events or cardiovascular death. Sleep Breath 2009. [Epub ahead of print].

91. Drager LF, Bortolotto LA, Figueiredo AC, et al. Obstructive sleep apnea, hypertension, and their interaction on arterial stiffness and heart remodeling. Chest 2007;131(5):1379–86.

92. Becker H, Jerrentrup A, Ploch T, et al. Effect of nasal continuous positive airway pressure treatment on blood pressure in patients with obstructive sleep apnea. Circulation 2003;107:68–73.

93. Pepperell J, Ramdassingh-Dow S, Crosthwaite N, et al. Ambulatory blood pressure after therapeutic and subtherapeutic nasal continuous positive airway pressure for obstructive sleep apnoea: a randomised parallel trial. Lancet 2002;359:204–10.

94. Faccenda J, Mackay T, Boon N, et al. Randomized placebo-controlled trial of continuous positive airway pressure on blood pressure in the sleep apnea-hypopnea syndrome. Am J Respir Crit Care Med 2001;163:344–8.

95. Barbe F, Mayoralas LR, Duran J, et al. Treatment with continuous positive airway pressure is not effective in patients with sleep apnea but no daytime sleepiness. a randomized, controlled trial. Ann Intern Med 2001;134(11):1015–23.

96. Monasterio C, Vidal S, Duran J, et al. Effectiveness of continuous positive airway pressure in mild sleep apnea-hypopnea syndrome. Am J Respir Crit Care Med 2001;164(6):939–43.

97. Giles T, Lasserson T, Smith B, et al. Continuous positive airways pressure for obstructive sleep apnoea in adults. Cochrane Database Syst Rev 2006;(3):CD001106.

98. Bazzano LA, Khan Z, Reynolds K, et al. Effect of nocturnal nasal continuous positive airway pressure on blood pressure in obstructive sleep apnea. Hypertension 2007;50(2):417–23.

99. Haentjens P, Van Meerhaeghe A, Moscariello A, et al. The impact of continuous positive airway pressure on blood pressure in patients with obstructive sleep apnea syndrome: evidence from a meta-analysis of placebo-controlled randomized trials. Arch Intern Med 2007;167(8):757–64.

100. MacMahon S, Peto R, Cutler J, et al. Blood pressure, stroke, and coronary heart disease. Part 1, prolonged differences in blood pressure: prospective observational studies corrected for the regression dilution bias. Lancet 1990;335(8692):765–74.

101. Drager LF, Bortolotto LA, Figueiredo AC, et al. Effects of continuous positive airway pressure on early signs of atherosclerosis in obstructive sleep

apnea. Am J Respir Crit Care Med 2007;176(7): 706–12.

102. Bayram NA, Ciftci B, Keles T, et al. Endothelial function in normotensive men with obstructive sleep apnea before and 6 months after CPAP treatment. Sleep 2009;32(10):1257–63.

103. Marti S, Sampol G, Munoz X, et al. Mortality in severe sleep apnoea/hypopnoea syndrome patients: impact of treatment. Eur Respir J 2002; 20:1511–8.

104. Doherty LS, Kiely JL, Swan V, et al. Long-term effects of nasal continuous positive airway pressure therapy on cardiovascular outcomes in sleep apnea syndrome. Chest 2005;127(6):2076–84.

105. Martinez-Garcia MA, Soler-Cataluna JJ, Ejarque-Martinez L, et al. Continuous positive airway pressure treatment reduces mortality in patients with ischemic stroke and obstructive sleep apnea: a 5-year follow-up study. Am J Respir Crit Care Med 2009;180(1):36–41.

106. Javaheri S, Parker TJ, Wexler L, et al. Occult sleep-disordered breathing in stable congestive heart failure. Ann Intern Med 1995;122(7):487–92.

107. Sin DD, Fitzgerald F, Parker JD, et al. Risk factors for central and obstructive sleep apnea in 450 men and women with congestive heart failure. Am J Respir Crit Care Med 1999;160(4):1101–6.

108. MacDonald M, Fang J, Pittman SD, et al. The current prevalence of sleep disordered breathing in congestive heart failure patients treated with beta-blockers. J Clin Sleep Med 2008;4(1):38–42.

109. Yumino D, Wang H, Floras JS, et al. Prevalence and physiological predictors of sleep apnea in patients with heart failure and systolic dysfunction. J Card Fail 2009;15(4):279–85.

110. Javaheri S, Parker TJ, Liming JD, et al. Sleep apnea in 81 ambulatory male patients with stable heart failure. Types and their prevalences, consequences, and presentations. Circulation 1998; 97(21):2154–9.

111. Bursi F, Weston SA, Redfield MM, et al. Systolic and diastolic heart failure in the community. JAMA 2006;296(18):2209–16.

112. Chan J, Sanderson J, Chan W, et al. Prevalence of sleep-disordered breathing in diastolic heart failure. Chest 1997;111(6):1488–93.

113. Partinen M, Telakivi T. Epidemiology of obstructive sleep apnea syndrome. Sleep 1992;15(Suppl 6): S1–4.

114. O'Connor GT, Caffo B, Newman AB, et al. Prospective study of sleep-disordered breathing and hypertension: the Sleep Heart Health Study. Am J Respir Crit Care Med 2009;179(12):1159–64.

115. Dursunoglu N, Dursunoglu D, Kilic M. Impact of obstructive sleep apnea on right ventricular global function: sleep apnea and myocardial performance index. Respiration 2005;72(3):278–84.

116. Sanner BM, Konermann M, Sturm A, et al. Right ventricular dysfunction in patients with obstructive sleep apnoea syndrome. Eur Respir J 1997;10(9): 2079–83.

117. Dursunoglu D, Dursunoglu N, Evrengul H, et al. Impact of obstructive sleep apnoea on left ventricular mass and global function. Eur Respir J 2005; 26(2):283–8.

118. Otto ME, Belohlavek M, Romero-Corral A, et al. Comparison of cardiac structural and functional changes in obese otherwise healthy adults with versus without obstructive sleep apnea. Am J Cardiol 2007;99(9):1298–302.

119. Gami AS, Hodge DO, Herges RM, et al. Obstructive sleep apnea, obesity, and the risk of incident atrial fibrillation. J Am Coll Cardiol 2007;49(5): 565–71.

120. Levy D, Garrison RJ, Savage DD, et al. Prognostic implications of echocardiographically determined left ventricular mass in the Framingham Heart Study. N Engl J Med 1990;322(22):1561–6.

121. Guidry UC, Mendes LA, Evans JC, et al. Echocardiographic features of the right heart in sleep-disordered breathing: the Framingham Heart Study. Am J Respir Crit Care Med 2001;164(6):933–8.

122. Bixler EO, Vgontzas AN, Ten Have T, et al. Effects of age on sleep apnea in men: I. Prevalence and severity. Am J Respir Crit Care Med 1998;157(1): 144–8.

123. Lanfranchi PA, Somers VK, Braghiroli A, et al. Central sleep apnea in left ventricular dysfunction: prevalence and implications for arrhythmic risk. Circulation 2003;107(5):727–32.

124. Bradley TD, Floras JS. Sleep apnea and heart failure: Part II: central sleep apnea. Circulation 2003;107(13):1822–6.

125. Solin P, Roebuck T, Johns DP, et al. Peripheral and central ventilatory responses in central sleep apnea with and without congestive heart failure. Am J Respir Crit Care Med 2000; 162(6):2194–200.

126. Javaheri S, Shukla R, Zeigler H, et al. Central sleep apnea, right ventricular dysfunction, and low diastolic blood pressure are predictors of mortality in systolic heart failure. J Am Coll Cardiol 2007; 49(20):2028–34.

127. Usui K, Bradley TD, Spaak J, et al. Inhibition of awake sympathetic nerve activity of heart failure patients with obstructive sleep apnea by nocturnal continuous positive airway pressure. J Am Coll Cardiol 2005;45(12):2008–11.

128. Mansfield DR, Gollogly NC, Kaye DM, et al. Controlled trial of continuous positive airway pressure in obstructive sleep apnea and heart failure. Am J Respir Crit Care Med 2004;169(3):361–6.

129. Kaneko Y, Floras JS, Usui K, et al. Cardiovascular effects of continuous positive airway pressure in

patients with heart failure and obstructive sleep apnea. N Engl J Med 2003;348(13):1233–41.

130. Ryan CM, Usui K, Floras JS, et al. Effect of continuous positive airway pressure on ventricular ectopy in heart failure patients with obstructive sleep apnoea. Thorax 2005;60(9):781–5.

131. Gilman MP, Floras JS, Usui K, et al. Continuous positive airway pressure increases heart rate variability in heart failure patients with obstructive sleep apnoea. Clin Sci (Lond) 2008;114(3): 243–9.

132. Wang H, Parker JD, Newton GE, et al. Influence of obstructive sleep apnea on mortality in patients with heart failure. J Am Coll Cardiol 2007;49(15): 1625–31.

133. Roebuck T, Solin P, Kaye DM, et al. Increased long-term mortality in heart failure due to sleep apnoea is not yet proven. Eur Respir J 2004; 23(5):735–40.

134. Alchanatis M, Tourkohoriti G, Kakouros S, et al. Daytime pulmonary hypertension in patients with obstructive sleep apnea: the effect of continuous positive airway pressure on pulmonary hemodynamics. Respiration 2001;68(6):566–72.

135. Sin DD, Logan AG, Fitzgerald FS, et al. Effects of continuous positive airway pressure on cardiovascular outcomes in heart failure patients with and without Cheyne-Stokes respiration. Circulation 2000;102(1):61–6.

136. Bradley TD, Logan AG, Kimoff RJ, et al. Continuous positive airway pressure for central sleep apnea and heart failure. N Engl J Med 2005;353(19): 2025–33.

137. Philippe C, Stoica-Herman M, Drouot X, et al. Compliance with and effectiveness of adaptive servoventilation versus continuous positive airway pressure in the treatment of Cheyne-Stokes respiration in heart failure over a six month period. Heart 2006;92(3):337–42.

138. Hastings PC, Vazir A, Meadows GE, et al. Adaptive servo-ventilation in heart failure patients with sleep apnea: a real world study. Int J Cardiol 2010; 139(1):17–24.

139. Zwillich C, Devlin T, White D, et al. Bradycardia during sleep apnea. Characteristics and mechanism. J Clin Invest 1982;69(6):1286–92.

140. Bonsignore MR, Romano S, Marrone O, et al. Different heart rate patterns in obstructive apneas during NREM sleep. Sleep 1997;20(12):1167–74.

141. Mehra R, Stone KL, Varosy PD, et al. Nocturnal arrhythmias across a spectrum of obstructive and central sleep-disordered breathing in older men: outcomes of sleep disorders in older men (MrOS sleep) study. Arch Intern Med 2009;169(12): 1147–55.

142. Guilleminault C, Connolly SJ, Winkle RA. Cardiac arrhythmia and conduction disturbances during sleep in 400 patients with sleep apnea syndrome. Am J Cardiol 1983;52(5):490–4.

143. Becker HF, Koehler U, Stammnitz A, et al. Heart block in patients with sleep apnoea. Thorax 1998; 53(Suppl 3):S29–32.

144. Grimm W, Koehler U, Fus E, et al. Outcome of patients with sleep apnea-associated severe bradyarrhythmias after continuous positive airway pressure therapy. Am J Cardiol 2000;86(6):688–92, A9.

145. Harbison J, O'Reilly P, McNicholas WT. Cardiac rhythm disturbances in the obstructive sleep apnea syndrome: effects of nasal continuous positive airway pressure therapy. Chest 2000;118(3): 591–5.

146. Fuster V, Ryden LE, Cannom DS, et al. ACC/AHA/ESC 2006 guidelines for the management of patients with atrial fibrillation—executive summary: a report of the American College of Cardiology/American Heart Association Task Force on Practice Guidelines and the European Society of Cardiology Committee for Practice Guidelines (Writing Committee to Revise the 2001 Guidelines for the Management of Patients With Atrial Fibrillation). J Am Coll Cardiol 2006;48(4):854–906.

147. Coromilas J. Obesity and atrial fibrillation: is one epidemic feeding the other? JAMA 2004;292(20): 2519–20.

148. Vgontzas AN, Papanicolaou DA, Bixler EO, et al. Sleep apnea and daytime sleepiness and fatigue: relation to visceral obesity, insulin resistance, and hypercytokinemia. J Clin Endocrinol Metab 2000; 85(3):1151–8.

149. Wang TJ, Parise H, Levy D, et al. Obesity and the risk of new-onset atrial fibrillation. JAMA 2004; 292(20):2471–7.

150. Gami AS, Pressman G, Caples SM, et al. Association of atrial fibrillation and obstructive sleep apnea. Circulation 2004;110(4):364–7.

151. Kanagala R, Murali NS, Friedman PA, et al. Obstructive sleep apnea and the recurrence of atrial fibrillation. Circulation 2003;107(20):2589–94.

152. Hoffstein V, Mateika S. Cardiac arrhythmias, snoring, and sleep apnea. Chest 1994;106(2):466–71.

153. Serizawa N, Yumino D, Kajimoto K, et al. Impact of sleep-disordered breathing on life-threatening ventricular arrhythmia in heart failure patients with implantable cardioverter-defibrillator. Am J Cardiol 2008;102(8):1064–8.

154. Pogwizd SM, Schlotthauer K, Li L, et al. Arrhythmogenesis and contractile dysfunction in heart failure: roles of sodium-calcium exchange, inward rectifier potassium current, and residual beta-adrenergic responsiveness. Circ Res 2001;88(11):1159–67.

155. Koshino Y, Satoh M, Katayose Y, et al. Association of sleep-disordered breathing and ventricular arrhythmias in patients without heart failure. Am J Cardiol 2008;101(6):882–6.

156. Garrigue S, Bordier P, Jais P, et al. Benefit of atrial pacing in sleep apnea syndrome. N Engl J Med 2002;346(6):404–12.

157. Garrigue S, Barold SS, Cazeau S, et al. Prevention of atrial arrhythmias during DDD pacing by atrial overdrive. Pacing Clin Electrophysiol 1998;21(9): 1751–9.

158. Simantirakis EN, Schiza SE, Chrysostomakis SI, et al. Atrial overdrive pacing for the obstructive sleep apnea-hypopnea syndrome. N Engl J Med 2005;353(24):2568–77.

159. Sharafkhaneh A, Sharafkhaneh H, Bredikus A, et al. Effect of atrial overdrive pacing on obstructive sleep apnea in patients with systolic heart failure. Sleep Med 2007;8(1):31–6.

160. Podszus T, Mayer J, Penzel T, et al. Nocturnal hemodynamics in patients with sleep apnea. Eur J Respir Dis Suppl 1986;146:435–42.

161. Hawrylkiewicz I, Palasiewicz G, Plywaczewski R, et al. [Pulmonary hypertension in patients with pure obstructive sleep apnea]. Pol Arch Med Wewn 2004;111(4):449–54 [in Polish].

162. Chaouat A, Weitzenblum E, Krieger J, et al. Pulmonary hemodynamics in the obstructive sleep apnea syndrome. Results in 220 consecutive patients. Chest 1996;109(2):380–6.

163. Bradley TD, Rutherford R, Grossman RF, et al. Role of daytime hypoxemia in the pathogenesis of right heart failure in the obstructive sleep apnea syndrome. Am Rev Respir Dis 1985;131(6):835–9.

164. Weitzenblum E, Krieger J, Apprill M, et al. Daytime pulmonary hypertension in patients with obstructive sleep apnea syndrome. Am Rev Respir Dis 1988;138(2):345–9.

165. Chaouat A, Weitzenblum E, Krieger J, et al. Association of chronic obstructive pulmonary disease and sleep apnea syndrome. Am J Respir Crit Care Med 1995;151(1):82–6.

166. Schulz R, Schmidt D, Blum A, et al. Decreased plasma levels of nitric oxide derivatives in obstructive sleep apnoea: response to CPAP therapy. Thorax 2000;55(12):1046–51.

167. Ip MS, Lam B, Chan LY, et al. Circulating nitric oxide is suppressed in obstructive sleep apnea and is reversed by nasal continuous positive airway pressure. Am J Respir Crit Care Med 2000;162(6):2166–71.

168. Sajkov D, Wang T, Saunders NA, et al. Continuous positive airway pressure treatment improves pulmonary hemodynamics in patients with obstructive sleep apnea. Am J Respir Crit Care Med 2002; 165(2):152–8.

169. Arias MA, Garcia-Rio F, Alonso-Fernandez A, et al. Pulmonary hypertension in obstructive sleep apnoea: effects of continuous positive airway pressure: a randomized, controlled cross-over study. Eur Heart J 2006;27(9):1106–13.

170. Kessler R, Chaouat A, Schinkewitch P, et al. The obesity-hypoventilation syndrome revisited: a prospective study of 34 consecutive cases. Chest 2001;120(2):369–76.

171. Berger KI, Ayappa I, Sorkin IB, et al. CO(2) homeostasis during periodic breathing in obstructive sleep apnea. J Appl Physiol 2000; 88(1):257–64.

172. Becker HF, Piper AJ, Flynn WE, et al. Breathing during sleep in patients with nocturnal desaturation. Am J Respir Crit Care Med 1999;159(1):112–8.

173. Bednarek M, Plywaczewski R, Jonczak L, et al. There is no relationship between chronic obstructive pulmonary disease and obstructive sleep apnea syndrome: a population study. Respiration 2005;72(2):142–9.

174. Radwan L, Maszczyk Z, Koziorowski A, et al. Control of breathing in obstructive sleep apnoea and in patients with the overlap syndrome. Eur Respir J 1995;8(4):542–5.

175. Bradley TD, Rutherford R, Lue F, et al. Role of diffuse airway obstruction in the hypercapnia of obstructive sleep apnea. Am Rev Respir Dis 1986;134(5):920–4.

176. Fletcher EC, Schaaf JW, Miller J, et al. Long-term cardiopulmonary sequelae in patients with sleep apnea and chronic lung disease. Am Rev Respir Dis 1987;135:525–33.

177. Krieger J, Sforza E, Apprill M, et al. Pulmonary hypertension, hypoxemia, and hypercapnia in obstructive sleep apnea patients. Chest 1989;96: 729–37.

178. Sajkov D, Cowie RJ, Thornton AT, et al. Pulmonary hypertension and hypoxemia in obstructive sleep apnea syndrome. Am J Respir Crit Care Med 1994;149:416–22.

179. Shinozaki T, Tatsumi K, Sakuma T, et al. [Daytime pulmonary hypertension in the obstructive sleep apnea syndrome]. Nihon Kyobu Shikkan Gakkai Zasshi 1995;33:1073–9 [in Japanese].

180. Laks L, Lehrhaft B, Grunstein RR, et al. Pulmonary hypertension in obstructive sleep apnoea. Eur Respir J 1995;8:537–41.

181. Sanner BM, Doberauer C, Konermann M, et al. Pulmonary hypertension in patients with obstructive sleep apnea syndrome. Arch Intern Med 1997;157:2483–7.

182. Bady E, Achkar A, Pascal S, et al. Pulmonary arterial hypertension in patients with sleep apnoea syndrome. Thorax 2000;55:934–9.

Pediatric Obstructive Sleep Apnea Syndrome

Eliot S. Katz, MD[a,b,*], Carolyn M. D'Ambrosio, MD[c,d]

KEYWORDS

- Children • Sleep-disordered breathing
- Obstructive sleep apnea syndrome • Sleep homeostasis

Obstructive sleep apnea (OSA) is a common and serious cause of metabolic, cardiovascular, and neurocognitive morbidity in children. The essential feature of OSA is increased upper airway resistance during sleep, resulting in intermittent partial or complete airway closure, associated with increased respiratory effort, sleep fragmentation, and/or gas exchange abnormalities. Consequently, children with OSA encounter a combination of oxidative stress, inflammation, autonomic activation, and/or disruption of sleep homeostasis. Causes of airway narrowing include soft tissue hypertrophy, craniofacial abnormalities, and/or neuromuscular deficits. There appears to be important individual genetic susceptibility and environmental factors that influence the expression of OSA sequelae.

The spectrum of *obstructive* sleep-disordered breathing ranges from persistent *primary snoring* to the frank, intermittent occlusion seen in *obstructive sleep apnea*. In most cases, partial obstructive events are also present, which share the pathophysiology and consequences of complete obstruction. Thus, the more inclusive term, *obstructive sleep apnea syndrome (OSAS)*, is used in this article. Although primary snoring was traditionally defined as a benign condition, recent evidence suggests that snoring per se may be associated with adverse neurobehavioral outcomes.[1,2] In this review, the authors aim to encapsulate the salient features of pediatric OSAS, and focus on recent data regarding adverse consequences and treatment options.

EPIDEMIOLOGY

The epidemiology of pediatric OSAS has not been precisely established due to methodological limitations regarding diagnostic criteria and the paucity of population-based studies. OSAS occurs in children from neonates to adolescents, with little evidence of a systematic variability with age. Habitual snoring is nearly universally observed in pediatric OSAS, though the reliability of a negative clinical history of snoring is poor, particularly in older children. The prevalence of snoring and OSAS is predicated on the questionnaire phrasing and whether objective testing was performed. Considering representative questionnaire-based studies with a sample size of at least 1000, 4.2% "always snored"[3]; 10.9% "almost always" snored[4]; 11.7% snored "greater than or equal to 3 times per week"[5]; and 27% snored "sometimes."[6] The incidence of OSAS determined objectively in population-based studies was 2.2 to 3.8%.[7,8] The primary risk factors for pediatric

Dr Katz was supported by NIH/NHLBI HL073238 and by grant #MO1 RR02172 to Children's Hospital, Boston.
[a] Division of Respiratory Diseases, Department of Medicine, Children's Hospital, Mailstop 208, 300 Longwood Avenue, Boston, MA 02115, USA
[b] Division of Respiratory Diseases, Department of Pediatrics, Harvard Medical School, 300 Longwood Avenue, Boston, MA 02115, USA
[c] Division of Pulmonary Diseases, Department of Medicine, Tufts-New England Medical Center, 800 Washington Street, Boston, MA 02111, USA
[d] Division of Pulmonary Diseases, Department of Medicine, Tufts Medical School, 800 Washington Street, Boston, MA 02111, USA
* Corresponding author. Division of Respiratory Diseases, Department of Medicine, Children's Hospital, Mailstop 208, 300 Longwood Avenue, Boston, MA 02115.
E-mail address: eliot.katz@childrens.harvard.edu

Clin Chest Med 31 (2010) 221–234
doi:10.1016/j.ccm.2010.02.002

OSAS and the putative mechanisms are listed in **Table 1.**

CLINICAL AND POLYSOMNOGRAPHIC FINDINGS IN PEDIATRIC OSAS

The principal symptoms and physical examination findings in children with OSAS are listed in **Boxes 1** and **2.** However, clinical history/questionnaires alone have poor sensitivity and specificity for the diagnosis of OSAS,[9] leading a consensus panel to recommend objective testing for snoring children.[10] Polysomnography represents the gold standard for establishing the presence and severity of sleep-disordered breathing in children, and can be performed in children of all ages. A comprehensive review of methodological considerations in pediatric polysomnography has recently been published.[11] There is minimal night-to-night variability in the respiratory variables during polysomnography.[12] Normative data from several large samples of nonsnoring, normal children after infancy (**Table 2**) indicate that (a) obstructive apneas and hypopneas very rarely occur; (b) inspiratory flow limitation and respiratory effort-related arousals are uncommon; and (c) oxygen saturation rarely drops below 90%, even during normal 10- to 15-second respiratory pauses following sighs or movements.[13–15]

Arousal from sleep is a protective reflex mechanism that restores airway patency, but is associated with sleep fragmentation. Although visible electroencephalographic arousals are present in only 51% of obstructive events in children, frequency domain analysis demonstrates additional evidence of sleep disruption.[16] Autonomic activation is present at the end of nearly all obstructive events, as measured by heart rate variability, blood pressure elevations, pulse transit time, and peripheral arterial tonometry. Children with OSAS have increases in slow wave sleep (23.5 vs 28.8%), decreases in rapid eye movement (REM) sleep (22.3 vs 17.3%), and decreases in spontaneous arousals.[17] Together, these observations provide evidence for a subtle disruption in sleep architecture, with increased sleep pressure and a homeostatic elevation in the arousal threshold.

PATHOPHYSIOLOGY OF OSAS IN CHILDREN

Children with OSAS have increased upper airway resistance during sleep due to a combination of soft tissue hypertrophy, craniofacial dysmorphology, neuromuscular weakness, or obesity. However, most children with OSAS obtain long periods of stable breathing during sleep, indicating a role for other determinants of airway patency such as neuromuscular activation, ventilatory control, and arousal threshold.

Anatomy

Children with OSAS have narrower pharyngeal airways and increased nasal resistance compared with control children.[18,19] Adenotonsillar hypertrophy, maxillary constriction, and retro-/micrognathia are the most common anatomic abnormalities in OSAS. However, the correlation between apnea severity and adenotonsillar size is surprisingly variable.[20,21] Mouth breathing children habitually lower their mandible resulting in a high-arched palate, narrow maxilla, retrognathia,

Table 1
Epidemiologic risk factors for pediatric obstructive sleep apnea syndrome

Adenotonsillar hypertrophy	Increased airway resistance
Obesity	Fatty infiltration of airway, abnormal ventilatory control
Race (African American)	Craniofacial structure, socioeconomic
Gender (male)	Slight male predominance in prepubertal children, which increases markedly after puberty
Prematurity	Neurologic impairment, adverse craniofacial growth, abnormal ventilatory control
Craniofacial dysmorphology	Increased airway resistance
Neurologic disorders	Abnormal motor control of the upper airway
Nasal/pharyngeal inflammation	Allergy or infection increasing airway resistance
Socioeconomic/environmental	Neighborhood disadvantage, passive cigarette smoke, indoor allergens, sleep quality (noise, stress)
Family history of OSAS	Heritable craniofacial structure, neuromuscular compensation, arousal threshold, ventilatory control

Box 1
Symptoms of pediatric obstructive sleep apnea syndrome

Diurnal Symptoms

Sleep

- Excessive daytime sleepiness
- Napping
- Morning headaches
- Difficult arousing from sleep

Neurocognitive

- Aggressive behavior
- Poor school performance
- Depression
- Attention deficit
- Hyperactivity
- Moodiness

Upper Airway

- Mouth breathing
- Nasal congestion
- Frequent otitis media, sinusitis
- Nasal speech

Nocturnal Symptoms

Snoring

Witnessed apnea

Choking/snorting noises

Increased work of breathing

Paradoxic respirations

Enuresis

Restless sleep

Diaphoresis

Hyperextended neck

Frequent awakenings

Mouth breathing/dry mouth

Parasomnias

Box 2
Physical examination in pediatric obstructive sleep apnea syndrome

General

Obesity

Increased neck circumference

Failure to thrive

Sleepiness

Head

Nose

- Swollen nasal mucous membranes
- Deviated septum

Mouth

- Tonsillar hypertrophy
- High-arched palate
- Elongated soft palate
- Posterior buccal cross-bite
- Overbite
- Crowded oropharynx
- Macroglossia
- Glossoptosis

Face

- Midfacial hypoplasia
- Micrognathia/retrognathia
- Long face syndrome
  - Infraorbital darkening
  - Mouth breathing
  - Elongated midface
  - Nasal atrophy

Cardiovascular

Systemic hypertension

Loud P2

Extremities

Edema

Clubbing

and increased lower facial height. This constellation of findings has been termed the "long face syndrome," and is associated with OSAS.[22,23] Thus not only does upper airway obstruction predispose to OSAS, but it also has an adverse effect on craniofacial development, posing an increased future risk of OSAS. Relief of upper airway obstruction during periods of rapid facial growth may at least partially normalize dentofacial abnormalities that predispose to OSAS.

Airway Mechanics

The upper airway is a highly compliant tube in which small changes in pressure produces large changes in airway cross-sectional area. The luminal pressure at which airway collapse occurs is termed the *critical closing pressure* (Pcrit). The Pcrit is an index of both the viscoelastic and neuromuscular properties of the pharynx. Children

Table 2
Polysomnographic data in normal children

Sleep	
EEG arousal index (per h TST)	9 ± 3
Sleep efficiency (%)	89 ± 7
Stage 1 (% TST)	5 ± 3
Stage 2 (% TST)	42 ± 8
Slow wave sleep (% TST)	26 ± 8
REM sleep (% TST)	20 ± 5
REM cycles	4 ± 1
Periodic leg movement index (per h TST)	1 ± 1
Respiratory	
Obstructive apnea index (per h TST)	0.0 ± 0.1
Obstructive apnea/hypopnea index (per h TST)	0.1 ± 0.1
Central apnea index (per h TST)	0.5 ± 0.5
$P_{ET}CO_2 \geq 50$ mm Hg (% TST)	2.8 ± 11.3
Peak $P_{ET}CO_2$ (mm Hg)	46 ± 3
$S_pO_2 > 95\%$ (% TST)	99.6 ± 1
S_pO_2 90%–95% (% TST)	0.4 ± 1
$S_pO_2 < 90\%$ (% TST)	0.05 ± 0.2
Desaturation index ($\geq 4\%$, per h TST)	0.4 ± 0.8
S_pO_2 Nadir (%)	93 ± 4

Data are presented as mean $\pm$ SD.
Abbreviations: EEG, electroencephalograph; REM, rapid eye movement; TST, total sleep time.
Data from Refs.[14,17,125–128]

with OSAS have a higher Pcrit than control subjects[24] and children with habitual snoring.[25] Pcrit correlates with the severity of OSAS, and decreases following adenotonsillectomy.[25] Of note, the Pcrit in OSAS patients after adenotonsillectomy does not decrease to level of control subjects[24] or even primary snorers,[25] suggesting that subtle abnormalities of anatomy or neuromuscular control remain after treatment.

Neuromuscular Compensation, Arousal, and Ventilatory Control

Upper airway muscles that are phasically activated during inspiration, such as the genioglossus, increase both the luminal size and stiffness of the airway. During wakefulness, children with OSAS have increased genioglossus activity compared with control children.[26] At sleep onset, pharyngeal dilator activity is reduced, ventilatory variability increases, and an apneic threshold slightly below eupneic levels is observed in non-REM sleep. Airway collapse is offset by increased pharyngeal dilator activity in response to hypercapnia and negative luminal pressure. Respiratory control mechanisms modulate ventilation and, therefore,

pharyngeal dilator activation, in non-REM sleep. Arousal from sleep immediately opens the airway and normalizes gas exchange abnormalities. However, arousal may also be considered an adverse epiphenomenon that potentiates obstructive cycling by augmenting ventilatory overshoot, interfering with sleep homeostasis.[27] Paroxysmal reductions in pharyngeal dilator activity related to central REM processes likely account for the disproportionate severity of OSAS observed during REM sleep.

Obesity

The prevalence of childhood obesity has tripled in the last 25 years, and is presently estimated to be 17% to 18%. Obese children are more likely to snore than lean children.[28] The incidence of OSAS in obese children is high at 36%,[29] and may exceed 60% if habitual snoring is present.[30] The risk of having moderate OSAS increases 12% for each 1 kg/m^2 of body mass index (BMI; calculated as the child's weight in kilograms divided by height in meters squared) above the mean.[31] Nevertheless, the relationship between BMI and OSAS severity is often poor, suggesting that *fat distribution* is of considerable importance.[32] Obesity can contribute to the severity of OSAS by influencing the dimension and collapsibility of the upper airway, as well as altering ventilatory control. Both OSAS and obesity are considered chronic, low-grade systemic inflammatory states and may act synergistically to produce cardiovascular, metabolic, and neurocognitive morbidities (**Box 3**). Obesity and OSAS are also associated with an impaired quality of life and sleepiness.[33–35]

Most obese children with OSAS will also have adenotonsillar hypertrophy.[30] However, when obese and lean children with OSAS are matched for disease severity, the obese children have less adenotonsillar hypertrophy, but significantly higher Mallampati scores (indicating more crowding of the oropharynx).[32] This finding also supports the concept that a central distribution of adiposity

---

Box 3
Sequelae of pediatric obstructive sleep apnea

Metabolic

    Elevated C-reactive protein

    Insulin resistance

    Hypercholesterolemia

    Elevated transaminases

    Decreased insulinlike growth factor

    Decreased/altered growth hormone secretion

Neurocognitive

    Decreased quality of life

    Aggressive behavior

    Poor school performance

    Depression

    Attention deficit

    Hyperactivity

    Moodiness

Cardiovascular

    Autonomic dysfunction

    Systemic hypertension

    Absent blood pressure "dipping" during sleep

    Left ventricular dysfunction

    Pulmonary hypertension

    Abnormal heart rate variability

    Elevated vascular endothelial growth factor

---

poses the greatest risk for OSAS. Obese children with OSAS have more obstructive events in the supine position, whereas nonobese children with OSAS are more severe in the prone or side positions.[36] This result suggests that there are important physiologic differences between obese and nonobese airways.

Adenotonsillectomy in obese children with OSAS results in a marked reduction in apnea/hypopnea index (AHI; expressed as the number of apneas and hypopneas per hour of sleep), but 76% have residual OSAS.[37,38] One series reported that 56% of obese children with OSAS required continuous positive airway pressure (CPAP) following adenotonsillectomy.[39] Weight loss in obese children of 18.7 kg over 20 weeks resulted in a reduction in the AHI from 14.1 to 1.6 per hour.[40] However, another study reported that 38% of obese children had an AHI of more than 2/h after a 24-kg weight loss over 5 months.[41] Bariatric surgery in adolescents resulting in an average 58 kg weight loss over 5 months resulted in a reduction in the AHI from a median of 9.1 to 0.7 per hour, with only 1 child with residual OSAS.[42] Postoperative respiratory complications are higher in obese children with suspected OSAS.

SEQUELAE OF PEDIATRIC OBSTRUCTIVE SLEEP APNEA
Metabolic Sequelae

Failure to thrive was reported in 27 to 62% of cases in early case series of pediatric OSAS.[43,44] The probable origin is a reduction of insulinlike growth factor (IGF) and growth hormone secretion. IGF binding protein 3 (IGFBP-3), which is correlated to growth hormone secretion, is decreased in children with OSAS. Also, both IGF-1 and IGFBP-3 were observed to increase following adenotonsillectomy, and catch-up growth, including height and weight, occurs.[45,46] In fact, increases in BMI z-scores occur in both lean and obese children following OSAS treatment.[46,47] More recently, the increased awareness of the adverse consequences of OSAS has made the presentation of failure to thrive rare, and indeed, obesity is present in nearly half of cases.[48] Leptin is an adipocyte-secreted peptide secreted that regulates metabolism, hunger, and inflammation, and stimulates ventilation. Leptin levels are increased in children with OSAS,[49] and decrease after treatment with CPAP.[50]

Obesity in children is associated with insulin resistance, dyslipidemia, and hypertension, termed the "metabolic syndrome," which is associated with adverse cardiovascular outcomes into adulthood.[51] Other factors that may influence the expression of the metabolic syndrome include genetics, diet, physical activity, and possibly, OSAS. The role of OSAS in the development of the metabolic syndrome in children is complex and is limited by cross-sectional data. In *obese* children, OSAS has been independently associated with insulin resistance,[52–54] dyslipidemia,[52,54] and blood pressure dysregulation.[52,55] By contrast, OSAS does not appear to increase the risk of insulin resistance in *lean* children[56] or *morbidly obese* children. The combination of obesity and OSAS likely magnify the proinflammatory comorbidities observed in both conditions.

Cardiovascular Sequelae

Children with OSAS have cardiovascular abnormalities ranging from autonomic dysfunction to structural heart disease (see **Box 3**), and may be predisposed toward more serious morbidity and mortality as adults. The pathophysiology is multifactorial including altered sympathovagal balance, oxidative stress, production of inflammatory cytokines, vascular remodeling, and endothelial cell dysfunction. In children with OSAS, urinary levels of catecholamines are elevated,[57] and sympathetic drive is increased based on heart rate variability, peripheral arterial tonometry, pulse transit time, and beat-to-beat blood pressure. Of importance is that these abnormalities are present in OSAS patients during both wakefulness[58] and sleep,[59] suggesting generalized autonomic dysfunction. Complicating the role of OSAS in the genesis of cardiovascular morbidity is the profound effect of obesity, genetic susceptibility factors, and the environment.

Blood pressure (BP) dysregulation has been reported in children with OSAS compared with controls during wakefulness[55,60] and sleep,[55] though frank hypertension is rare.[55,61] Children with severe OSAS (AHI >5 events/h) have an increased morning BP surge, elevated mean 24-hour BP, and lack the normal "dipping" of BP at sleep onset (**Fig. 1**).[55,62] The sensitivity of the baroreflex system is reduced in children with OSAS, impairing their ability to maintain cardiovascular homeostasis.[63] Of note, BP dysregulation and lower baroreflex gain is observed even in children with mild OSAS (AHI 1–5 events/h), supporting the need to intervene at early stages in the disease.[55] Paradoxically, some children with OSAS develop orthostatic hypotension and therefore are reported to have low systemic blood pressure and orthostatic hypotension.[61]

Children with OSAS have been reported to have echocardiographic evidence for left ventricular hypertrophy,[64] right ventricular hypertrophy,[64]

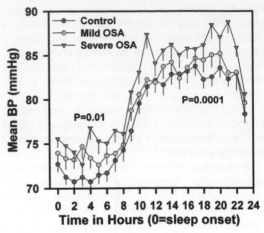

Fig. 1. Group mean 24-hour ambulatory BP recording for children with mild OSA (AHI 1–5/h), severe OSA (>5/h), and a control population. Sleep onset is at time 0. Children with severe OSA have significantly greater mean BP during wakefulness and sleep. (*From* Amin R, Somers VK, McConnell K, et al. Activity-adjusted 24-hour ambulatory blood pressure and cardiac remodeling in children with sleep-disordered breathing. Hypertension 2008;51:84–91; with permission.)

and decreased left ventricular function,[65] without clinical symptoms. The increase in systolic BP, morning BP surge, and BP variability has been associated with increasing left ventricular wall thickness.[55,63] Thus, the subtle changes in BP homeostasis observed in children with OSAS may be an intermediate phenotype, leading to significant cardiovascular morbidity over time. Improvement of left ventricular function has been observed following treatment of OSAS.[65] Right and left ventricular hypertrophy has been associated with an increased risk of postoperative complications in children with OSAS, and is suspected to be a risk factor for adverse cardiovascular outcomes in adulthood.

The recurrent episodes of hypoxemia and arousal associated with OSAS are associated with oxidative stress and systemic inflammation, independent of obesity. Children with OSAS have elevated serum levels of tumor necrosis factor α (TNF-α), C-reactive protein (CRP),[66] interferon-γ (INF-γ),[67] interleukin (IL)-6,[68] and IL-8.[67] Pathology studies of tonsillar tissue from children with OSAS demonstrate increased expression of TNF-α and IL-6, compared with children with recurrent tonsillitis.[69] In addition, levels of IL-8,[70] IL-6,[66,68] and CRP[54,71] decline following treatment of OSAS. Of note, children with a family history of premature cardiovascular disease were more likely to have residual endothelial cell dysfunction following treatment.[72]

Neuropsychological Sequelae

Children with symptoms of OSAS have been reported to have a wide range of neuropsychological dysfunction, including cognition,[73] hyperactivity,[74] sleepiness,[33] memory,[75] executive function,[76] attention,[77] school performance,[78,79] and behavior.[77] Parents and teachers both report disruptive behavior including aggression, conduct, and emotional control.[80] Even mild OSAS or primary snoring (increased respiratory effort without discrete obstructive events) is associated with adverse neurodevelopmental outcomes.[2,75,76,81] Children with attention-deficit hyperactivity disorder (ADHD) have a high incidence of OSAS both subjectively and objectively.[82] In contrast, the incidence of ADHD by DSM-IV-R (*Diagnostic and Statistical Manual of Mental Disorders* Fourth Edition—Text Revised) criteria was 28% in a population of children undergoing adenotonsillectomy for predominantly obstructive indications.[83] Treatment of OSAS with adenotonsillectomy has been shown to improve hyperactive behavior,[83] inattention,[84] sleepiness,[84] behavior,[85] school performance,[78] and cognition.[86,87] However, a history of frequent or loud snoring between 2 and 6 years of age was associated with lower academic performance at 13 to 14 years old, suggesting that OSAS-induced deficits incurred during periods of brain development may not be fully reversible.[88]

Excessive daytime sleepiness (EDS) is rarely reported by children with OSAS themselves. Parental reports vary with the type of questionnaire used, from 7% ("moderate/severe EDS") using a single question,[9] to 49% ("problematic subjective sleepiness") using the more comprehensive 4-item Pediatric Sleep Questionnaire-Sleepiness Subscale (PSQ-SS).[89] There was a good correlation between the subjective PSQ-SS questionnaire and the objective Multiple Sleep Latency Test (MSLT).[89] Objective sleepiness in children with OSAS evaluated with an MSLT varies between approximately 13% and 40%.[33,89] Of importance is that parents will not report EDS in over 50% of cases in which the mean MSLT sleep is less than 12 minutes, indicating pathologic sleepiness. Objective sleepiness is positively associated with AHI, oxygen desaturation, respiratory arousal index (number of arousals per hour of sleep), and BMI.[33] Obese children with OSAS are more likely to have objective sleepiness than lean children with OSAS, at all levels of OSAS severity.[33]

DIAGNOSTIC AND TREATMENT PARADIGM

The optimal methodology and criteria for the diagnosis of OSAS in children has not been established. Previous efforts to define OSAS severity with threshold levels of the AHI (mild 1–5/h, moderate 5–10/h, severe >10/h), gas exchange abnormalities, or sleep fragmentation have proven unsatisfactory, because they fail to account for the individual trait susceptibility to the neurocognitive, cardiovascular, and metabolic sequelae of OSAS. Thus the threshold amount of OSAS associated with adverse consequences varies widely among children. Therefore, current efforts to diagnose and classify OSAS are using the *personalized medicine* paradigm, in which the genomic and molecular profile of an individual is combined with clinical and polysomnographic phenotyping. Toward this end, a hybrid approach to the diagnosis and treatment of OSAS in children has been proposed, combining polysomnographic indices, symptoms, and biomarkers,[90] but this has not been rigorously studied.

Despite advances in the recognition of abnormal respiratory patterns during sleep, there is no clear consensus on the severity of childhood OSAS that warrants treatment. The choice of therapy is predicated on the etiology, severity, natural history, and therapeutic options available for the increased upper airway resistance. Most clinicians consider adenotonsillectomy as the first line of treatment in the setting of adenotonsillar hypertrophy. However, with a compatible clinical history and physical examination of allergies, the threshold level of OSAS necessary for treatment with intranasal steroids and leukotriene antagonists is low. By contrast, it is recognized that the initiation of *CPAP* is fraught with difficulties in tolerance and may itself be disruptive of sleep. Thus, initiating CPAP therapy requires more polysomnographic evidence of obstruction (usually AHI >5 events/h), more profound gas exchange abnormalities (SpO_2 <90%), increased sleep fragmentation (arousal index >15/h), or neurobehavioral symptoms. Finally, children with severe OSAS polysomnographically, and severe manifestations including failure to thrive, pulmonary hypertension, and marked aberrations in daytime functioning, would mandate consideration of all available therapies, including medically supervised weight loss and, if life-threatening, tracheotomy.

Pharmacologic Therapy

Leukotrienes and their receptors are increased in adenotonsillar tissue[91] and exhaled condensate[92] of children with OSAS. Topical intranasal steroids have been shown to decrease adenoidal hypertrophy and improve symptom scores of obstructed breathing.[93] Aqueous beclomethasone decreased the adenoid/choanae ratio from 91%

at baseline, to 77% at 1 month, and 62% after 6 months.[93] Several studies have documented reduction in the AHI following a course of nasal steroids: (1) 5 weeks of intranasal fluticasone decreased the AHI from 11 to 6/h[94]; (2) 6 weeks of intranasal budesonide decreased the AHI from 3.7 to 1.3/h[95]; (3) 4 weeks of intranasal budesonide reduced the AHI from 5.2 to 3.2/h.[96] The improvement in OSAS severity after discontinuing intranasal steroid therapy appears to be stable after at least 2 months polysomnographically,[95] and after at least 9 months symptomatically.[96] Children whose symptoms improve with nasal steroids are less likely to have an adenotonsillectomy within 2 years, compared with nonresponders (54% vs 83%).[97] The combination of budesonide and montelukast in children with mild residual OSAS following adenotonsillectomy resulted in a reduction in the AHI from 3.9 to 0.3 per hour after 3 months of therapy.[98] The long-term success of anti-inflammatory therapy has not been established.

Positive Pressure/Oxygen Therapy

CPAP delivered noninvasively through nasal or oronasal interface is a highly efficacious therapy for pediatric OSAS, though long-term compliance is often problematic.[99–101] CPAP is typically reserved for moderate to severe OSAS not amenable to surgical or pharmacologic treatment. A properly fitted mask and adequate age-appropriate behavioral training is crucial to the success of CPAP therapy.[102,103] The minimum daily duration of CPAP therapy required to mitigate the adverse effects of OSAS is unknown. In a prospective study of children with severe OSAS, CPAP compliance monitored electronically after approximately 1 month of therapy revealed that CPAP usage of longer than 4 hours, longer than 5 hours, and longer than 6 hours per night was observed in only 54%, 48%, and 31% of patients, respectively.[104] The reported side effects of CPAP in children include skin erythema, eye irritation, congestion, rhinorrhea, and maxillary growth impairment.[105] CPAP was reported to be equally as efficacious as bilevel ventilation for the treatment of OSAS in children.[105]

Oxygen therapy has a limited role in the treatment of children with OSAS. Two studies have evaluated the effect of supplemental oxygen in children with OSAS, with disappointing results. Improvements in oxygen saturation are evident, but there is no significant decrease in OSAS severity.[106,107] In addition, 2 children with OSAS developed a marked increase in P_{CO_2} on supplemental oxygen (>75 torr).[106] Thus, oxygen therapy

will not alleviate the sleep fragmentation or hypoventilation associated with OSAS.

Surgical Therapy

Successful treatment of children with OSAS is predicated on identifying the origin of the increased upper airway resistance. In most children with documented OSAS and adenotonsillar hypertrophy, an adenotonsillectomy is the recommended first-line therapy. Following adenotonsillectomy, children with OSAS have reported improvements in quality of life,[108] behavior,[85] attention,[83] growth,[109] cognitive scores,[86,87] and school performance.[78] However, residual OSAS may be present polysomnographically in more than 40% of cases postoperatively.[37,38] Moreover, there is no consensus on whether the adenoids, tonsils, or both need to be removed. A retrospective study in children undergoing adenoidectomy for obstructive symptoms reported that 27% subsequently had a tonsillectomy.[110] Selected patients may benefit from treatments of additional sites of obstruction, such as turbinectomy, deviated septum repair, maxillary expansion, mandibular distraction, maxillary distraction, tongue reduction/advancement, or lingual tonsillar removal.[111]

Parental reports of OSAS symptomatology post adenotonsillectomy are usually favorable, though objective testing often reveals considerable residual obstruction. Complete normalization of OSAS (AHI<1) following adenotonsillectomy was observed in only 25% of patients, with 46% having persistent mild OSAS (1<AHI<5), and 29% having at least moderate OSAS (AHI>5).[37] Children with residual OSAS following adenotonsillectomy are most likely to have obesity, severe OSA, enlarged turbinates, deviated septum, neurologic disorders, or craniofacial malformations.[37,38] Together, these studies indicate that adenotonsillar hypertrophy is only one of several important determinants of OSAS in children. A recent meta-analysis of the cure rate of adenotonsillectomy for OSAS (defined as an AHI <1) was only 60%, though there was a marked improvement in OSAS in the majority of children.[112]

Adenotonsillectomy for OSAS is associated with postoperative bleeding (3% of cases), pain, and respiratory decompensation (20% of cases), including pulmonary edema, upper airway obstruction and, rarely, death.[113–115] Adenoidectomy alone has a lower risk of postoperative bleeding (<0.5%). The first postoperative night may be associated with significant OSAS, resulting in profound desaturation.[116] However, the majority of children with mild OSAS will improve on the first postoperative night.[117] Patients at high risk for postoperative complications include children younger than 3 years, or those with prematurity, craniofacial abnormalities, obesity, neuromuscular weakness, cerebral palsy, cor pulmonale, or severe OSAS.[118,119] Careful postoperative monitoring of high-risk patients in a pediatric intensive care unit is recommended. Children experiencing respiratory distress postoperatively have been reported to benefit from positive airway pressure.[118]

Dental Therapy

Craniofacial growth in children is determined by both genetic and environmental factors. Chronic mouth breathing results in aberrant facial development, including maxillary constriction. Rapid maxillary expansion, using an orthodontic appliance to deliver a lateral force to the upper posterior molars, opens the midpalatal suture transversely and therefore widens the nasal cavity. Over a period of about 3 weeks, the intermolar distance increases approximately 3.9 mm, and the nasal pyriform opening increases 1.3 mm.[120] After 4 months of therapy, rapid maxillary expansion decreases nasal resistance[120] and improves OSAS in children with maxillary constriction.[120–122] Children with OSAS due to both maxillary constriction and adenotonsillar hypertrophy generally require both rapid maxillary expansion and adenotonsillectomy to resolve the OSAS.

Children with OSAS and dysgnathia (87% deep/retrusive bite, 13% cross-bite) were randomized into a 6-month trial of a custom mandibular advancement device versus an untreated control group.[123] Twenty-six percent of the children in the treatment group discontinued therapy for unknown reasons. As a group, follow-up polysomnography revealed a decrease in the AHI from 7.1 to 2.6 events per hour, but 20% of the patients had a residual AHI above 5 events/h.[123] Another pediatric study similarly demonstrated that mandibular advancement devices reduced the AHI from 8 to 4 events per hour.[124] Nevertheless, there are insufficient long-term efficacy data using mandibular advancement devices to treat OSAS in children with dysgnathia.

SUMMARY

OSAS is a common and serious cause of metabolic, cardiovascular, and neurocognitive morbidity in children. The essential feature of OSAS is increased upper airway resistance during sleep, resulting in intermittent partial or complete airway closure, increased respiratory effort, sleep fragmentation, or gas exchange abnormalities.

Consequently, children with OSAS encounter a combination of oxidative stress, inflammation, autonomic activation, and disruption of sleep homeostasis. Causes of airway narrowing include soft tissue hypertrophy, craniofacial abnormalities, or neuromuscular deficits. Most children with OSAS obtain long periods of stable breathing during sleep, indicating a role for other determinants of airway patency such as neuromuscular activation, ventilatory control, and arousal threshold. There appear to be important individual genetic susceptibility and environmental factors that influence the expression of OSAS sequelae. In some children even mild OSAS can result in adverse neurocognitive and cardiovascular sequelae. The choice of therapy is predicated on the etiology, severity, natural history, and therapeutic options available for the increased upper airway resistance. Most clinicians consider adenotonsillectomy the first-line treatment in the setting of adenotonsillar hypertrophy. However, anti-inflammatory therapy with intranasal steroids and leukotriene antagonists is helpful in many cases. CPAP is generally reserved for children without surgically correctable obstruction, or significant residual OSAS following other treatments. Preliminary data suggest that the consequences of pediatric OSAS are at least partially reversible with appropriate therapy. However, there is concern that exposure to OSAS during critical developmental intervals may result in lasting neurocognitive deficits.

REFERENCES

1. Urschitz MS, Guenther A, Eggebrecht E, et al. Snoring, intermittent hypoxia and academic performance in primary school children. Am J Respir Crit Care Med 2003;168:464–8.
2. O'Brien LM, Mervis CB, Holbrook CR, et al. Neurobehavioral implications of habitual snoring in children. Pediatrics 2004;114:44–9.
3. Kaditis AG, Finder J, Alexopoulos EI, et al. Sleep-disordered breathing in 3,680 Greek children. Pediatr Pulmonol 2004;37:499–509.
4. Ng DK, Kwok KL, Cheung JM, et al. Prevalence of sleep problems in Hong Kong primary school children. A community-based telephone survey. Chest 2005;128:1315–23.
5. O'Brien LM, Holbrook CR, Mervis CB, et al. Sleep and neurobehavioral characteristics of 5- to 7-year-old children with parentally reported symptoms of attention-deficit/hyperactivity disorder. Pediatrics 2003;111(3):554–63.
6. Owen GO, Canter RJ, Robinson A. Snoring, apnoea, and ENT symptoms in the paediatric community. Acta Paediatr 2003;92:425–9.

7. Rosen CL, Larkin EK, Kirchner HL, et al. Prevalence and risk factors for sleep-disordered breathing in 8- to 11-year-old children: association with race and prematurity. J Pediatr 2003; 142:383–9.

8. Schlaud M, Urschitz MS, Urschitz-Duprat PM, et al. The German study on sleep-disordered breathing in primary school children: epidemiological approach, representativeness of study sample, and preliminary screening results. Paediatr Perinat Epidemiol 2004;18:431–40.

9. Carroll J, McColley S, Marcus C, et al. Inability of clinical history to distinguish primary snoring from obstructive sleep apnea syndrome in children. Chest 1995;108:610–8.

10. Section on Pediatric Pulmonology. Clinical practice guideline: diagnosis and management of childhood obstructive sleep apnea syndrome. Pediatrics 2002;109:704–12.

11. Muzumdar H, Arens R. Diagnostic issues in pediatric obstructive sleep apnea. Proc Am Thorac Soc 2008;5:263–73.

12. Katz ES, Greene MG, Carson KA, et al. Night-to-night variability of polysomnography in children with symptoms of sleep-disordered breathing. J Pediatr 2002;140:589–94.

13. Montgomery-Downs HE, O'Brien LM, Gulliver TE, et al. Polysomnographic characteristics in normal preschool and early school-aged children. Pediatrics 2006;117:741–53.

14. Uliel S, Tauman R, Greenfeld M, et al. Normal polysomnographic respiratory values in children and adolescents. Chest 2004;125:872–8.

15. Verhulst SL, Schrauwen N, Haentjens D, et al. Reference values for sleep-related respiratory variables in asymptomatic European children and adolescents. Pediatr Pulmonol 2007;42:159–67.

16. Bandla HP, Gozal D. Dynamic changes in EEG spectra during obstructive apnea in children. Pediatr Pulmonol 2000;29:359–65.

17. Tauman R, O'Brien LM, Holbrook CR, et al. Sleep pressure score: a new index of sleep disruption in snoring children. Sleep 2004;27:274–8.

18. Monahan KJ, Larkin EK, Rosen CL, et al. Utility of noninvasive pharyngometry in epidemiologic studies of childhood sleep-disordered breathing. Am J Respir Crit Care Med 2002;165:1499–503.

19. Isono S, Shimada A, Utsugi M, et al. Comparison of static mechanical properties of the passive pharynx between normal children and children with sleep-disordered breathing. Am J Respir Crit Care Med 1998;157:1204–12.

20. Arens R, McDonough JM, Costarino AT, et al. Magnetic resonance imaging of the upper airway structure of children with obstructive sleep apnea syndrome. Am J Respir Crit Care Med 2001;164: 698–703.

21. Fregosi RF, Quan SF, Kaemingk KL, et al. Sleep-disordered breathing, pharyngeal size and soft tissue anatomy in children. J Appl Phys 2003;95: 2030–8.

22. Kawashima S, Niikuni N, Chia-hung L, et al. Cephalometric comparisons of craniofacial and upper airway structures in young children with obstructive sleep apnea syndrome. Ear Nose Throat J 2000;79: 499–506.

23. Zettergren-Wijk L, Forsberg CM, Linder-Aronson S. Changes in dentofacial morphology after adeno-/tonsillectomy in young children with obstructive sleep apnoea—a 5-year follow-up study. Eur J Orthod 2006;28:319–26.

24. Marcus CL, Katz ES, Lutz J, et al. Upper airway dynamic responses in children with the obstructive sleep apnea syndrome. Pediatr Res 2005;57(1): 99–107.

25. Marcus CL, McColley SA, Carroll JL, et al. Upper airway collapsibility in children with obstructive sleep apnea syndrome. J Appl Phys 1994;77: 918–24.

26. Katz ES, White DP. Genioglossus activity in children with obstructive sleep apnea during wakefulness and sleep onset. Am J Respir Crit Care Med 2003;168:664–70.

27. Younes M. Role of arousals in the pathogenesis of obstructive sleep apnea. Am J Respir Crit Care Med 2004;169:623–33.

28. Urschitz MS, Guenther A, Eitner S, et al. Risk factors and natural history of habitual snoring. Chest 2004;126:790–800.

29. Marcus CL, Curtis S, Koerner CB, et al. Evaluation of pulmonary function and polysomnography in obese children and adolescents. Pediatr Pulmonol 1996;21:176–83.

30. Silvestri JM, Weese-Meyer DE, Bass MT, et al. Polysomnography in obese children with a history of sleep-associated breathing disorders. Pediatr Pulmonol 1993;16:124–9.

31. Redline S, Tishler PV, Schluchter M, et al. Risk factors for sleep-disordered breathing in children: associations with obesity, race, and respiratory problems. Am J Respir Crit Care Med 1999;159: 1527–32.

32. Dayyat E, Kheirandish-Gozal L, Capdevila OS, et al. Obstructive sleep apnea in children. Relative contributions of body mass index and adenotonsillar hypertrophy. Chest 2009;136:137–44.

33. Gozal D, Kheirandish-Gozal L. Obesity and excessive daytime sleepiness in prepubertal children with obstructive sleep apnea. Pediatrics 2009; 123:13–8.

34. Crabtree VM, Varni JW, Gozal D. Health-related quality of life and depressive symptoms in children with suspected sleep-disordered breathing. Sleep 2004;27:1131–8.

35. Tsiros MD, Olds T, Buckley JD, et al. Health-related quality of life in obese children and adolescents. Int J Obes 2009;33:387–400.

36. Dayyat E, Maarafeya MM, Capdevila OS, et al. Nocturnal body position in sleeping children with and without obstructive sleep apnea. Pediatr Pulmonol 2007;42:374–9.

37. Tauman R, Gulliver TE, Krishna J, et al. Persistence of obstructive sleep apnea syndrome in children after adenotonsillectomy. J Pediatr 2006;149:803–8.

38. Guilleminault C, Huang Y, Glamann C, et al. Adenotonsillectomy and obstructive sleep apnea in children: a prospective survey. Otolaryngol Head Neck Surg 2007;136:169–75.

39. Shine NP, Lannigan FJ, Coates HL, et al. Adenotonsillectomy for obstructive sleep apnea in obese children: effects on respiratory parameters and clinical outcome. Arch Otolaryngol Head Neck Surg 2006;132:1123–7.

40. Willi SM, Oexmann MJ, Wright NM, et al. The effects of a high protein, low-fat, ketogenic diet on adolescents with morbid obesity: body compensation, blood chemistries, and sleep abnormalities. Pediatrics 1998;10:161–7.

41. Verhulst SL, Franckx H, Van Gaal L, et al. The effect of weight loss on sleep-disordered breathing in obese teenagers. Obesity (Silver Spring) 2009;17:1178–83.

42. Kalra M, Inge T, Garcia V, et al. Obstructive sleep apnea in extremely overweight adolescents undergoing bariatric surgery. Obes Res 2005;13:1175–9.

43. Guilleminault C, Eldridge FL, Simmons FB, et al. Sleep apnea in eight children. Pediatrics 1976;58(1):23–30.

44. Brouillette RT, Fernbach SK, Hunt CE. Obstructive sleep apnea in infants and children. J Pediatr 1982;100:31–40.

45. Bonuck KA, Freeman K, Henderson J. Growth and growth biomarker changes after adenotonsillectomy: systematic review and meta-analysis. Arch Dis Child 2009;94:83–91.

46. Bar A, Tarasiuk A, Segev Y, et al. The effect of adenotonsillectomy on serum insulin-like growth factor-I and growth in children with obstructive sleep apnea syndrome. J Pediatr 1999;135:76–80.

47. Soultan Z, Wadowski S, Rao M, et al. Effect of treating obstructive sleep apnea by tonsillectomy and/or adenoidectomy on obesity in children. Arch Pediatr Adolesc Med 1999;153:33–7.

48. Gozal D, Simakajornboon N, Holbrook CR, et al. Secular trends in obesity and parentally-reported daytime sleepiness among children referred to a pediatric sleep center for snoring and suspected sleep-disordered breathing (SDB). Sleep 2006;29:A74.

49. Tauman R, Serpero LD, Capdevila OS, et al. Adipokines in children with sleep disordered breathing. Sleep 2007;30:443–9.

50. Nakra N, Bhargava S, Dzuira J, et al. Sleep-disordered breathing in children with metabolic syndrome: the role of leptin and sympathetic nervous system activity and the effect of continuous positive airway pressure. Pediatrics 2008;122:e634–42.

51. Sinaiko AR, Steinberger J, Moran A, et al. Influence of insulin resistance and body mass index at age 13 on systolic blood pressure, triglycerides, and high-density lipoprotein cholesterol at age 19. Hypertension 2006;48:730–6.

52. Redline S, Storfer-Isser A, Rosen CL, et al. Association between metabolic syndrome and sleep-disordered breathing in adolescents. Am J Respir Crit Care Med 2007;176:401–8.

53. de la Eva RC, Baur LA, Donaghue KC, et al. Metabolic correlates with obstructive sleep apnea in obese subjects. J Pediatr 2002;140:654–9.

54. Gozal D, Capdevila OS, Kheirandish-Gozal L. Metabolic alterations and systemic inflammation in obstructive sleep apnea among nonobese and obese prepubertal children. Am J Respir Crit Care Med 2008;177:1142–9.

55. Amin R, Somers VK, McConnell K, et al. Activity-adjusted 24-hour ambulatory blood pressure and cardiac remodeling in children with sleep-disordered breathing. Hypertension 2008;51:84–91.

56. Tauman R, O'Brien LM, Ivanenko A, et al. Obesity rather than severity of sleep-disordered breathing as the major determinant of insulin resistance and altered lipidemia in snoring children. Pediatrics 2005;116:e66–73.

57. Kaditis AG, Alexopoulos EI, Damani E, et al. Urine levels of catecholamines in Greek children with obstructive sleep-disordered breathing. Pediatr Pulmonol 2009;44:38–45.

58. Chaicharn J, Lin Z, Chen ML, et al. Model-based assessment of cardiovascular autonomic control in children with obstructive sleep apnea. Sleep 2009;32:927–38.

59. Aljadeff G, Gozal D, Schechtman VL, et al. Heart rate variability in children with obstructive sleep apnea. Sleep 1997;20:151–7.

60. Enright PL, Goodwin JL, Sherrill DL, et al. Blood pressure elevation associated with sleep-related breathing disorder in a community sample of white and Hispanic children. The Tucson children's assessment of sleep apnea study. Arch Pediatr Adolesc Med 2003;157:901–4.

61. Guilleminault C, Khramstov A, Stoohs RA, et al. Abnormal blood pressure in prepubertal children with sleep-disordered breathing. Pediatr Res 2004;55:76–84.

62. Amin RS, Carroll JL, Jeffries JL, et al. Twenty-four-hour ambulatory blood pressure in children with sleep-disordered breathing. Am J Respir Crit Care Med 2004;169:950–6.

63. McConnell K, Somers VK, Kimball T, et al. Baroreflex gain in children with obstructive sleep apnea. Am J Respir Crit Care Med 2009;180:42–8.

64. Amin RS, Kimball TR, Bean JA, et al. Left ventricular hypertrophy and abnormal ventricular geometry in children and adolescents with obstructive sleep apnea. Am J Respir Crit Care Med 2002; 165(10):1395–9.

65. Amin RS, Kimball TR, Kalra M, et al. Left ventricular function in children with sleep-disordered breathing. Am J Cardiol 2005;95:801–4.

66. Tauman R, O'Brien LM, Gozal D. Hypoxemia and obesity modulate plasma C-reactive protein and interleukin-6 levels in sleep-disordered breathing. Sleep Breath 2008;11:77–84.

67. Tam CS, Wong M, McBain R, et al. Inflammatory measures in children with obstructive sleep apnoea. J Paediatr Child Health 2006; 42:277–82.

68. Gozal D, Serpero LD, Capdevila OS, et al. Systemic inflammation in non-obese children with obstructive sleep apnea. Sleep Med 2008;9: 254–9.

69. Kim J, Bhattacharjee R, Dayyat E, et al. Increased cellular proliferation and inflammatory cytokines in tonsils derived from children with obstructive sleep apnea. Pediatr Res 2009;66:423–8.

70. Li AM, Lam HS, Chan MH, et al. Inflammatory cytokines and childhood obstructive sleep apnea. Ann Acad Med Singapore 2008;37:649–54.

71. Kheirandish-Gozal L, Capdevila OS, Tauman R, et al. Plasma C-reactive protein in nonobese children with obstructive sleep apnea before and after adenotonsillectomy. J Clin Sleep Med 2006;15: 301–4.

72. Gozal D, Kheirandish-Gozal L, Serpero LD, et al. Obstructive sleep apnea and endothelial function in school-aged nonobese children. Circulation 2007;116:2307–14.

73. Carvalho LB, Prado LF, Silva L, et al. Cognitive dysfunction in children with sleep-disordered breathing. J Child Neurol 2005;20:400–4.

74. Rosen CL, Storfer-Isser A, Taylor JR, et al. Increased behavioral morbidity in schoolaged children with sleep-disordered breathing. Pediatrics 2004;114:1640–8.

75. Kennedy JD, Blunden S, Hirte C, et al. Reduced neurocognition in children who snore. Pediatr Pulmonol 2004;37(4):330–7.

76. Gottlieb DJ, Chase C, Vezina RM, et al. Sleep-disordered breathing symptoms are associated with poorer cognitive function in 5-year-old children. J Pediatr 2004;145:458–64.

77. Gottlieb DJ, Vezina RM, Chase C, et al. Symptoms of sleep-disordered breathing in 5-year-old children are associated with sleepiness and problem behaviors. Pediatrics 2003;112:870–7.

78. Gozal D. Sleep-disordered breathing and school performance in children. Pediatrics 1998;102: 616–20.

79. Urschitz MS, Wolff J, Sokollik C, et al. Nocturnal arterial oxygen saturation and academic performance in a community sample of children. Pediatrics 2005;115:e204–9.

80. Beebe DW, Wells CT, Jeffries J, et al. Neuropsychological effects of pediatric obstructive sleep apnea. J Int Neuropsychol Soc 2004;10:962–75.

81. Blunden S, Lushington K, Kennedy D, et al. Behavior and neurocognitive performance in children aged 5-10 years who snore compared to controls. J Clin Exp Neuropsychol 2000;22: 554–68.

82. Cortese S, Faraone SV, Konofal E, et al. Sleep in children with attention-deficit/hyperactivity disorder: meta-analysis of subjective and objective studies. J Am Acad Child Adolesc Psychiatry 2009; 48:894–908.

83. Dillon JE, Blunden S, Ruzicka DL, et al. DSM-IV diagnoses and obstructive sleep apnea in children before and 1 year after adenotonsillectomy. J Am Acad Child Adolesc Psychiatry 2007;46: 1425–36.

84. Chervin RD, Ruzicka DL, Giordani BJ, et al. Sleep-disordered breathing, behavior, and cognition in children before and after adenotonsillectomy. Pediatrics 2006;117:e769–78.

85. Wei JL, Bond J, Mayo MS, et al. Improved behavior and sleep after adenoidectomy in children with sleep-disordered breathing: long-term follow-up. Arch Otolaryngol Head Neck Surg 2009;135:642–6.

86. Montgomery-Downs HE, Crabtree VM, Gozal D. Cognition, sleep and respiration in at-risk children treated for obstructive sleep apnea. Eur Respir J 2005;25:216–7.

87. Friedman BC, Hendeles-Amitai A, Kozminsky E, et al. Adenotonsillectomy improves neurocognitive function in children with obstructive sleep apnea syndrome. Sleep 2003;15:999–1005.

88. Gozal D, Pope DW. Snoring during early childhood and academic performance at ages thirteen to fourteen years. Pediatrics 2001;107:1394–9.

89. Chervin RD, Weatherly RA, Ruzicka DL, et al. Subjective sleepiness and polysomnographic correlates in children scheduled for adenotonsillectomy vs. other surgical care. Sleep 2006;29: 495–503.

90. Kheirandish-Gozal L, Gozal D. The multiple challenges of obstructive sleep apnea in children: diagnosis. Curr Opin Pediatr 2008;20:650–3.

91. Goldbart AD, Goldman JL, Li RC, et al. Differential expression of cysteinyl leukotriene receptors 1 and 2 in tonsils of children with obstructive sleep apnea syndrome or recurrent infection. Chest 2004;12: 613–8.

92. Goldbart AD, Krishna J, Li RC, et al. Inflammatory mediators in exhaled condensate of children with obstructive sleep apnea syndrome. Chest 2006; 130:143–8.

93. Demain JG, Goetz DW. Pediatric adenoidal hypertrophy and nasal airway obstruction: reduction with aqueous nasal beclomethasone. Pediatrics 1995; 95:355–64.

94. Brouillette RT, Manoukian JJ, Ducharme FM, et al. Efficacy of fluticasone nasal spray for pediatric obstructive sleep apnea. J Pediatr 2001;138: 838–44.

95. Kheirandish-Gozal L, Gozal D. Intranasal budesonide treatment for children with mild obstructive sleep apnea syndrome. Pediatrics 2008;122: e149–55.

96. Alexopoulos EI, Kaditis AG, Kalampouka E, et al. Nasal corticosteroids for children with snoring. Pediatr Pulmonol 2004;38:161–7.

97. Criscuoli G, D'Amora S, Ripa G, et al. Frequency of surgery among children who have adenotonsillar hypertrophy and improve after treatment with nasal beclomethasone. Pediatrics 2003;111:e236–8.

98. Kheirandish L, Goldbart AD, Gozal D. Intranasal steroids and oral leukotriene modifier therapy in residual sleep-disordered breathing after tonsillectomy and adenoidectomy in children. Pediatrics 2006;117:e61–6.

99. Waters KA, Everett FM, Bruderer JW, et al. Obstructive sleep apnea: The use of nasal CPAP in 80 children. Am J Respir Crit Care Med 1995; 152:780–5.

100. Marcus C, Ward SL, Mallory GM, et al. Use of nasal continuous positive airway pressure as treatment of childhood obstructive sleep apnea. J Pediatr 2002; 127:88–94.

101. Downey R III, Perkin RM, MacQuarrie J. Nasal continuous positive airway pressure use in children with obstructive sleep apnea younger than 2 years of age. Chest 2000;117:1608–12.

102. Rains J. Treatment of obstructive sleep apnea in pediatric patients. Behavioral intervention for compliance with nasal continuous positive airway pressure. Clin Pediatr 1995;34:535–41.

103. Koontz KL, Slifer KJ, Cataldo MD, et al. Improving pediatric compliance with positive airway pressure therapy: the impact of behavioral intervention. Sleep 2003;26:1010–5.

104. Castorena-Maldonado A, Torre-Bouscoulet L, Meza-Vargas S, et al. Preoperative continuous positive airway pressure compliance in children with obstructive sleep apnea syndrome: assessed by a simplified approach. Int J Pediatr Otorhinolaryngol 2008;72:1795–800.

105. Marcus CL, Rosen G, Davidson-Ward SL, et al. Adherence to and effectiveness of positive airway pressure in children with obstructive sleep apnea. Pediatrics 2006;117:e442–51.

106. Marcus CL, Carroll JL, Bamford O, et al. Supplemental oxygen during sleep in children with sleep-disordered breathing. Am J Respir Crit Care Med 1995;152:1297–301.

107. Aljadeff G, Gozal D, Bailey-Wahl SL, et al. Effects of overnight supplemental oxygen in obstructive sleep apnea in children. Am J Respir Crit Care Med 1996;153:51–5.

108. Colen TY, Seidman C, Weedon J, et al. Effect of intracapsular tonsillectomy on quality of life for children with obstructive sleep-disordered breathing. Arch Otolaryngol Head Neck Surg 2008;134:124–7.

109. Nieminen P, Lopponen T, Tolonen U, et al. Growth and biochemical markers of growth in children with snoring and obstructive sleep apnea. Pediatrics 2002;109:e55–61.

110. Brietzke S, Kenna M, Katz ES, et al. Pediatric adenotonsillectomy: what is the effect of obstructive symptoms on the likelihood of future surgery? Int J Pediatr Otorhinolaryngol 2006;70:1467–72.

111. Cohen S, Simms C, Burstein F, et al. Alternatives to tracheostomy in infants and children with obstructive sleep apnea. J Pediatr Surg 1999; 34:182–7.

112. Friedman M, Wilson M, Lin HC, et al. Updated systemic review of tonsillectomy and adenoidectomy for treatment of pediatric obstructive sleep apnea/hypopnea syndrome. Otolaryngol Head Neck Surg 2009;140:800–8.

113. Tami TA, Parker GS, Taylor RE. Post-tonsillectomy bleeding: an evaluation of risk factors. Laryngoscope 1987;97:1307–11.

114. Wilkinson AR, McCormick MS, Freeland AP, et al. Electrocardiographic signs of pulmonary hypertension in children who snore. BMJ 1981;282: 1579–81.

115. Yates DW. Adenotonsillar hypertrophy and cor pulmonale. Br J Anaesth 1988;61:355–9.

116. Nixon GM, Kermack AS, McGreagor CD, et al. Sleep and breathing on the first night after adenotonsillectomy for obstructive sleep apnea. Pediatr Pulmonol 2005;39:332–8.

117. Helfaer MA, McColley SA, Pyzik PL, et al. Polysomnography after adenotonsillectomy in mild pediatric obstructive sleep apnea. Crit Care Med 1996;24:1323–7.

118. Rosen GM, Muckle RP, Abboud FM, et al. Postoperative respiratory compromise in children with obstructive sleep apnea syndrome: can it be anticipated? Pediatrics 1994;93:784–8.

119. Ruboyianes JM, Cruz RM. Pediatric adenotonsil-lectomy for obstructive sleep apnea. Ear Nose Throat J 1996;75:430–3.

120. Pirelli P, Saponara M, Guilleminault C. Rapid maxil-lary expansion in children with obstructive sleep apnea syndrome. Sleep 2004;27:761–6.

121. Pirelli P, Saponara M, Attanasio G. Obstructive sleep apnoea syndrome (OSAS) and rhino-tubaric dysfunction in children: therapeutic effects of RME therapy. Prog Orthod 2005;6:48–61.

122. Villa MP, Malagola C, Pagani J, et al. Rapid maxil-lary expansion in children with obstructive sleep apnea syndrome: 12-month follow-up. Sleep Med 2007;8:128–34.

123. Villa MP, Bernkopf E, Pagani J, et al. Randomized controlled study of an oral jaw-positioning appli-ance for the treatment of obstructive sleep apnea in children with malocclusion. Am J Respir Crit Care Med 2002;165:123–7.

124. Cozza P, Gatto R, Ballanti F, et al. Management of obstructive sleep apnoea in children with modified monobloc appliances. Eur J Pediatr Dent 2004;5: 24–9.

125. Goh DY, Galster P, Marcus CL. Sleep architecture and respiratory disturbances in children with obstructive sleep apnea. Am J Respir Crit Care Med 2000;162:682–6.

126. Marcus CL, Omlin KJ, Basinski DJ, et al. Normal polysomnographic values for children and adoles-cents. Am Rev Respir Dis 1992;146:1235–9.

127. Witmans MB, Keens TG, Ward SLD, et al. Obstruc-tive hypopneas in children and adolescents: normal values. Am J Respir Crit Care Med 2003; 168:1540.

128. Traeger N, Schultz B, Pollock AN, et al. Polysomno-graphic values in children 2-9 years old: additional data and review of the literature. Pediatr Pulmonol 2005;40:22–30.

Central Sleep Apnea

S. Javaheri, MD[a,b,*]

KEYWORDS

• Central sleep apnea • Mechanisms • Causes • Prevalence

Central apnea is caused by temporary failure in the pontomedullary pacemaker generating breathing rhythm. This results in the loss of ventilatory effort, and if it lasts 10 seconds or more it is defined as central apnea. During central apnea, there is no brainstem inspiratory neural output and the nerves innervating the inspiratory thoracic pump muscles are silent. Therefore, on the polysomnogram, central apnea is characterized by the absence of naso-oral airflow and thoracoabdominal excursions.

Central apnea as a polysomnographic finding could be either physiologic (normal) or have one of many pathologic causes (**Box 1**). The author and others have used a central apnea index (CAI) greater than or equal to 5 per hour of sleep as abnormal. However, the minimum number of events (apneas and hypopneas) required during sleep to represent a distinct disorder or syndrome (a condition associated with consequences; eg, insomnia, excessive daytime sleepiness, impaired quality of life, morbidity or mortality) is not known. The issue of a clinically significant threshold of central disordered breathing events is compounded by lack of inclusion of the number of hypopneas in the index (in contrast to the use of the obstructive apnea-hypopnea index [AHI], which is used to define the threshold), in part because of the difficulty in accurately distinguishing central hypopneas and obstructive hypopneas. In addition, the presence of central and obstructive apneas and hypopneas (mixed pattern of breathing) in the polysomnogram complicates accurate scoring. Examples of this mixed pattern of breathing include neuromuscular disorders,

systolic heart failure, and opioid-associated sleep apnea. For these reasons, in patients with systolic heart failure, the author has used arbitrary polysomnographic criteria[1–3] to classify disordered breathing into either predominant central or obstructive sleep apnea. However, what the minimum central AHI should be to define the presence of a clinically significant sleep-related breathing disorder is not clear. In our studies of patients with heart failure, an AHI of 15 per hour or greater has been used arbitrarily, but this does not mean that it is the appropriate threshold. Further studies using outcomes are necessary to answer this question.

Box 1 shows the various physiologic and pathologic conditions associated with central sleep apnea.[4] The classification is in part based on the mechanisms and in part on the pathologic disorders associated with central sleep apnea. There is considerable overlap in disorders in which the pathologic process is diffuse, involving multiple sites. The mechanisms generating central sleep apnea are known in some but not all the disorders listed.

THE MECHANISMS OF GENESIS OF CENTRAL APNEA DURING SLEEP: THE APNEIC THRESHOLD AND DIMINISHED P_{CO_2} RESERVE

The mechanisms involved in the genesis of central apnea in sleep primarily relate to the removal of wakefulness drive to breathe and unmasking of a P_{CO_2}-sensitive apneic threshold,[5–8] a P_{CO_2} level below which rhythmical breathing ceases resulting in central apnea. Normally at onset sleep,

[a] Department of Medicine, University of Cincinnati College of Medicine, 4780 Socialville Fosters Road, Mason, OH 45040, USA
[b] Sleepcare Diagnostics, 4780 Socialville Fosters Road, Mason, OH 45040, USA
* Department of Medicine, University of Cincinnati College of Medicine, 4780 Socialville Fosters Road, Mason, OH 45040.
E-mail address: Javaheri@snorenomore.com

Clin Chest Med 31 (2010) 235–248
doi:10.1016/j.ccm.2010.02.013
0272-5231/10/$ – see front matter © 2010 Elsevier Inc. All rights reserved.

chestmed.theclinics.com

Box 1
Central sleep apnea

I. Physiologic CSA

    1. Sleep onset
    2. Postarousal/postsigh
    3. Phasic REM sleep

II. Hypopcapnic (nonhypercapnic) CSA[a]

    1. Systolic heart failure
    2. Idiopathic
    3. Idiopathic pulmonary arterial hypertension
    4. High altitude
    5. Poststroke

III. Hypercapnic CSA[a]

    1. Alveolar hypoventilation with normal pulmonary function

       a. Congenital central hypoventilation syndrome
       b. Primary chronic alveolar hypoventilation syndrome

    2. Brainstem and spinal cord disorders encephalitis; tumors; infarcts; cervical cordotomy; anterior cervical spinal artery syndrome; neurodegenerative disorders; amyotrophic lateral sclerosis; multiple sclerosis; Chiari malformation
    3. Muscular disorders; myotonic and Duchenne dystrophies; acid maltase deficiency; Guillain-Barré syndrome
    4. Opioids

IV. CSA with endocrine disorders

    1. Acromegaly
    2. Hypothyrodism

V. CSA with OSA

    1. A minor component of OSA
    2. With CPAP therapy (complex sleep apnea)
    3. Posttracheotomy

VI. CSA with upper airway disorders

Abbreviations: CPAP, continuous positive airway pressure; CSA, central sleep apnea; OSA, obstructive sleep apnea; REM, rapid eye movement.
  [a] Pco_2, however, may be normal at times.
Data from Javaheri S. Central sleep apnea. In: Lee-Chiong T, editor. Sleep medicine essentials. Hoboken (NJ): Wiley-Blackwell; 2009. p. 81–9.

---

ventilation decreases and Pco_2 increase by few a millimeters of mercury.

With removal of wakefulness drive to breathe, breathing during sleep is dominated by the metabolic control system, which is sensitive to small changes in Pco_2. As long as the level of the prevailing Pco_2, referred to as the eupneic Pco_2, is more than the apneic Pco_2, rhythmical breathing is maintained. However, if eupneic Pco_2 decreases below the apneic threshold Pco_2, for example, after an arousal-related hyperventilation, breathing ceases. As a result of central apnea, Pco_2 increases and after it exceeds the apneic threshold Pco_2, breathing resumes.

The difference between 2 Pco_2 set points, the eupneic Pco_2 minus the Pco_2 at the apneic threshold, referred to as the Pco_2 reserve, is a critical factor for development of central apnea. The less the Pco_2 reserve, the greater the likelihood of occurrence of central apnea. This is because small increases in ventilation could lower the eupneic Pco_2 to less than the apneic threshold. On the contrary, when apneic threshold Pco_2 is far away from the eucapnic Pco_2, large ventilatory changes are necessary to lower the Pco_2 below the apneic threshold Pco_2 and therefore the likelihood of developing central apnea decreases.

CAUSES OF CENTRAL SLEEP APNEA

In this article, only selective causes of central sleep apnea are reviewed in detail (see **Box 1**). For other disorders, please see Ref.[4]

Physiologic Central Apnea

The conditions causing or associated with central sleep apnea in this category are considered normal sleep phenomena and, not surprisingly, the frequency of occurrence of such central apneas is normally minimal. Such central apneas are observed with onset of sleep, after an arousal or a sigh and occasionally during phasic rapid eye movement (REM) sleep.[9]

Eucapnic-hypocapnic (Nonhypercapnic) Central Sleep Apnea

These disorders are characterized by (1) an awake steady-state $Paco_2$ which is either within the low range of or less than the normal value (<36 mm Hg at sea level), and (2) increased ventilatory response to changes in Pco_2 and perhaps also to Po_2.

During sleep, the prevailing Pco_2 may decrease to less than the apneic threshold (resulting in a central apnea), either because of inability to increase the Pco_2 or because the apneic threshold Pco_2 increases (eg, as a result of hypoxemia), or a combination of the 2. In addition, in these disorders (see **Box 1**), the hypercapnic ventilatory response is invariably increased above and below eupnoea. The increase in ventilatory response above eupnoea increases the likelihood of developing central apnea because any time an arousal occurs, the immediate prearousal sleeping P_{CO_2} becomes hypercapnic for the aroused brain, and therefore, intense hyperventilation occurs that could drive the prevailing P_{CO_2} below the apneic threshold, causing a central apnea as sleep is resumed. Following central apnea, P_{CO_2} increases until an arousal recurs. In this way, the cycle of apnea-hyperpnea is perpetuated. The increase in CO_2 chemosensitivity below eupnoea is critical and has been best studied in systolic heart failure and during hypoxemia to explain the mechanism of high-altitude periodic breathing.

Systolic heart failure

Heart failure is a highly prevalent syndrome; it is estimated that about 5 to 6 million Americans, about 2% of the population, and 10% of those more than 65 years of age have heart failure. The approximate annual incidence is half a million.[10] Because heart failure is highly prevalent and central sleep apnea is common in the setting of the failing heart, heart failure is the most common cause of central sleep apnea in the general population (see later).

There is a distinct pattern of periodic breathing in systolic heart failure in that the breathing cycle has long crescendo decrescendo arms, as a result of a long arterial circulation time, a pathophysiologic feature of systolic heart failure. This pattern of periodic breathing is referred to as Hunter-Cheyne-Stokes breathing. John Hunter, a British surgeon, described it 37 years before John Cheyne's description.[11–14]

Prevalence of central apnea in systolic heart failure Studies[1–3,15–26] of patients with stable heart failure and left ventricular systolic dysfunction show that 40% to 80% have an AHI of 15 per hour or more. These indices include central and obstructive sleep apnea, events that commonly occur together during sleep in a patient with heart failure.

The largest and most systematic study[17] involved 100 ambulatory male patients with stable, treated heart failure. In this study, 114 consecutive eligible patients who were followed in a cardiology and a primary care clinic were asked to participate (88% recruitment) without regard to any symptom of sleep apnea. Using an AHI of 15 per hour or greater as the threshold, 49 patients (49% of all patients) had moderate to severe sleep apnea-hypopnea with an average index of 44 per hour. This index included central and obstructive events. In our studies about 10% of the patients were on β-blockers; however, the results of recent studies[23–26] that used an AHI of 15/h or more as the threshold are consistent with our report showing a high prevalence of sleep apnea, both central sleep apnea and obstructive sleep apnea despite use of β-blockers (up to 80% of the patients were on a β-blocker). Combining the results of these recent series[23–26] and our study[17] and using an AHI of 15/h of sleep as the threshold, there are 1250 consecutive patients with systolic heart failure, of which 52% have moderate to severe sleep apnea, 31% have central sleep apnea, and 21% have obstructive sleep apnea (**Fig 1**).

Mechanisms of central sleep apnea and periodic breathing in heart failure For simplicity, I make a distinction between mechanisms of central sleep apnea in heart failure (which have to do with increased CO_2 chemosensitivity below eupnoea, the P_{CO_2} reserve, and the lack of increase in P_{CO_2} with sleep onset) and the mechanisms mediating periodic breathing (which have to do with pathologic processes of heart failure).

Lack of increase in P_{CO_2} at sleep onset in systolic heart failure Normally, with onset of sleep, ventilation decreases and P_{CO_2} increases. This maintains the prevailing P_{CO_2} above the apneic threshold P_{CO_2}, and rhythmical breathing occurs. However, in some patients with heart failure, the prevailing awake P_{CO_2} does not increase at sleep onset.[27,28] This sets the stage for developing central apnea because of the proximity of the prevailing P_{CO_2} to the exposed apneic threshold.[8,27] The reason for the lack of increase in P_{CO_2} could be because of the lack of decrease in ventilation that normally occurs at sleep onset. Presumably, in patients with heart failure with severe left ventricular diastolic dysfunction (and stiff left ventricle which invariably accompanies systolic dysfunction), when in supine position venous return increases and pulmonary capillary pressure could increase. This results in a small increase in respiratory rate and ventilation, preventing the increase in P_{CO_2} normally observed.

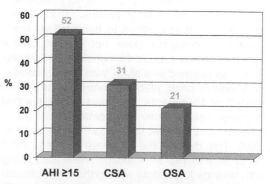

Fig. 1. Worldwide prevalence of sleep apnea in systolic heart failure (n = 1250 consecutive patients).

Increased CO_2 chemosensitivity below eupnea Several studies[29–31] have shown that patients with heart failure and low awake steady-state arterial Pco_2 have a high probability of developing central sleep apnea during sleep. It has been misinterpreted that it is this low awake Pco_2 that predisposes patients to central sleep apnea. In contrast, in the absence of an increase in CO_2 chemosensitivity below eupnoea, low awake Pco_2 per se should be protective in the sense that it decreases the likelihood of developing central apnea during sleep.

Why in the absence of increased CO_2 chemosensitivity below eupnoea, is low awake arterial Pco_2 per se protective? With nonhypoxic chemoreceptor stimulation such as metabolic acidosis or administration of almitrine (which stimulates carotid bodies), ventilation increases and Pco_2 decreases, without changing the chemosensitivity below eupnoea.[8] Under such conditions, the hyperbolic nature of the alveolar ventilation curve dictates a considerable increase in ventilation to decrease an already low Pco_2 below the apneic threshold Pco_2. This is referred to as decreased plant gain (which is dictated by where $Paco_2$ resides on the alveolar ventilation equation curve) with an increase in $\triangle Pco_2$ making development of central sleep apnea less probable.

In 1 study,[32] polysomnograms of 13 hypocapnic ($Paco_2$ <36 mm Hg, mean = 33 mm Hg) patients with heart failure, mean left ventricular ejection fraction of 23% were compared with those of 10 age-, gender-, and $Paco_2$-matched hypocapnic ($Paco_2$ <36 mm Hg, mean = 32 mm Hg) patients with cirrhosis of the liver and normal ejection fraction (60%). In the former group, the mean apnea-hypopnea index was 28/h and central sleep apnea accounted for most of the breathing disorders; in the goup with cirrhosis, the mean AHI was 2/h and maximum CAI was 0.2/h. There were no significant differences in age, demographics, pulmonary function tests, Pao_2, $Paco_2$, minute and alveolar ventilation, and ventilatory responses to CO_2 between the 2 groups. The authors concluded that in contrast to heart failure, presence of hypocapnia does not predict central apnea in cirrhosis. A similar conclusion regarding Pco_2 was reached in a study with acetazolamide. In a double-blind placebo-controlled crossover study[33] of 12 patients with heart failure, the CAI decreased significantly with acetazolamide (49 ± 28 vs 23 ± 21, mean ± standard deviation, P = .004). This despite the decrease in $Paco_2$, from 38 to 34 mm Hg, P = .0003. These data along with findings in patients with cirrhosis emphasize that it is not the absolute value of the steady state that increases the likelihood of developing central

apnea. Rather, it is the difference between the prevailing Pco_2 and the apneic threshold Pco_2 that is important.[8,27] As noted earlier, in the face of background increased stimulus to breathing, the difference between the prevailing Pco_2 minus apneic threshold Pco_2 widens.[8] This widening decreases the likelihood of developing central sleep apnea.

Then why in systolic heart failure is a low awake steady-state $Paco_2$ highly predictive for the development of central sleep apnea? In systolic heart failure, the low $Paco_2$ has to do with the severity of the ventricular diastolic dysfunction. Heart failure patients with hypocapnia have a more severe left ventricular diastolic dysfunction and a higher wedge pressure than patients with eucapnia patients.[19] Wedge pressure further increases in the supine position with the increase in venous return, stimulating J receptors. Consequently, such patients are not able to appropriately decrease their ventilation with sleep onset and their Pco_2 remains close to the apneic threshold.

Furthermore, via mechanisms yet to be discovered, pulmonary congestion increases the CO_2 chemosensitivity below eupnea and decreases the Pco_2 reserve increasing the likelihood of developing central sleep apnea.[34]

Although a low awake $Paco_2$ is highly predictive of central sleep apnea, it is not a prerequisite. Many patients with heart failure and central sleep apnea have normal awake $Paco_2$.[15,35] What is important is the proximity of the apneic threshold to the $Paco_2$.[8,27]

Another mechanism that increases the likelihood of developing central apnea during sleep and periodic breathing is enhanced ventilatory response to CO_2[36] which is discussed later.

Mechanisms of periodic breathing in systolic heart failure In systolic heart failure, central sleep apnea occurs in the background of periodic breathing characterized by long cresendo-decresendo ventilation arms, a reflection of prolonged circulation time. Increased arterial circulation time (which delays the transfer of information regarding changes in pulmonary capillary blood Po_2 and Pco_2 to the chemoreceptors), enhanced gain of the chemoreceptors (enhanced CO_2/O_2 chemosensitivity), and enhanced plant gain (a large change in $Paco_2$ for a small change in ventilation) collectively increase the likelihood of periodic breathing.[36–46]

In systolic heart failure, effective arterial circulation time is increased (as a result of pulmonary congestion, left atrial and ventricular enlargement, and diminished stroke volume); plant gain is also increased because of a low functional residual capacity (as a result of the presence of pleural effusion, cardiomegaly, pulmonary congestion, or edema). In some patients hypercapnic ventilatory response is increased[36] and the chemoreceptors elicit a large ventilatory response whenever the partial pressure of carbon dioxide increases. The consequent intense hyperventilation, by driving the P_{CO_2} below the apneic threshold, results in central apnea. As a result of central apnea, P_{CO_2} increases and the cycles of hyperventilation and hypoventilation are maintained.

Because the aforementioned alterations are not sleep/wake specific, periodic breathing may occur during both states, although most frequently during sleep. During sleep, cardiac output decreases (further prolonging arterial circulation time), and functional residual capacity (supine position) and metabolic rate decrease enhancing the plant gain.

Treatment of central sleep apnea in heart failure is reviewed elsewhere[1–3,47–56] and is not discussed in this article.

Idiopathic central sleep apnea

This is a rare disorder[57,58] and a diagnosis of exclusion; other causes of central apnea noted in **Box 1**, including asymptomatic left ventricular dysfunction and multiple small infarcts that otherwise may be silent, should be excluded.

On the polysomnograph, idiopathic central sleep apnea is characterized by repetitive episodes of central apnea. However, the cycles of periodic breathing are shorter than those in systolic heart failure. Patients with idiopathic central sleep apnea are commonly older men, and may present with complaints of restless sleep, insomnia, and/or daytime symptoms such as sleepiness and fatigue related to insomnia, sleep fragmentation, and arousals.

Idiopathic central apnea in patients with idiopathic central apnea commonly have a low arterial P_{CO_2}, and increased hypercapnic ventilatory response[58,59] during wakefulness, which facilitates development of central apnea during sleep.

Although there are no randomized therapeutic trials, 2 nonrandomized open studies[59,60] have shown efficacy of acetazolamide in the treatment of idiopathic central sleep apnea. These results are consistent with the results of the double-blind placebo-controlled study on systolic heart failure showing the efficacy of acetazolamide in the treatment of central sleep apnea.[33]

Bilevel positive airway pressure devices are not recommended for treatment of central sleep apnea of any cause because by lowering the prevailing P_{CO_2} below the apneic threshold these devices could worsen central apnea.[61] New generation servo ventilators, however, should be effective.

Idiopathic pulmonary arterial hypertension

This disorder is characterized by pulmonary arterial hypertension with normal pulmonary capillary pressure. Genetic associations have been found.[62]

In the more advanced hemodynamic state of this disorder, there is severe pulmonary arterial hypertension, right ventricular failure, and diminished cardiac output. In 1 study[63] of 20 patients with idiopathic pulmonary artery hypertension (3 men and 17 women), 6 had moderately severe sleep apnea with an AHI of 37/h resulting in desaturation. The mean Pa_{CO_2} did not significantly differ between the 2 groups, but patients with periodic breathing had significantly more hemodynamic abnormalities than those without. Presumably, diminished stroke volume and increased arterial circulation time were the underlying mechanisms in mediating periodic breathing in this disorder.

In the study of Schultz and colleagues,[63] 3 out of the 3 men, but only 3 of 17 women had periodic breathing. This gender distribution is similar to that in systolic heart failure, and may have to do with gender differences in apneic threshold P_{CO_2}.[64,65]

For the treatment of central sleep apnea in idiopathic pulmonary arterial hypertension, the author recommends nocturnal supplemental nasal oxygen.[63] In 1 patient with idiopathic pulmonary hypertension, hypocapnia, and low cardiac output, central sleep apnea was eliminated after lung transplantation.[66] In another case report[67] use of bilevel positive airway pressure therapy was associated with death, although cause and effect cannot be proved, several possibilities including worsening of central sleep apnea and reduction in cardiac output with use of a bilevel device may be speculated. In general, the author does not recommend use of bilevel device to treat central sleep apnea.[68]

However, obstructive sleep apnea is a known cause of secondary pulmonary hypertension (for review see Ref.[69]). Therefore, in patients with pulmonary arterial hypertension, obstructive sleep apnea should be ruled out by polysomnography. If obstructive sleep apnea is present, use of a continuous positive airway pressure (CPAP) device is the treatment of choice. Pulmonary arterial hypertension may improve with effective treatment of obstructive sleep apnea with CPAP.[69]

High altitude

Periodic breathing commonly occurs at high altitude.[70] The cycle of periodic breathing is short in contrast to the long cycle of periodic breathing in heart failure.

The underlying mechanism of high-altitude periodic breathing is hypoxemia, which narrows the difference between eupneic Pco_2 minus apneic threshold Pco_2, and increases hypocapnic chemosensitivity below the apneic threshold.[8] Furthermore, the quantity of periodic breathing during sleep at high altitude tends to be more in individuals with enhanced ventilatory response to hypercapnia and hypoxia.[71] The relation with hypercapnic ventilatory response resembles that reported in patients with heart failure.[36]

Inhalation of supplemental oxygen or a small amount of CO_2 decreases periodic breathing. Furthermore, administration of acetazolamide improves desaturation and ameliorates the symptoms of acute mountain sickness in man at high altitude.[72,73] As discussed earlier, acetazolamide[8] widens the difference between the 2 Pco_2 set points (in contrast to hypoxemia) resulting in improvement of periodic breathing at high altitude.

Poststroke

Several studies[74–82] have shown that patients with stroke (acute, chronic, ischemic, nonischemic) have obstructive and central sleep apnea. Although obstructive sleep apnea could either precede (cause or contribute to the development of) or be caused by stroke, central apneas are most probably caused by the stroke and may decrease with time.[79]

A pattern of breathing similar to Hunter-Cheyne-Stokes breathing has also been reported in patients with stroke.[80–83] This pattern of breathing seems to have no relation to the site of pathology. Systolic heart failure should be considered in such patients.

Hypercapnic Central Sleep Apnea

These heterogeneous disorders are characterized by daytime steady-state hypercapnia or a Pco_2 level close to the upper normal limit. According to the alveolar ventilation equation, $Paco_2$ is directly proportional to CO_2 production and inversely proportional to alveolar ventilation. In these disorders, the increase in $Paco_2$ is caused by decreased global ventilation, and therefore the term hypoventilation is appropriate.[4] However, hypoventilation and hypercapnia become profound during sleep. Normally with the removal of the wakefulness drive to breathe, ventilation decreases with sleep onset and Pco_2 rises slightly. However, such a small physiologic decrease in ventilation results in a large increase in Pco_2, if hypercapnia is already present; this is dictated by the alveolar ventilation equation and has to do with the hyperbolic relation of Pco_2 with alveolar ventilation.[4] Furthermore, in the presence of hypercapnia, if an arousal occurs, because

of return of the wakefulness drive to breathe, ventilation increases somewhat but Pco_2 decreases considerably (this is referred to as increased plant gain). The increased plant gain increases the probability of developing central apnea if the apneic threshold Pco_2 is also increased.[84]

Another pathophysiologic consequence of sleep-induced hypercapnia is the development of severe desaturation. When Pco_2 rises considerably, severe hypoxemia ensues, given the reciprocal relation between alveolar Pco_2 and Po_2.

In some of the disorders in this category, the pathologic process involves brainstem medullary respiratory centers responsible for automatic breathing (either for anatomic or functional reasons, eg, use of opioids). Consequently, when the wakefulness drive to breathe is absent, central apneas occur during sleep.

REM sleep may be associated with central sleep apnea in neuromuscular disorders involving the diaphragm. During REM sleep, there is costal muscle atonia and the diaphragm is the only inspiratory thoracic pump muscle active. Therefore, with diaphragmatic weakness or paralysis, during REM sleep, airflow ceases, and thoracoabdominal tracings look like central apnea. This is a pseudo central apnea and may occur in a variety of disorders associated with diaphragmatic paralysis.

Alveolar hypoventilation syndromes with normal pulmonary function

These central nervous system disorders are characterized by chronic alveolar hypoventilation with daytime hypercapnia, diminished or absent CO_2 chemosensitivity, and normal pulmonary function.

These disorders could be either genetic (congenital central hypoventilation syndrome and perhaps primary hypoventilation syndrome) or acquired (a variety of brainstem and spinal cord disorders). The unique feature of all of these disorders, however, is the failure of automatic/metabolic control of breathing that becomes manifest during sleep (Ondine curse) when breathing is controlled by the automatic/metabolic pathway. If this pathway is defective, ventilation decreases dramatically and hypoventilation and central apneas could occur.

Congenital central hypoventilation syndrome Congenital central hypoventilation syndrome (CCHS), a rare genetic disorder,[85–94] has gained considerable attention because of the recent discovery of its genetic basis.[89–92] The disorder is associated with other neurocristopathies such as Hirschsprung disease, which is caused by segmental colonic aganglionosis. The disorder manifests itself after birth.

Primary (idiopathic) alveolar hypoventilation syndrome Primary (idiopathic) alveolar hypoventilation syndrome is usually a disorder of adult men diagnosed in the third or fourth decade. This disorder is characterized by chronic hypercapnia without any demonstrable neuromuscular, thoracic, pulmonary, or central nervous system pathology. The mechanisms leading to chronic hypercapnia in primary alveolar hypoventilation syndrome are not understood and they could have a genetic basis, similar to CCHS.

There are several therapeutic options for the treatment of CCHS and idiopathic chronic alveolar hypoventilation syndrome. These include nocturnal oxygen therapy, diaphragmatic pacing and mechanical ventilation by mask, via tracheotomy, or by negative pressure ventilation.[86,95–106] Respiratory stimulants are generally ineffective.[107]

Oxygen therapy may further increase P_{CO_2}, diaphragmatic pacing or negative pressure ventilation may unmask or result in upper airway occlusion during sleep necessitating tracheotomy. However, a positive airway pressure device should be the first choice. Although no trials have been performed, the new generation noninvasive adaptive servoventilation devices should be effective in treating hypoventilation and central sleep apneas.

Brainstem and spinal cord disorders

Brainstem and spinal cord disorders constitute several heterogeneous pathologic processes that could result in severe hypoventilation and central apnea during sleep. With regard to brain stem pathology, this is not surprising, because central chemoreceptors and respiratory centers are located in this region. Various pathologic processes such as compression, edema, ischemia, infarct, tumor, encephalitis, neurodegenerative disorders and Chiari malformation have been associated with central sleep apnea.[108–115]

Cervical cordotomy[116] and anterior cervical spinal artery syndrome[117] result in automatic failure of breathing. In these 2 conditions, the process involves the descending pathways subservient to the automatic control of breathing with preservation of the voluntary pathway. Therefore, during sleep when the wakefulness drive to breathe ceases, hypoventilation and central apnea occur (Ondine curse). This phenomenon is in a way similar to CCHS.

For treatment of central apneas and hypoventilation in this category, therapy should be individualized. Several modalities including bilevel ventilation

in time mode, tracheostomy with mechanical ventilation, or diaphragm pacing could be used.

Neuromuscular disorders

This category (see **Box 1**) includes a large number of neuromuscular disorders that may affect respiratory muscles (muscular dystrophies such as myotonic dystrophy, idiopathic diaphragmatic paralysis), the neuromuscular junction (myasthenia gravis), and phrenic and intercostal nerves (amyotrophic lateral sclerosis).[118]

Depending on the site of pathology, a specific pathophysiologic breathing disorder could occur during sleep. With diaphragmatic involvement, however, breathing is particularly compromised in REM sleep when hypoventilation and what appears to be a central apnea on a polysomnograph (discussed earlier) may occur. In disorders that involve the pharyngeal muscles, obstructive apneas and hypopneas may occur during sleep.

In neuromuscular disorders, as respiratory muscle weakness progresses and daytime hypercapnia develops, sleep-related breathing disorders present with more severe hypoventilation hypercapnia, more severe desaturation, and perhaps more central apneas. These phenomena have to do with where P_{CO_2} resides on the hyperbolic curve of the alveolar ventilation equation discussed earlier.

Treatment of sleep-related breathing disorders in neuromuscular diseases should be individualized.[118–122] Two important factors determining the modality of therapy include the presence of impaired rhythmogenesis and upper airway obstruction during sleep. Use of bilevel ventilation could be extremely helpful for patients with hypercapnia if the brainstem is not involved. If rhythmogenesis is impaired and upper airway obstruction is present during sleep, tracheostomy with assisted ventilation may become necessary. However, bilevel ventilation with back up rate and new generation pressure support servoventilators should be extremely effective.

Opioids

Ventilatory depression during wakefulness is a well-known effect of opioid drugs. However, with chronic use, daytime hypoventilation is generally mild, but sleep apnea is quite prevalent.[123–127] In a case-control study[125] of 60 patients taking opioids for pain management, matched for age, gender, and body mass with 60 patients not taking opioids, the former group had a significantly higher AHI than the control group, primarily because of an increase in the number of central apneas. In a large study of patients in a pain clinic, Webster and associates[126] routinely recommended polysomnography to 392 consecutive subjects. Of the 140 subjects who underwent polysomnography in their institution, 75% had an AHI of 5/h or more, 50% had an AHI of 15/h or more, and 36% had severe sleep apnea with an AHI of 30/h or more. Opioids use is associated with a mixed pattern of sleep-disordered breathing (presence of central and obstructive events) although central apneas commonly predominate.

In the last few years, there has been a dramatic change in the management of chronic pain associated with a marked acceleration in the use of opioids. Given the high prevalence of sleep apnea in this population, a large number may suffer from significant unrecognized sleep apnea. Sleep apnea probably contributes to excess unexplained mortality associated with the use of opioids as many are discovered dead in the morning or in bed during the day.

The mechanisms of opioid-induced sleep apnea are best explained by the model of 2 respiratory rhythm generators that are anatomically distinct but coupled.[127] The inspiratory rhythm generator is located in the pre-Botzinger complex, whereas the expiratory rhythm generator is located in the retrotrapezoid nucleus/parafacial respiratory group. In this model, the pre-Botzinger complex neurons are inhibited by opioids but the expiratory motor neurons remain unaffected. Opioids inhibit discharge of inspiratory neurons in the pre-Botzinger complex, resulting in central apneas. In these experiments, genioglossus muscle activity also decreased consistent with the observation that opioids can cause obstructive sleep-disordered breathing events.

Treatment of opioid-induced sleep apnea is difficult because of the simultaneous presence of obstructive sleep apnea and central sleep apnea, with the latter being resistant to CPAP.[128] A preliminary study[129] showed that a new generation pressure support servoventilator could be promising.

Central Sleep Apnea in Endocrine Disorders

Central sleep apnea has been observed in 2 endocrine disorders: acromegaly and hypothyroidism. In both disorders, obstructive sleep apnea is the predominant form.

Acromegaly
Several studies have reported a relatively high prevalence of sleep apnea in patients with acromegaly.[130–132] Obstructive and central sleep apneas occur. Excess pharyngeal soft tissue (caused by cellular hyperplasia, excess connective tissue, and extracellular water) and macroglossia could account for obstructive sleep apnea, which may contribute to the high prevalence and progression of cardiovascular disease of acromegaly.[132]

Obstructive sleep apnea should be treated with CPAP, although treatment with octreotide (a somatastatin analogue) could result in tissue regression and improvement in sleep apnea.[130,133,134] However, this may take several months, and sleep apnea may persist in spite of therapy for acromegaly.

Studies have shown that patients with acromegaly also suffer from central sleep apnea, and this correlated with the levels of human growth hormone, insulinlike growth factor 1, and hypercapnic ventilatory response.[130,133,135] The enhanced ventilatory response could increase the likelihood of developing central sleep apnea. Treatment with octreotide also improved central sleep apnea.[133]

Hypothyroidism
Similar to acromegaly, obstructive and central sleep apneas occur in patients with hypothyroidism, although central sleep apnea is much less frequent than obstructive apneas.[136,137] The mechanisms of central sleep apnea are not understood, but excess pharyngeal soft tissue, similar to acromegaly could account for obstructive sleep apnea.

Central Sleep Apnea with Obstructive Sleep Apnea

Few central apneas are observed in polysomnograms of patients with obstructive sleep apnea and are appropriately ignored because they are of no clinical significance. However, some patients referred for evaluation of obstructive sleep apnea may have excess central apneas or develop central sleep apnea during initiation of CPAP therapy. These include patients with severe obstructive sleep apnea, those with systolic heart failure, atrial fibrillation, neuromuscular disorders, or on opioids.

The presence of central sleep apnea (CAI ≥ 5/h) on CPAP could therefore be emergent (ie, not present on a diagnostic polysomnograph) or considered persistent (central sleep apnea is present on a diagnostic polysomnograph). Such patients commonly continue to have obstructive and central sleep apnea on CPAP and this has been referred to as complex sleep apnea with an estimated prevalence of 5% to 20%[129,138–140]; most recent studies[129,141,142] show a prevalence of about 5% to 6%.

In our study,[129] which included 1286 patients referred for evaluation of obstructive sleep apnea, the monthly incidence of central sleep apnea during initial CPAP titration (CPAP1) varied from 3% to 10% during a 1-year period, with an average of 6.5%. An important part of this study has to do with determination of the natural history of central sleep apnea on CPAP. Of the 42 patients who developed CPAP1, central sleep apnea was eliminated in most of them with long-term use of CPAP (average time/night = 5.6 hours). However, 9 of the 42 patients (an estimated 1.5% of 1286 patients with obstructive sleep apnea) had persistent central sleep apnea with long-term use of CPAP. This observation is consistent with the results of 2 long-term studies[143,144] with tracheotomy. Guilleminault and colleagues[143] noted that patients with obstructive sleep apnea who underwent tracheostomy initially had central sleep apnea. However, a repeat polysomnograph after a period of time showed the number of central apneas had decreased. Coccagna and colleagues[144] reported a similar observation. In the study of Dernaika and colleagues[139] most of the central sleep apneas resolved in 12 of the 14 patients with CPAP1 who had a repeat titration polysomnogram 9 weeks after their initial polysomnogram, resulting in a prevalence of CPAP-persistent central sleep apnea of about 1.5%, the prevalence observed in our study.[129]

Central Sleep Apnea with Upper Airway Disorders

The nose, larynx, and pharynx are replete with receptors[145,146] and animal and preterm infants studies[146–150] have shown that stimulation of upper airway receptors may cause central apnea. Apnea may be produced by water, chemical, or mechanical stimulation of these receptors.

Studies in normal adults[151,152] have shown that nasal obstruction results in central apneas. This finding has not been reproduced in allergic rhinitis, however. McNicholas and colleagues[153] studied 7 subjects when asymptomatic and during exacerbation of allergic rhinitis; CAI did not change significantly, although the obstructive apnea index increased significantly.

High-frequency (30 Hz) low-pressure ventilation[154] and CPAP[155,156] have been shown to improve central sleep apnea suggesting that upper airway receptors and closure may induce central apnea in humans.

REFERENCES

1. Javaheri S. Heart failure. In: Kryger MH, Roth T, Dement WC, editors. Principles and practices of sleep medicine. 5th edition. Philadelphia: WB Saunders; 2010, in press.
2. Javaheri S. Sleep dysfunction in heart failure. Curr Treat Options Neurol 2008;10:323–5.
3. Javaheri S. Sleep-related breathing disorders in heart failure. In: Mann DL, editor. Heart failure. A companion to Braunwald's heart disease. Philadelphia: WB Saunders; 2010, in press.
4. Javaheri S. Central sleep apnea. In: Lee-Chiong T, editor. Sleep medicine essentials. Hoboken (NJ): Wiley-Blackwell; 2009. p. 81–9.
5. Dempsey JA, Skatrud JB. Fundamental effects of sleep state on breathing. Curr Opin Pulm Med 1988;9:267–304.
6. Skatrud JB, Dempsey JA. Interaction of sleep state and chemical stimuli in sustaining rhythmical ventilation. J Appl Physiol 1983;55:813–22.
7. Dempsey JA, Skatrud JB. A sleep-induced apneic threshold and its consequences. Am Rev Respir Dis 1986;133:1163–70.
8. Nakayama H, Smith CA, Rodman JR, et al. Effect of ventilatory drive on CO_2 sensitivity below eupnea during sleep. Am J Respir Crit Care Med 2002; 165:1251–8.
9. Orem J, Kubin L. Respiratory physiology: central neural control. In: Kryger MH, Roth T, Dement WC, editors. Principles and practices of sleep medicine. 3rd edition. Philadelphia: WB Saunders; 2000. p. 205–28.
10. Heart disease and stroke statistics— 2009 update. Circulation 2009;119:e1–161.
11. Ward M. Periodic respiration. A short historical note. Ann R Coll Surg Engl 1973;52:330–4.
12. Allen E, Turk JL, Murley R. The case books of John Hunter FRS. New York: Parthenon Publishing; 1993. p. 29–30.
13. Cheyne J. A case of apoplexy, in which the fleshy part of the heart was converted into fat. Dublin Hospital Reports 1818;2:216–23.
14. Stokes W. Observations on some cases of permanently slow pulse. Dublin Q J Med Sci 1846;2: 73–85.
15. Javaheri S, Parker TJ, Wexler L, et al. Occult sleep-disordered breathing in stable congestive heart failure. Ann Intern Med 1995;122:487–92 [Erratum, Ann Intern Med 1995;123:77].
16. Javaheri S, Parker TJ, Liming JD, et al. Sleep apnea in 81 ambulatory male patients with stable heart failure: types and their prevalences, consequences, and presentations. Circulation 1998;97: 2154–9.
17. Javaheri S. Sleep disorders in 100 male patients with systolic heart failure. A prospective study. Int J Cardiol 2006;106:21–8.
18. Solin P, Bergin P, Richardson M, et al. Influence of pulmonary capillary wedge pressure on central apnea in heart failure. Circulation 1999;99:1574–9.
19. Sin DD, Fitzgerald F, Parker JD, et al. Risk factors for central and obstructive sleep apnea in 450 men and women with congestive heart failure. Am J Respir Crit Care Med 1999;160:1101–6.
20. Lofaso F, Verschueren P, Rande JLD, et al. Prevalence of sleep-disordered breathing in patients on

a heart transplant waiting list. Chest 1994;106: 1689–94.

21. Ferrier K, Campbell A, Yee B, et al. Sleep-disordered breathing occurs frequently in stable outpatients with congestive heart failure. Chest 2005; 128:2116–22.

22. Lanfranchi PA, Braghiroli A, Bosimini E, et al. Prognostic value of nocturnal Cheyne-Stokes respiration in chronic heart failure. Circulation 1999;99: 1435–40.

23. Vazir A, Hastings PC, Dayer M, et al. A high prevalence of sleep disorder breathing in men with mild symptomatic chronic heart failure due to left ventricular systolic dysfunction. Eur J Heart Fail 2007;9:243–50.

24. Oldenburg O, Lamp B, Faber L, et al. Sleep disordered breathing in patients with symptomatic heart failure: a contemporary study of prevalence in and characteristics of 700 patients. Eur J Heart Fail 2007;9:251–7.

25. MacDonald M, Fang J, Pittman SD, et al. The current prevalence of sleep disordered breathing in congestive heart failure patients treated with beta-blockers. J Clin Sleep Med 2008;4:38–42.

26. Wang H, Parker JD, Newton GE, et al. Influence of obstructive sleep apnea on mortality in patients with heart failure. J Am Coll Cardiol 2007;49: 1625–31.

27. Xie A, Skatrud JB, Puleo DS, et al. Apnea-hypopnea threshold for CO_2 in patients with congestive heart failure. Am J Respir Crit Care Med 2002;165: 1245–50.

28. Tkacova R, Hall ML, Luie PP, et al. Left ventricular volume in patients with heart failure and Cheyne-Stokes respiration during sleep. Am J Respir Crit Care Med 1997;156:1549–55.

29. Hanly P, Zuberi N, Gray R. Pathogenesis of Cheyne-Stokes respiration in patients with congestive heart failure. Relationship to arterial PCO_2. Chest 1993;104:1079–84.

30. Naughton M, Bernard D, Tam A, et al. Role of hyperventilation in the pathogenesis of central sleep apneas in patients with congestive heart failure. Am Rev Respir Dis 1993;148:330–8.

31. Javaheri S, Corbett WS. Association of low $PaCO_2$ with central sleep apnea and ventricular arrhythmias in ambulatory patients with stable heart failure. Ann Intern Med 1998;128:204–7.

32. Javaheri S, Almoosa K, Saleh K, et al. Hypocapnia is not a predictor of central sleep apnea in patients with cirrhosis. Am J Respir Crit Care Med 2005; 171:908–11.

33. Javaheri S. Acetazolamide improves central sleep apnea in heart failure: a double-blind prospective study. Am J Respir Crit Care Med 2006;173:234–7.

34. Chenuel B, Smith C, Skatrud J, et al. Increased propensity of apnea in response to acute elevations

in left atrial pressure during sleep in the dog. J Appl Physiol 2006;101:76–83.

35. Javaheri S. Central sleep apnea and heart failure [letter to the editor]. Circulation 2000;342:293–4.

36. Javaheri S. A mechanism of central sleep apnea in patients with heart failure. N Engl J Med 1999;341: 949–54.

37. Cherniack NS. Respiratory dysrhythmias during sleep. N Engl J Med 1981;305:325–30.

38. Khoo MC, Kronauer RE, Strohl KP, et al. Factors inducing periodic breathing in humans: a general model. J Appl Physiol 1982;53:644–59.

39. Cherniack NS, Longobardo GS. Cheyne-Stokes breathing: an instability in physiologic control. N Engl J Med 1973;288:952–7.

40. Carley DW, Shannon DC. A minimal mathematical model of human periodic breathing. J Appl Physiol 1988;65:1400–9.

41. Cherniack NS. Apnea and periodic breathing during sleep. N Engl J Med 1999;341:985–7.

42. Khoo MC. Theoretical models of periodic breathing in sleep apnea. In: Bradley TD, Floras JS, editors. Implications in cardiovascular and cerebrovascular disease. New York: Marcel Dekker; 2000. p. 335–84.

43. Guyton AC, Crowell JW, Moore JW. Basic oscillating mechanisms of Cheyne-Stokes breathing. Am J Phys 1956;187:395–8.

44. Younes M. The physiologic basis of central apnea and periodic breathing. Curr Opin Pulm Med 1989;10:265–326.

45. Millar TW, Hanly PJ, Hunt B, et al. The entrainment of low frequency breathing periodicity. Chest 1990; 98:1143–8.

46. Hall MJ, Xie A, Rutherford R, et al. Cycle length of periodic breathing in patients with and without heart failure. Am J Respir Crit Care Med 1996; 154:376–81.

47. Javaheri S. Treatment of obstructive and central sleep apnoea in heart failure: practical options. Eur Respir Rev 2007;16:183–8.

48. Javaheri S, Abraham WT, Brown C, et al. Prevalence of obstructive sleep apnea and periodic limb movement in 45 subjects with heart transplantation. Eur Heart J 2004;25:260–6.

49. Javaheri S. Pembrey's dream: the time has come for a long-term trial of nocturnal supplemental nasal oxygen to treat central sleep apnea in congestive heart failure. Chest 2003;123:322–5.

50. Javaheri S, Parker TJ, Wexler L, et al. Effect of theophylline on sleep-disordered breathing in heart failure. N Engl J Med 1996;335:562–7.

51. Javaheri S. Effects of continuous positive airway pressure on sleep apnea and ventricular irritability in patients with heart failure. Circulation 2000;101: 392–7.

52. Naughton MT, Liu PP, Benard DC, et al. Treatment of congestive heart failure and Cheyne-Stokes

respiration during sleep by continuous positive airway pressure. Am J Respir Crit Care Med 1995;151:92–7.

53. Sin DD, Logan AG, Fitzgerald FS, et al. Effects of continuous positive airway pressure on cardiovascular outcomes in heart failure patients with and without Cheyne-Stokes respiration. Circulation 2000;102:61–6.

54. Teschler H, Döhring J, Wang YM, et al. Adaptive pressure support servo-ventilation. Am J Respir Crit Care Med 2001;164:614–9.

55. Javaheri S. Heart failure and sleep apnea: emphasis on practical therapeutic options. Clin Chest Med 2003;24:207–22.

56. Garrigue S, Bordier P, Jaïs P, et al. Benefit of atrial pacing in sleep apnea syndrome. N Engl Med 2002;346:404–12.

57. Bradley TD, McNicholas WT, Rutherford R, et al. Clinical and physiologic heterogeneity of the central sleep apnea syndrome. Am Rev Respir Dis 1986;134:217–21.

58. Bradley TD, Phillipson EA. Central sleep apnea. Clin Chest Med 1992;13:493–505.

59. White DP, Zwillich CW, Pickett CK, et al. Central sleep apnea. Improvement with acetazolamide therapy. Arch Intern Med 1982;142:1816–9.

60. DeBacker WA, Verbraecken J, Willemen M, et al. Central apnea index decreases after prolonged treatment with acetazolamide. Am J Respir Crit Care Med 1995;151:87–91.

61. Hommura F, Nishimura M, Oguri M, et al. Continuous versus bilevel positive airway pressure in a patient with idiopathic central sleep apnea. Am J Respir Crit Care Med 1997;155:1482–5.

62. Farber HW, Loscalzo J. Pulmonary arterial hypertension. N Engl J Med 2004;351:1655–65.

63. Schulz R, Baseler G, Ghofrani HA, et al. Nocturnal periodic breathing in primary pulmonary hypertension. Eur Respir J 2002;19:658–63.

64. Zhou XS, Shahabuddin S, Zahn BR, et al. Effect of gender on the development of hypocapnic apnea/hypopnea during NREM sleep. J Appl Physiol 2000;89:192–9.

65. Zhou XS, Rowley JA, Demirovic F, et al. Effect of testosterone on the apnea threshold in women during NREM sleep. J Appl Physiol 2003;94:101–7.

66. Schulz R, Fegbeutel C, Olschewski H, et al. Reversal of nocturnal periodic breathing in primary pulmonary hypertension after lung transplantation. Chest 2004;125:344–7.

67. Shiomi T, Guilleminault C, Sasanabe R, et al. Primary pulmonary hypertension with central sleep apnea – sudden death after bilevel positive airway pressure therapy. Jpn Circ J 2000;64:723–6.

68. Johnson KG, Johnson DC. Bilevel positive airway pressure worsens central apnea during sleep. Chest 2005;128:2141–50.

69. Young T, Nieto J, Javaheri S. Systemic and pulmonary hypertension in obstructive sleep apnea. In: Kryger MH, Roth T, Dement WC, editors. Principles and practices of sleep medicine. 5th edition. Philadelphia: WB Saunders; 2010, in press.

70. Weil JV. Sleep at high altitude. In: Kryger MH, Roth T, Dement WC, editors. Principles and practices of sleep medicine. 3rd edition. Philadelphia: WB Saunders; 2000. p. 204–53.

71. White DP, Gleeson K, Pickett CK, et al. Altitude acclimatization: influence on periodic breathing and chemoresponsiveness during sleep. J Appl Physiol 1987;63:401–12.

72. Sutton JR, Houstion CS, Mansell AL, et al. Effect of acetazolamide on hypoxemia during sleep at high altitude. N Engl J Med 1979;301:1329–31.

73. Greene MK, Kerr AM, McIntosh IB, et al. Acetazolamide in prevention of acute mountain sickness: a double-blind controlled cross-over study. Br Med J 1981;283:811.

74. Yaggi H, Mohsenin V. Obstructive sleep apnoea and stroke. Lancet Neurol 2004;3:333–42.

75. Hermann DM, Bassetti CL. Sleep-disordered breathing and stroke. Curr Opin Neurol 2003;16:87–90.

76. Yaggi H, Mohsenin V. Sleep-disordered breathing and stroke. Clin Chest Med 2003;24:223–37.

77. Dyken ME, Somers VD, Yamada T, et al. Investigating the relationship between stroke and obstructive sleep apnea. Stroke 1996;27:401–7.

78. Shahar E, Whitney CW, Redline S, et al. Sleep-disordered breathing and cardiovascular disease: cross-sectional results of the Sleep Heart Health Study. Am J Respir Crit Care Med 2001;163:19–25.

79. Parra O, Arboix A, Bechich S, et al. Time course of sleep-related breathing disorders in first-ever stroke or transient ischemic attack. Am J Respir Crit Care Med 2000;161:375–80.

80. Brown HW, Plum F. The neurologic basis of Cheyne-Stokes respiration. Am J Med 1961;30:849–60.

81. Nachtmann A, Siebler M, Rose G, et al. Cheyne-Stokes respiration in ischemic stroke. Neurology 1995;45:820–1.

82. North JB, Jennett S. Abnormal breathing patterns associated with acute brain damage. Arch Neurol 1974;31:338–44.

83. Heyman A, Birchfield RI, Sieker HO. Effects of bilateral cerebral infarction on respiratory center sensitivity. Neurology 1958;8:694–700.

84. Boden AG, Harris MC, Parkes MJ. Apneic threshold for CO_2 in the anesthetized rat: fundamental properties under steady-state conditions. J Appl Physiol 1998;85:898–907.

85. Mellins RB, Balfour HH, Turino GM, et al. Failure of automatic control of ventilation (Ondine's curse). Medicine 1970;49:487–504.

86. Vanderlaan M, Holbrook CR, Wang M, et al. Epidemiologic survey of 196 patients with congenital central hypoventilation syndrome. Pediatr Pulmonol 2004;37:217–29.

87. Trochet D, O'Brien LM, Gozal D, et al. PHOX2B genotype allows for prediction of tumor risk in congenital central hypoventilation syndrome. Am J Hum Genet 2005;76:421–6.

88. Trang H, Dehan M, Beaufils F, et al. The French congenital central hypoventilation syndrome registry. General data, phenotype, and genotype. Chest 2005;127:72–9.

89. Blanchi B, Sieweke MH. Mutations of brainstem transcription factors and central respiratory disorders. Trends Mol Med 2005;11:23–30.

90. Amiel J, Laudier B, Attié-Bitach J, et al. Polyalanine expansion and frameshift mutations of the paired-like homeobox gene PHOX2B in congenital central hypoventilation syndrome. Nat Genet 2003;33:459–61.

91. Sasaki A, Kanai M, Kijima K, et al. Molecular analysis of congenital central hypoventilation syndrome. Hum Genet 2003;114:22–6.

92. Weese-Mayer DE, Berry-Kravis EM, Zhou L, et al. Idiopathic congenital central hypoventilation syndrome: analysis of genes pertinent to early autonomic nervous system embryologic development and identification of mutations in PHOX2B. Am J Med Genet 2003;123:267–78.

93. Dauger S, Pattyn A, Lofaso F, et al. PHOX2B controls the development of peripheral chemoreceptors and afferent visceral pathways. Development 2003;130:6635–42.

94. Blanchi B, Kelly LM, Viemari JC, et al. MafB deficiency causes defective respiratory rhythinogenesis and fatal central sleep apnea at birth. Nat Neurosci 2003;6:1091–100.

95. Cirignotta F, Schiavina M, Mondini S, et al. Central alveolar hypoventilation (Ondine's curse) treated with negative pressure ventilation. Monaldi Arch Chest Dis 1996;51:22–6.

96. Flageole H, Adolph VR, Davis GM, et al. Diaphragmatic pacing in children with congenital central alveolar hypoventilation syndrome. Surgery 1995;118:25–8.

97. Garrido-Garcia H, Alvarez JM, Escribono PM, et al. Treatment of chronic ventilatory failure using a diaphragmatic pacemaker. Spinal Cord 1998;36:310–4.

98. Oren J, Newth CJL, Hung CE, et al. Ventilatory effects of almitrine bismesylate in congenital central hypoventilation syndrome. Am Rev Respir Dis 1986;134:917–9.

99. Reichel J. Primary alveolar hypoventilation. Clin Chest Med 1980;1:119–24.

100. Bubis MJ, Anthonisen NR. Primary alveolar hypoventilation treated by nocturnal administration of O_2. Am Rev Respir Dis 1978;118:947–53.

101. McNicholas WT, Carter JL, Rutherford R, et al. Beneficial effect of oxygen on primary alveolar hypoventilation with central sleep apnea. Am Rev Respir Dis 1982;125:773–5.

102. Guilleminault C, Stoohs R, Schneider H, et al. Central alveolar hypoventilation and sleep: treatment by intermittent positive-pressure ventilation through nasal mask in an adult. Chest 1989;96:1210–2.

103. Man GC, Jones RL, MacDonald GF, et al. Primary alveolar hypoventilation managed by negative-pressure ventilators. Chest 1979;76:219–21.

104. Garay SM, Turino GM, Goldring RM. Sustained reversal of chronic hypercapnia in patients with alveolar hypoventilation syndromes. Am J Med 1981;70:269–74.

105. Farmer WC, Glenn WW, Gee JBL. Alveolar hypoventilation syndrome: studies of ventilatory control in patients selected for diaphragm pacing. Am J Med 1978;64:39–49.

106. Glenn WWL, Gee JBL, Cole DR, et al. Combined central alveolar hypoventilation and upper airway obstruction. Am J Med 1978;64:50–60.

107. Cohn JE, Kuida H. Primary alveolar hypoventilation associated with Western equine encephalitis. Ann Intern Med 1962;56:633–44.

108. White DP, Miller F, Erickson RW. Sleep apnea and nocturnal hypoventilation after western equine encephalitis. Am Rev Respir Dis 1983;127:132–3.

109. Devereaux MW, Keane JR, Davis RL. Automatic respiratory failure associated with infarction of the medulla: report of two cases with pathologic study of one. Arch Neurol 1973;29:46–52.

110. Levin BE, Margolis G. Acute failure of automatic respirations secondary to a unilateral brainstem infarct. Ann Neurol 1977;1:583–6.

111. Kraus J, Heckmann JG, Druschky A, et al. Ondine's curse in association with diabetes insipidus following transient vertebrobasilar ischemia. Clin Neurol Neurosurg 1999;101:196–8.

112. Manning HL, Leiter JC. Respiratory control and respiratory sensation in a patient with a ganglioglioma within the dorsocaudal brain stem. Am J Respir Crit Care Med 2000;161:2100–6.

113. Cummiskey J, Guilleminault C, Davis R, et al. Automatic respiratory failure: sleep studies and Leigh's disease. Neurology 1987;37:1876–8.

114. Schulz R, Fegbeutel C, Althoff A, et al. Central sleep apnoea and unilateral diaphragmatic paralysis associated with vertebral artery compression of the medulla oblongata. J Neurol 2003;250:503–5.

115. Yglesias A, Narbona J, Vanaclocha V, et al. Chiari type 1 malformation, glossopharyngeal neuralgia and central sleep apnea in a child. J Child Neurol 1996;38:1126–30.

116. Severinghaus JW, Mitchell RA. Onidine's curse: failure of respiratory center automacity while awake. Clin Res 1962;10:122.

117. Manconi M, Mondini S, Fabiani A, et al. Anterior spinal artery syndrome complicated by the Ondine Curse. Arch Neurol 2003;60:1787–90.

118. George CF. Neuromuscular disorders. In: Kryger MH, Roth T, Dement WC, editors. Principles and practices of sleep medicine. 3rd edition. Philadelphia: WB Saunders; 2000. p. 1087–92.

119. Kerby GR, Mayer LS, Pingleton SK. Nocturnal positive pressure ventilation via nasal mask. Am Rev Respir Dis 1987;135:738–40.

120. Ellis ER, Bye PTP, Bruderer JW, et al. Treatment of respiratory failure during sleep in patients with neuromuscular disease: positive-pressure ventilation through a nose mask. Am Rev Respir Dis 1987;135:148–52.

121. Newson-Davis IC, Lyall RA, Leigh PN, et al. The effect of non-invasive positive pressure ventilation (NIPPV) on cognitive function in amyotrophic lateral sclerosis: a prospective study. J Neurol Psychiatr 2001;71:482–7.

122. Goldstein RS, Molotiu N, Skrastins R, et al. Reversal of sleep-induced hypoventilation and chronic respiratory failure by nocturnal negative pressure ventilation in patients with restrictive ventilatory impairment. Am Rev Respir Dis 1987;135:1049–55.

123. Teichtahl H, Prodromidis A, Miller B, et al. Sleep-disordered breathing in stable methadone programme patients: a pilot study. Addiction 2001; 96:395–403.

124. Fareny RJ, Walker JM, Cloward RS. Sleep-disordered breathing associated with long-term opioid therapy. Chest 2003;123:632–9.

125. Walker M, Farney J, et al. Chronic opioid use a risk factor for the development of central sleep apnea and ataxic breathing. J Clin Sleep Med 2007;3: 455–61.

126. Webster L, Choi Y, Desai H, et al. Sleep disordered breathing and chronic opioid therapy. Panminerva Med 2008;9:425–32.

127. Feldman J, Del Negro C. Looking for inspiration: new perspectives on respiratory rhythm. Nat Rev 2006;7:232–42.

128. Javaheri S, Smith J, Chung J. The prevalence and natural history of complex sleep apnea. J Clin Sleep Med 2009;5:205–11.

129. Javaheri S, Malik A, Smith J, et al. Adaptive pressure support servoventilation: a novel treatment for sleep apnea associated with use of opioids. J Clinic Sleep Med 2008;4:305–10.

130. Grunstein RR, Ho KK, Sullivan CE, et al. Sleep apnea in acromegaly. Ann Intern Med 1991;115: 527–32.

131. Colas A, Fergone D, Marzullo P, et al. Systemic complications of acromegaly: epidemiology, pathogenesis, and management. Endocr Rev 2004;25:102–52.

132. Rosenow F, McCarthy V, Caruso AC. Sleep apnea in endocrine diseases. J Sleep Res 1998;7:3–11.

133. Grunstein RR, Ho KK, Sullivan CE. Effect of octreotide, a somatostatin analog, on sleep apnea in acromegaly. Ann Intern Med 1994;121:478–87.

134. Herrmann BL, Wessendorf TE, Ajaj W, et al. Effects of octreotide on sleep apnea and tongue volume (magnetic resonance imaging) in patients with acromegaly. Eur J Endocrinol 2004;151:309–15.

135. Grunstein RR, Ho KK, Berthon-Jones M, et al. Central sleep apnea is associated with increased ventilatory response to carbon dioxide and hypersecretion of growth hormone in patients with acromegaly. Am J Respir Crit Care Med 1994;150:496–502.

136. Rajagopal KR, Abbrecht PH, Derderian SS, et al. Obstructive sleep apnea in hypothyroidism. Ann Intern Med 1984;101:991–4.

137. Meyrier A. Central sleep apnea in hypothyroidism. Am Rev Respir Dis 1983;127:504–7.

138. Morgenthaler T, Kagramanov V, Hanak V, et al. Complex sleep apnea syndrome: is it a unique clinical syndrome? Sleep 2006;29:1203–8.

139. Dernaika T, Tawk M, Nazir S, et al. The significance and outcome of continuous positive airway pressure-related central sleep apnea during split-night sleep studies. Chest 2007;132:81–8.

140. Lehman S, Anic N, Thompson C, et al. Central sleep apnea on commencement of continuous positive airway pressure in patient with primary diagnosis of obstructive sleep apnea-hyperpnoea. J Clin Sleep Med 2007;3:462–6.

141. Endo Y, Suzuki M, Inoue Y, et al. Prevalence of complex sleep apnea among Japanese patients with sleep apnea syndrome. Tohoku J Med 2008; 215:349–54.

142. Yaegashi H, Fujimoto K, Abe H, et al. Characteristics of Japanese patients with complex sleep apnea syndrome: a retrospective comparison with obstructive sleep apnea syndrome. Intern Med 2009;48:427–32.

143. Guilleminault C, Simmons B, Motta J, et al. Obstructive sleep apnea syndrome and tracheostomy. Arch Intern Med 1981;141:985–8.

144. Coccagna G, Mantovani M, Brignani F, et al. Tracheostomy in hypersomnia with periodic breathing. Physio Path Resp 1972;8:1217–27.

145. Widdicombe J. Airway receptors. Respir Physiol 2001;125:3–15.

146. Storey AT, Johnson P. Laryngeal receptors initiating apnea in lamb. Exp Neurol 1975;47:42–55.

147. James JE, Daly MB. Nasal reflexes. Proc R Soc Med 1969;62:1287–93.

148. Harms CA, Zeng YJ, Smith CA, et al. Negative pressure-induced deformation of the upper airway causes central apnea in awake and sleeping dogs. J Appl Physiol 1996;80:1528–39.

149. Lawson EE. Prolonged central respiratory inhibition following reflex-induced apnea. J Appl Physiol 1981;50:874–9.

150. Davis AM, Koenig JC, Thack BT. Upper airway che-moreflex responses to saline and water in preterm infants. J Appl Physiol 1988;64:1412–20.
151. Suratt PM, Turner BL, Wilhoit SC. Effect of intra-nasal obstruction on breathing during sleep. Chest 1986;90:324–9.
152. Zwillich CW, Pickett C, Hanson FN, et al. Disturbed sleep and prolonged apnea during nasal obstruction in normal man. Am Rev Respir Dis 1981;124:158–60.
153. McNicholas WT, Tavlo S, Cole P, et al. Obstructive apneas during sleep in patients with seasonal allergic rhinitis. Am Rev Respir Dis 1982;126: 625–8.
154. Henke KG, Sullivan CE. Effects of high-frequency pressure waves applied to upper airway on respira-tion in central apnea. J Appl Physiol 1992;73:1141–5.
155. Issa FG, Sullivan CE. Reversal of central sleep apnea using nasal CPAP. Chest 1986; 90:165–71.
156. Hoffstein V, Slutsky AS. Central sleep apnea reversed by continuous positive airway pressure. Am Rev Respir Dis 1987;135:1210–2.

Hypoventilation Syndromes

Lee K. Brown, MD[a,b,*]

KEYWORDS

- Hypoventilation • Hypoxia • Hypoxemia • Hypercapnia
- Chest wall disease • Neuromuscular disease
- Control of breathing

DEFINITION

Hypoventilation is conventionally said to exist when arterial pCO_2 ($PaCO_2$) exceeds the upper limit of normal. Data for the normal range of this parameter began to appear in the literature in about 1942, with most sources estimating a mean value of about 38 mm Hg and the upper 95% confidence limit to be about 45 mm Hg.[1] Consequently, a value of $PaCO_2$ greater than 45 mm Hg (presumably only applicable at or near sea level) is commonly used to define the presence of hypoventilation. Basic pulmonary physiology teaches us that arterial pCO_2 is proportional to CO_2 production divided by alveolar ventilation, and that alveolar ventilation is the product of tidal volume (V_t), respiratory rate (RR), and the dead space to tidal volume ratio (V_d/V_t).

MECHANISMS OF HYPOVENTILATION

Theoretically, elevated levels of $PaCO_2$ can result from either overproduction of carbon dioxide or reduced alveolar ventilation. In the real world, overproduction is rarely a factor except in situations whereby alveolar ventilation is already marginal.[2,3] For the purposes of this review, hypoventilation can therefore be attributed to reduced alveolar ventilation; in turn, this may be the result of reduced minute ventilation (decreased tidal volume and or respiratory rate) or increased V_d/V_t, or some combination of these factors. Yet another way of looking at hypoventilation pathophysiology holds that reduced alveolar ventilation can be attributed to either: (1) decreased ventilatory drive ("won't breathe"), or (2) worsening respiratory mechanics and/or severely deranged gas exchange. ("can't breathe").

Ventilatory Drive

In this age of polypharmacy, the administration of respiratory depressant medications (opiates; benzodiazepines or other sedative medications that depress ventilatory drive) may be the most common etiologic agent for reduced central ventilatory drive.[4] However, a variety of central nervous system (CNS) pathologies (usually involving the brainstem or diencephalic regions) can impair control of breathing and lead to hypoventilation; both congenital and acquired etiologies have been described.[5,6] In addition, impaired control of breathing may occur in some disorders that have a major component of abnormal respiratory mechanics, for example, obesity hypoventilation (Pickwickian) syndrome (OHS). It has been posited that depressed ventilatory drive in these conditions is an adaptive CNS response to the

Financial Disclosures: Dr Brown recently completed terms on the boards of directors of the American Academy of Sleep Medicine, Associated Professional Sleep Societies LLC, and American Sleep Medicine Foundation. He currently serves on the board of trustees of the Greater Albuquerque Medical Association. He receives no grant or commercial funding pertinent to the subject of this article.

[a] Division of Pulmonary, Critical Care, and Sleep Medicine, Department of Internal Medicine, University of New Mexico School of Medicine, 1101 Medical Arts Avenue NE, Building #2, Albuquerque, NM 87102, USA
[b] Program in Sleep Medicine, University of New Mexico Health Sciences Center, Albuquerque, NM 87102 , USA
* Corresponding author. Division of Pulmonary, Critical Care, and Sleep Medicine, Department of Internal Medicine, University of New Mexico School of Medicine, 1101 Medical Arts Avenue NE, Building #2, Albuquerque, NM 87102.
E-mail address: lkbrown@alum.mit.edu

Clin Chest Med 31 (2010) 249–270
doi:10.1016/j.ccm.2010.03.002

hypoventilation initially attributable to abnormal respiratory mechanics: increased $PaCO_2$ leads to elevated levels of cerebrospinal fluid bicarbonate, which then blunts the usually vigorous ventilatory response to elevated $PaCO_2$.[7] However, other possibilities include compensatory metabolic alkalosis from renal bicarbonate retention[8] or other factors as yet unknown.[9] Among these other possible factors is intriguing evidence concerning leptin's role as a ventilatory stimulant, and acquired resistance to this effect of leptin in some patients with OHS as a possible factor in mediating hypoventilation.[10] Finally, a small number of patients exhibit diurnal hypoventilation even after all other conditions (no apparent CNS lesion, primary lung disease, skeletal malformations, significant obesity, or neuromuscular disorder) have been excluded. Some of these patients exhibit other CNS abnormalities, particularly related to hypothalamic function, and it seems probable that many have anatomic or functional defects of central ventilatory control that have not yet been well characterized.[11,12]

Respiratory Mechanics

Altered respiratory mechanics can induce hypoventilation through several mechanisms. Hypoventilation in obstructive airways disease is readily explained; it is intuitively obvious that airflow limitation will necessarily constrain maximal minute ventilation and thus maximal alveolar ventilation, and this has been repeatedly demonstrated in such patients.[13] Only a fraction of maximal voluntary ventilation is sustainable over the long term (usually about 50%), and if airflow obstruction is profound enough to reduce this maximum sustainable ventilation below the threshold for maintaining eucapnia, hypoventilation will occur by definition. Restrictive ventilatory impairment from nonneuromuscular chest wall disease or interstitial lung disease usually does not impair maximum sustainable minute ventilation until late in the course of the disorder because compensation for reduced tidal volumes due to the restrictive disorder can usually be attained by increasing respiratory rate. However, shallow tidal volumes necessarily result in higher values of V_d/V_t, and at some point in the progression of disease the combination of elevated dead space fraction and reduced maximum sustainable minute ventilation will produce alveolar hypoventilation and hypercapnia.[14,15] A combination of these factors leads to hypoventilation in neuromuscular disorders affecting the ventilatory muscles. As in obstructive disorders, maximum sustainable ventilation is generally reduced in tandem with indices of vital capacity and airflow,[16,17] but in addition a rapid shallow breathing pattern is assumed, leading to higher V_d/V_t as seen in other restrictive chest wall diseases and interstitial lung disease.[18]

Gas Exchange

In addition to the effect of rapid shallow breathing on dead space ventilation, disorders that obliterate pulmonary vasculature will result in lung units that are ventilated but not well perfused, thus increasing V_d/V_t by increasing physiologic dead space. These disorders include pulmonary vascular diseases such as primary pulmonary hypertension, pulmonary hypertension caused by collagen-vascular disorders, and pulmonary hypertension from chronic pulmonary thromboembolic disease; and interstitial lung diseases such as usual interstitial pneumonia, sarcoidosis, or adult respiratory distress syndrome (ARDS). However, alveolar hypoventilation from this mechanism usually does not occur until very late in the course of disease because alveolar ventilation can usually be maintained by increasing minute ventilation (by using higher respiratory rates) as noted earlier. However, hypercapnia from this mechanism may be seen in end-stage ARDS patients receiving invasive positive pressure ventilation despite maintenance of normal or even elevated minute ventilation.[19]

HYPOVENTILATION DUE TO NEUROMUSCULAR AND CHEST WALL DISORDERS
Obesity Hypoventilation Syndrome

Burwell and colleagues[20] first used the term Pickwickian syndrome in 1956 to describe patients with obesity, awake hypercapnia and hypoxemia, sleepiness, polycythemia, and cor pulmonale. The eponym was based on the character "Joe" in Charles Dickens' The Posthumous Papers of the Pickwick Club who was described as "a natural curiosity," "...always asleep. Goes on errands fast asleep, and snores as he waits at table."[21] The disorder was later rechristened with the less literary, but probably more accurate, name of obesity hypoventilation syndrome (OHS) because it is more likely that Joe had obstructive sleep apnea syndrome rather than necessarily suffering from OHS. A diagnosis of OHS commonly requires awake alveolar hypoventilation ($PaCO_2$ >45 mm Hg) in an obese patient (body mass index [BMI; body weight divided by height squared] >30 kg/m^2; other investigators have used >35 kg/m^2) with no other identifiable cause of hypoventilation.[22]

It is well that OHS continues to carry the designation of a "syndrome" rather than achieving the category of a "disease," because it has become clear that OHS is not a homogeneous entity. In many (but not all) cases OHS is associated with obstructive sleep apnea syndrome (OSAS), an entity poorly recognized in Burwell's time, and improves when OSAS is effectively managed; in a minority of patients, it is not associated with OSAS or if OSAS is present does not respond to treating the OSAS alone. The importance of OHS derives in large part from the staggering increase in obesity in the population of developed countries, both in the United States and worldwide. The US Centers for Disease Control and Prevention Web site reports that in 2008, only one state (Colorado) had a prevalence of obesity less than 1 in 5; in 32 states more than 1 in 4 of their residents were obese, while in 6 of these states (Alabama, Mississippi, Oklahoma, South Carolina, Tennessee, and West Virginia) obesity prevalence exceeded 30%.[23] The public, as well as personal, health consequences of obesity are considerable, comprising an elevated risk of pulmonary, cardiovascular, gastrointestinal, metabolic, and joint disorders, all of which lead to high use of health care resources.[24] Those individuals who develop OHS add significantly to this burden.[25]

The secondary consequences of OHS are many, including disturbed sleep leading to hypersomnia, awakenings with headache or nausea (thought to be a consequence of hypercapnia-induced cerebrovascular dilation), depressive symptoms, polycythemia, and pulmonary hypertension with or without *cor pulmonale*.[26] The prevalence of OHS in the general population is still unknown. Ganesh and Alapat[27] (reported as an abstract only) reviewed the charts of all patients referred for pulmonary function testing and arterial blood gas determinations in an inner city hospital in Houston, Texas over the course of 2 years. One hundred and twenty of the 227 patients (53%) fulfilling entrance criteria were obese (BMI >30 kg/m^2) and of these, 21 had $PaCO_2$ greater than 45 mm Hg without other conditions known to result in hypercapnia (overall prevalence 9% and of obese subjects, 17.5%). It is clear that the rate of obesity in this population exceeded that which would be expected in the general population, and one would therefore suspect an overestimate of OHS prevalence; in addition, patients referred for pulmonary function testing are unlikely to be representative of the general population, and it is not stated whether the subjects were outpatients or also included inpatients. A study by Nowbar and colleagues[28] of 4332 consecutive admissions to a general medicine service reported that

approximately 1% met the definition of OHS among the 6% with BMI of or above 35 kg/m^2. However, 75 patients meeting the BMI criterion were excluded due to unwillingness to participate, and inpatients are clearly not representative of the general population. The largest body of literature reporting OHS prevalence focuses on patients with OSAS. For instance, Laaban and Chailleux[29] reported an 11% prevalence of diurnal hypercapnia in a database of 1141 French adults with OSAS, and Mokhlesi and colleagues[30] identified OHS in 20% of 270 OSAS patients in a prospective study of urban, mainly minority, individuals referred for evaluation of sleep-disordered breathing in the United States. A recent meta-analysis of published cohort studies, including those referenced above and encompassing 4250 subjects, estimated that 19% of patients with OSAS met standard criteria for OHS and found no difference in OHS prevalence by gender.[31] One could extrapolate from this estimate and the reported prevalence of apnea/hypopnea index (AHI; number of apneas and hypopneas per hour of sleep) greater than 5 in the adult population[32] to conclude that approximately 3% of adults have OHS, a figure that seems higher than clinical experience might suggest but is actually fairly close to the estimate (1%) from the inpatient study described here.[28] Factors that seem to predict the development of OHS in patients with obstructive sleep-disordered breathing include increasing AHI and BMI as well as more restrictive ventilatory impairment on pulmonary function testing.[31] Mortality in OHS is similarly difficult to estimate, and is probably changing as effective treatment becomes more commonly adopted; the report of inpatients with OHS previously cited suggests an 18-month mortality of 23%, although only 11 of their 47 subjects with OHS were recognized as such at discharge and considered for treatment.[28]

OHS is now believed to be a heterogeneous group of disorders in which diverse pathophysiological mechanisms produce the final common pathway of hypoventilation, hypoxemia, and the clinical sequelae described above. Early investigators speculated that morbid obesity altered pulmonary mechanics to such an extent that, in a holistic manner, hypercapnia became preferable to the radical increase in work of breathing that would be necessary to maintain eucapnia. Obesity is a mass load; that is, the mass of excess adipose tissue increases the inertance (tendency of a system to oppose being set in motion) of the respiratory pump; in addition, the weight of this adipose tissue compresses the respiratory apparatus with an effect that necessarily varies with body position.[33,34] Respiratory compliance declines, although some or all of this may be attributable to the mass load rather than an actual change in the elastic properties of the respiratory system.[35] More recent data suggest that obesity also results in a degree of fixed obstructive ventilatory impairment, although the mechanism is unclear and there have been inconsistent results with respect to gender; men may be more commonly affected than women.[36–38] An increasing body of literature points to an association between obesity and bronchial asthma, most frequently in women,[39] and a recent meta-analysis of prospective studies encompassing an extraordinarily large number of subjects (n = 333,102) demonstrated a higher incidence of asthma related to obesity in both genders.[40] These mechanical loads result in increased work of breathing, which is achieved by augmented ventilatory drive to the inspiratory muscles. It is interesting that the magnitude of the increase in ventilatory drive is out of proportion to the extra work subsumed by the respiratory pump, suggesting that a defect is also present in excitation/contraction coupling of the inspiratory muscles. This phenomenon of increased ventilatory drive without concomitant increased ventilation has been well-demonstrated in the eucapnic obese.[41]

Given the mechanical loads imposed by significant obesity, early thinking on OHS pathogenesis postulated that at some point in time the excessive work of breathing necessary to maintain eucapnia in the OHS patient becomes untenable, and a central mechanism of some sort alters control of breathing so as to accept a degree of hypercapnia to limit the work of breathing. Why this would occur in some individuals and not others of the same weight, and even in patients with fairly modest degrees of obesity, was not known until descriptions of OSAS as a prevalent sleep disorder became widely disseminated. Starting in the mid 1980s the significant demographic overlap between OSAS and OHS patients was recognized, and studies of nocturnal respiration in individuals with diurnal hypercapnia began to appear. Rapoport and colleagues[42] at New York University (NYU) School of Medicine reported on a group of 4 patients with OHS and severe OSAS, who became eucapnic when effectively treated for OSAS; 4 other similarly treated individuals did not achieve eucapnia. It was postulated that the first group developed diurnal hypercapnia from the loss of a "critical balance" between the time spent asleep and apneic versus the time spent awake, and that the second group represented "true Pickwickians" whose OHS was an intrinsic result of obesity rather than OSAS. Several possible mechanisms for the upset in "critical balance" of the 4 responders can be advanced: (1) inspiratory muscle fatigue related to the recurrent episodes of obstructed nocturnal breathing; (2) increased $PaCO_2$ from apneas leading to depression of respiratory muscle function and/or central control of breathing, as described above[7–9,43]; (3) depressed central ventilatory control due to the severe disruption in sleep quality. Later work by the NYU group has focused on mechanisms for the development of sustained hypercapnia during sleep in patients with severe OSAS, and how sleep-related hypercapnia could lead to diurnal hypercapnia. Mathematical modeling predicted, and human studies confirmed, that temporal mismatch between ventilation and perfusion during periodic breathing could lead to CO_2 retention if interevent time was short and/or interevent ventilation was inadequate.[44–47] Once sustained hypercapnia accompanies sleep, these investigators propose that renal bicarbonate retention then leads to depressed ventilatory drive and diurnal CO_2 retention.[8,48]

The heterogeneity of OHS based on whether treatment of OSAS corrects awake hypercapnia has subsequently been confirmed by other investigators, along with the identification of a third group of OHS patients: those who do not exhibit significant OSAS. These patients presumably can be lumped into the "true Pickwickian" category because their OSAS does not seem to be a significant factor in the development of their OHS.[49,50]

Another line of investigation for OHS pathogenesis centers on recent developments concerning the humoral effects of obesity, primarily involving leptin. Leptin is a protein of 167 amino acids that is produced in white adipose tissue and therefore increases in direct proportion to the degree of obesity. Leptin was originally studied with respect to energy homeostasis, because it acts in the hypothalamus to inhibit appetite.[51] However, leptin-deficient mice exhibit not only severe obesity but also hypoventilation and decreased ventilatory responsiveness to hypercapnia that corrects after exogenous leptin replacement.[52] Obese humans generally produce very high levels of leptin consistent with their high mass of adipose tissue, but these elevated levels do not seem to create the expected negative energy balance; CNS leptin resistance has been postulated to explain this. It is therefore conceivable that CNS leptin resistance may also contribute to depressed ventilatory drive and hypercapnia in OHS. However, data from human studies attempting to support this hypothesis are somewhat contradictory and confusing. Several groups have demonstrated that leptin levels, after controlling for the degree of obesity, are higher in obese OSAS patients with hypercapnia compared with those that are eucapnic[53,54]; however, one group has reported the opposite finding.[55] Yee and colleagues[56] demonstrated that serum leptin decreases in patients with OHS and OSAS when treated with noninvasive ventilation, but Redolfi and colleagues[57] found the opposite in patients with OHS not accompanied by OSAS. Finally, Campo and colleagues[10] obtained anthropometrics, leptin levels, polysomnography, end-tidal pCO_2, and hypercapnic P0.1 response on obese adults, and found that higher leptin predicted reduced hypercapnic response in men but not women. Leptin concentrations did not differ significantly when patients with and without OSAS were compared. Unfortunately, the investigators apparently did not analyze their end-tidal pCO_2 and AHI results in a manner that would have helped resolve the contradictory findings reported by other workers. Specifically, it may be that leptin and its relationships differ depending on whether an OHS patient is a "true Pickwickian" or has OHS due to OSAS.

Early diagnosis and appropriate therapy are essential to mitigate the morbidity and mortality associated with OHS. Diagnostic polysomnography must be performed to determine if OSAS is present, as this will profoundly affect the choice of treatment modality.[50] Weight loss obviously represents the most definitive therapy, and has proven efficacy in that a reduction of 5% to 10% of body weight can result in a significant improvement in hypercapnia.[58] Unfortunately, diet alone infrequently yields the desired result (a sustained reduction in BMI), and bariatric surgery has therefore been advocated. Data from Sugerman and colleagues[59] demonstrated that a decrease in BMI from 56 ± 13 to 38 ± 9 kg/m^2 after bariatric surgery in 31 patients with OHS was associated with a reduction in $PaCO_2$ from 53 ± 9 to 44 ± 8 mm Hg at 1 year. Patients analyzed in this study underwent a variety of bariatric surgical techniques, and overall within-30-day operative mortality was 4% in the 126 OHS patients compared with 0.2% in the 884 eucapnic patients. Boone and colleagues[60] reported the results of vertical banded gastroplasty performed on 35 patients, 19 with OHS + OSAS and 16 with OSAS alone, and achieved significant weight reductions. In the 7 patients with baseline and follow-up arterial blood gas determinations, group mean $PaCO_2$ decreased from 55 ± 4 to 41 ± 3 mm Hg; however, for the group as a whole mortality was 17%. Most recently, Martí-Valeri and colleagues[61] summarized the 1-year follow-up of 30 patients with OSAS undergoing open Roux-en-Y gastric bypass. Arterial pCO_2 declined

from 44.5 ± 5.7 to 40.6 ± 4.9 mm Hg, and only 4 patients continued to require positive airway pressure (PAP) therapy. Seven patients had respiratory complications postoperatively, but no mortality occurred. Of note, although individual studies and meta-analyses incorporating in total tens of thousands of patients have examined morbidity and mortality following bariatric surgery, the only information specific to OHS appears to be from these 3 reports. There are studies demonstrating that patients with OSAS incur elevated risk following weight loss surgery, and almost certainly, significant numbers of OHS subjects are included in such analyses.[62] It is possible that laparoscopic gastric banding may be more broadly, and safely, used; one meta-analysis found lower complication rates with this laparoscopic technique versus Roux-en-Y gastric bypass, although more profound weight loss was obtained with the latter procedure.[63]

For OHS associated with OSAS, the evidence consistently supports the effectiveness of PAP treatment, either continuous (CPAP)[42,43,49,50,64–69] or bilevel PAP.[50,57,67–70] The latter modality not only stabilizes the upper airway but also provides ventilatory support, and therefore may be preferable in the subgroup of patients that do not become eucapnic with effective treatment of their sleep-disordered breathing.[8,50] Bilevel PAP can also be continued into wakefulness if diurnal levels of $PaCO_2$ remain unacceptably high, which may well occur when OHS is not associated with significant OSAS or in individuals with the most severe mechanical derangements from obesity. When OHS is associated with OSAS, improvement in diurnal hypercapnia may be seen in as little as 24 hours.[43,66] Measures of central respiratory control (hypercapnic and hypoxic ventilatory drive) have been shown to improve in subgroups of patients with OHS plus OSAS treated with either modality,[42,43,71,72] and in the one published randomized prospective trial of CPAP versus bilevel PAP, outcome at 3 months did not differ significantly.[67] However, the latter study excluded patients that remained profoundly hypoxemic or exhibited significant increases in $PaCO_2$ during a screening CPAP titration night, a group of patients that would have almost certainly skewed the results to favor nocturnal bilevel PAP. Even when bilevel PAP is initially required in the patient with OHS and OSAS, it is often possible to transition the patient to CPAP alone once diurnal hypercapnia resolves.[68]

Budweiser and colleagues[73] retrospectively analyzed outcomes in 126 OHS patients treated with bilevel PAP, including 39 without OSAS. Compared with historical data on mortality,[28] this treated cohort exhibited lower mortality (97%, 92%, and 70% at 1, 2, and 5 years, respectively). Predictors of worse mortality included baseline awake PaO_2 less than 50 mm Hg, pH 7.44 or greater, and leukocyte count $7.8 \times 10^3/\mu L$, while a reduction in nocturnal $PaCO_2$ on bilevel PAP of more than 23% was predictive of improved survival. Because these investigators did not separately analyze treatment results in patients with and without OSAS, it remains unknown whether outcomes differ between these groups. In addition to bilevel PAP, it should be noted that other modalities have also been used for nocturnal ventilatory support in OHS patients, including volume-cycled ventilators[74] and, most recently, average volume-assured pressure support (AVAPS).[75,76] With respect to the latter modality, a small (n = 12) study of AVAPS versus patients' usual bilevel PAP treatment, one night of each in random order, demonstrated a slight but significant improvement in nocturnal transcutaneous pCO_2 with AVAPS, but patients complained of it being less comfortable.[75] The other study, also small (n = 10), was of a randomized crossover design and again demonstrated improved ventilation with AVAPS but no difference in sleep quality or health-related quality of life (HRQL) score.[76] The use of this newer, and doubtless more expensive, modality would best be reserved for patients not adequately responding to conventional CPAP or bilevel PAP. Furthermore, it is recommended that efficacy for each individual patient should first be demonstrated by employing the AVAPS device during overnight polysomnography.[77]

Progesterone is responsible for the hyperventilation associated with pregnancy, is known to stimulate ventilation when administered to normal subjects,[78] and can produce a modest improvement in hypercapnia in OHS patients.[79] However, the drug will not ameliorate coexisting OSAS, and bilevel PAP will more profoundly augment ventilation. Moreover, the side effects associated with this hormone almost certainly outweigh any putative benefits in these patients. Finally, oxygen treatment alone is not indicated as definitive treatment for OSAS, OHS with OSAS, or OHS without OSAS. However, oxygen is frequently a useful adjunct to PAP in patients with OHS when hypoxemia persists despite adequate resolution of OSAS and improvement in hypercapnia, particularly when inadequate oxygenation is a result of the gas exchange abnormalities known to accompany morbid obesity.[80]

Neuromuscular Disorders

Many neurologic or primary muscle diseases can produce weakness in the various muscles of respiration, and can afflict both adults and children. A comprehensive list of such disorders is beyond the scope of this article; in brief, these conditions include demyelinating diseases such as multiple sclerosis and Guillain-Barré syndrome; motor neuron disorders such as amyotrophic lateral sclerosis (ALS), acute poliomyelitis (now rarely seen), post-polio syndrome (more common), and spinal muscular atrophy; myelopathies such as spinal cord trauma, neoplasm, or transverse myelitis; peripheral nerve disorders such as phrenic nerve injury, critical illness polyneuropathy, and Charcot-Marie-Tooth disease; disorders of the neuromuscular junction such as myasthenia gravis and Eaton-Lambert syndrome; and primary muscle diseases such as the muscular dystrophies and the mitochondrial myopathies.[5,80,81] While the pathogenesis, treatment, and course of each of these conditions differ, the "final common pathway" with respect to pulmonary function is one of respiratory muscle weakness resulting in hypoventilation. Consequently, several observations can be made concerning clinical symptoms, evaluation, and treatment that in general hold for all of them.

Weakness of the major inspiratory muscle (the diaphragm) leads to a restrictive ventilatory defect with reduced tidal volumes, increased V_d/V_t, and inability to maintain alveolar ventilation at a level that will prevent hypercapnia. Accessory muscles of respiration (sternomastoids, scalenes, intercostals) are pressed into action as the diaphragmatic weakness progresses, but they too are affected by most of the disorders noted here and eventually are unable to sustain minute ventilation. In addition, the combination of reduced vital capacity from inspiratory muscle weakness and inability to generate a forced expiration due to expiratory muscle weakness (abdominal muscles, internal intercostals) leads to inadequate cough and insufficient clearance of secretions. Weakness of upper airway dilator muscles can result in failure to maintain an adequate airway and add an obstructive component to the ventilatory impairment. Symptoms include dyspnea (that sometimes may occur only on exertion as an early manifestation), weak cough, and inability to speak in full sentences. Hypoventilation during sleep may be the most prominent manifestation, causing symptoms such as headache or nausea on awakening or arousals with breathlessness.[82] During sleep, the recumbent position places the diaphragm at a mechanical disadvantage and respiratory drive declines. The latter phenomenon is most prominent in rapid eye movement (REM) sleep, the same sleep state in which skeletal muscle atonia normally occurs. The combination of the lost contribution to ventilation by the accessory muscles of respiration and reduced respiratory drive leads to the most profound degree of sleep-related hypoventilation. On physical examination in the clinic, findings include rapid shallow breathing, use of the accessory muscles of respiration, and paradoxic movement of the chest and abdomen.[83]

In addition to arterial blood gas determinations to identify frank hypercapnia, pulmonary function testing has proven to be of great use in predicting the likelihood of ventilatory failure. Spirometric measurement of forced vital capacity (FVC) can be useful in that values less than about 50% of predicted usually herald the onset of ventilatory failure.[84] The relationship between FVC and $PaCO_2$ is curvilinear, with little change in $PaCO_2$ until approximately half of predicted FVC has been lost, following which hypercapnia worsens at an increasingly faster rate as FVC continues to decline. Similar relationships hold for forced expiratory volume in 1 second (FEV_1)[85] and maximal voluntary ventilation (MVV).[86] A possibly more sensitive spirometric test consists of measuring FVC in the upright and supine positions, because in the normal individual FVC will not decline by more than about 10% when recumbent despite the additional inspiratory work required to displace the abdominal viscera. A decline of 25% or more correlated with maximal sniff transdiaphragmatic pressure (Pdi) of greater than −30 cm H_2O in one study of patients with various neuromuscular disorders,[87] but in a study of patients with ALS the supine FVC as a percentage of predicted was a better predictor of abnormal Pdi, and the postural change in FVC was not particularly useful.[88]

More direct measures of respiratory muscle strength include maximal inspiratory mouth pressure (MIP) and maximal expiratory mouth pressure (MEP). These maneuvers are usually performed at residual volume (RV) and total lung capacity (TLC), respectively; however, either or both may be measured at functional residual capacity (FRC). Assessment of MIP at FRC carries the advantage of eliminating the contribution of chest wall elastic recoil, which may vary depending on whether expiratory muscle strength is sufficient to achieve exhalation to RV. Both MIP and MEP are highly effort dependent, and therefore issues of motivation and patient cooperation may complicate the assessment. In addition, MEP in particular may be difficult to obtain in the patient with facial weakness that prevents adequate seal around a mouthpiece. Finally, both measurements carry a fairly high degree of variability that is inherent in the technique even in normal subjects.[89,90] Inspiratory muscle and expiratory muscle strength are reflected in MIP and MEP, respectively and, depending on the specific neurologic impairment, one may be affected more than the other. For instance, in pure diaphragmatic paralysis one would not expect MEP to be particularly abnormal while MIP will be significantly attenuated.[91] In general, MIP and MEP are more sensitive for the early detection of respiratory muscle involvement in neurologic disease than spirometric indices. Usually MIP will be greater than −60 cm H_2O before FVC falls to abnormal values, and MIP values greater than −30 cm H_2O will correlate with the onset of hypercapnia.[84,92,93] Maximal expiratory pressures lower than 45 cm H_2O often indicate the patient who is at risk for retention of secretions because of inability to generate an effective cough.[94]

Inspiratory pressure may also be assessed during a maximal inspiratory sniff maneuver, with a pressure transducer sampling at the nares (with one naris occluded), the mouth with the nares occluded, or with an esophageal catheter.[95–99] This method is said to be particularly useful in ALS or other diseases with prominent bulbar involvement. Isolated diaphragmatic function can also be assessed by passing a catheter with esophageal and gastric balloons so as to measure transdiaphragmatic pressure (Pdi_{max}) during an inspiratory sniff maneuver. This parameter is most useful in isolated diaphragmatic paralysis, but may also be the most sensitive and specific predictor of hypoventilation in other neuromuscular disorders such as ALS.[100] Finally, there are several techniques that must currently be considered best suited to the research laboratory, including measurement of Pdi_{max} with transcutaneous phrenic nerve stimulation. Either an electrical or magnetic technique may be employed, with electrical stimulation more specifically affecting the phrenic nerve, while magnetic stimulation will also activate the accessory muscles of respiration via the cervical nerve roots.[101] One recent investigation demonstrated that phrenic nerve studies had high sensitivity, specificity, and negative predictive value for hypoventilation in ALS patients, but low positive predictive value.[102]

Of importance is that abnormalities in respiratory muscle strength do not necessarily correlate with manifestations of nonrespiratory muscle weakness in many neuromuscular diseases. Therefore, the clinician should maintain a high index of suspicion for respiratory muscle involvement and the need for direct assessment of ventilatory function despite functional status otherwise being satisfactory.[103,104]

Some disorders in the category of neuromuscular disease have known causes for which effective treatment is available (eg, myasthenia gravis), and this should obviously be pursued where possible. With respect to supportive management for hypoventilation, supplemental oxygen alone may be appropriate for milder cases but noninvasive positive pressure ventilation (NPPV) has become the treatment of choice, particularly since the advent of nasal, oronasal, and oral interfaces as well as bilevel PAP and other ventilatory devices that are readily obtained for home use.[100,105] These modalities have also greatly increased in popularity because they avoid the ethical dilemmas and potential medical complications of positive pressure ventilation via tracheotomy, and because home ventilation using negative pressure devices (cuirass, and so forth) require bulky, uncomfortable interfaces and do not guarantee that the inspiratory effort will be synchronous with maintenance of a patent upper airway. With respect to chronic, progressive neuromuscular disorders, NPPV has been shown to improve quality of life and enhance survival.[100,105–107] This modality also may have a role in the care of acute, reversible ventilatory failure due to neuromuscular diseases; successful management of myasthenia gravis crisis has been reported,[108] but less sanguine results have been the case with respect to Guillain-Barré syndrome.[109]

Neurologic disorders may also cause hypoventilation on a central basis rather than by impairing ventilatory muscle function.[110,111] Loss of automatic control of ventilation is a rare complication of multiple sclerosis,[110–113] and has been reported to complicate brainstem stroke,[110,111,114–116] congenital brainstem malformations such as Arnold-Chiari malformation (both types I and II) with or without syringobulbia,[110,111,117–121] syringobulbia alone,[110,111,121,122] multiple system atrophies such as Shy-Drager syndrome,[110,111,123,124] and encephalitis of various etiologies.[110,111,125–128] The latter category includes paraneoplastic encephalitic syndromes and autoimmune encephalitis.[125] Apropos of the current H1N1 pandemic, there has been much made of the temporal relationship between an epidemic of von Economo encephalitis (encephalitis lethargica) and the H1N1 influenza pandemic centered around 1918.[128,129] A variety of breathing-control abnormalities accompanied the development of postencephalitic parkinsonism in these patients, including hypoventilation.[129,130] However, despite the temporal relationship with the influenza pandemic, the weight of evidence currently favors a pathogenesis not related to the influenza virus but rather involving a different, currently unidentified viral pathogen.[128,129] Most importantly, at the present time no cases of a similar encephalitis have been reported during the current novel H1N1 pandemic. Treatment of hypoventilation caused by CNS disease affecting ventilatory control generally follows the same management algorithm as for the neuromuscular disorders, most commonly with the use of NPPV.

Other Chest Wall Disorders

Patients with chest wall disorders impacting the ability of the thorax to expand such as kyphoscoliosis,[131,132] status post thoracoplasty,[133] ankylosing spondylitis,[134,135] or pleural conditions causing fibrothorax,[136,137] may develop hypoventilation. As described earlier, these patients assume a rapid, shallow breathing pattern to minimize the work of breathing, but the reduction in tidal volume leads to increased V_d/V_t and reduced alveolar ventilation. If the restrictive impairment progresses, the patient will eventually be unable to maintain adequate alveolar ventilation: first during sleep and then during wakefulness. As with many of the conditions discussed in this review, the relative atonia of the accessory muscles of respiration and the reduced ventilatory drive accompanying REM sleep often produce dramatic decompensation during this sleep stage. Individuals with chest wall disorders are also subject to developing atelectasis because of the shallow tidal volumes, further worsening hypoxemia. Finally, it has been postulated that kyphoscoliotic deformities may lead to changes in the length and orientation of the diaphragm, resulting in impairment of diaphragmatic function and force generation.[138,139] However, recent work using dynamic magnetic resonance imaging during respiration has failed to confirm this theory.[140,141] Pulmonary function testing in all of these disorders generally demonstrates restrictive ventilatory impairment with proportional reductions in FVC, TLC, and RV, the exceptions being ankylosing spondylitis in which increased chest wall elastic recoil tends to maintain normal or elevated RV,[14] and thoracoplasty for tuberculous disease, in which an additional obstructive impairment is said to be common.[142]

As in hypoventilation resulting from other causes of restrictive ventilatory impairment, NPPV has become the most common treatment modality employed.[143–149] Noninvasive positive pressure ventilation in patients with kyphoscoliosis and ventilatory failure improves daytime and nighttime oxyhemoglobin saturation, respiratory muscle performance, symptoms of hypoventilation, and quality of life.[145] The combination of NPPV plus oxygen leads to greater improvement and survival than oxygen alone.[146] Pulmonary hypertension secondary to respiratory insufficiency from chest wall restrictive disease has also been shown to improve with NPPV treatment.[147]

HYPOVENTILATION DUE TO LOWER AIRWAYS OBSTRUCTION
Chronic Obstructive Pulmonary Disease

Chronic obstructive pulmonary disease (COPD) is a generic term encompassing several different disease processes that cause airways obstruction that is not fully reversible. Except for disease due to inherited deficiency of α1-antitrypsin and inherited and acquired disorders causing bronchiectasis, COPD is closely associated with tobacco abuse. Some nosologies also include bronchial asthma under the COPD umbrella, although the "not fully reversible" requirement would seemingly exclude its membership in this group. This discussion is confined to the entities of chronic obstructive bronchitis and pulmonary emphysema.

Chronic obstructive bronchitis is clinically defined when a history of chronic cough and sputum production is obtained and pulmonary function testing demonstrates obstructive ventilatory impairment. The histopathology of the disease consists of an inflammatory process within small conducting airways that leads to epithelial remodeling, mucus gland hypertrophy, and thickened bronchial walls, thereby narrowing their lumen and impeding airflow.[150,151] The pathophysiology of the functional disability in these individuals involves obstruction to airflow that limits overall ventilation, and uneven distribution of ventilation throughout the lungs leading to ventilation-perfusion mismatch and impaired gas exchange. In contrast, pulmonary emphysema does not primarily affect the airways but rather is a destructive inflammatory process beginning in the respiratory bronchioles.[150,151] As the disease progresses, adjacent alveolar septae are obliterated and a centrilobular pattern of emphysema develops. The pathophysiological basis of the respiratory disability in pulmonary emphysema consists of the reduction in alveolar surface area and pulmonary capillary bed available for gas exchange, and the loss of lung elastic recoil that normally helps to maintain airway caliber, particularly with exhalation. It is uncommon for any given patient to present with pure chronic obstructive bronchitis or pure pulmonary emphysema; most commonly, patients will manifest both processes, with one or the other predominating. The historical description of patients as "blue bloaters" or "pink puffers" refers to whether the predominant pattern is one of chronic obstructive bronchitis or pulmonary

emphysema, respectively.[152–155] In addition to the clinical manifestations being somewhat different (early development of hypoxemia and cor pulmonale in the former; cachexia, worse quality of life, and late development of resting hypoxemia in the latter), the pattern of pulmonary function abnormality also varies. Patients with predominantly chronic obstructive bronchitis characteristically demonstrate an obstructive ventilatory defect without significant reduction in diffusing capacity, and may show an element of reversibility after administration of a bronchodilator medication, while those with predominantly pulmonary emphysema also have obstructive physiology but a prominent reduction in diffusing capacity. Arterial blood gas determinations are more likely to show hypoxemia and hypercapnia in the former phenotype. With respect to hypoventilation syndromes, both disorders can progress to sleep-associated, and then diurnal, hypercapnia as FEV_1 falls and the capacity to sustain adequate alveolar ventilation declines. Contributing to the mechanical limitation on minute ventilation is an increase in V_d/V_t,[156] a consequence of adopting a rapid, shallow breathing pattern,[157] as well as an increase in the magnitude of V_d caused by ventilation-perfusion mismatching and (in the case of pulmonary emphysema) attenuation of the pulmonary vascular bed.[158] It has long been known that the value of FEV_1 in any individual patient will not predict whether hypercapnia is present,[159,160] although most practitioners will increase their index of suspicion when FEV_1 falls below about 0.8 L. The main reason for variability in the FEV_1 to $PaCO_2$ relationship seems to be related to respiratory muscle strength rather than depressed ventilatory drive,[160,161] and inspiratory muscle strength most probably varies as a function of mechanical load,[162] hyperinflation leading to reduced mechanical advantage of the diaphragm,[163,164] and cachexia impairing diaphragmatic function.[165,166] Additional factors that have been implicated include the effects of inflammatory mediators on diaphragmatic contractility[163] and diaphragm myopathy from corticosteroid treatment.[167] Another factor in some patients may be the well-recognized phenomenon of hypercapnia induced by oxygen administration. The most definitive study to date suggests that a decrease in minute ventilation as well as increases in V_d/V_t from reversal of hypoxia-induced vasoconstriction play a role.[168] Finally, some patients with COPD also suffer from OSAS, a combination that has been termed by Flenley the "overlap syndrome."[169] It was originally hypothesized that some manner of causal relationship between COPD and OSAS existed, but it now seems clear that both of these disorders frequently co-occur because they are commonly seen in the same demographic group.[170] The overlap syndrome does have implications with respect to the development of hypoventilation, however. Overlap syndrome patients have been reported to exhibit diurnal hypercapnia more frequently,[171] and concomitant COPD appears to be an important cause of acute-on-chronic ventilatory failure in patients with severe OSA, so-called critical care syndrome.[172]

In addition to optimizing medical management, oxygen remains the mainstay of treatment for the hypoxemia of stable COPD patients, including those with hypoxemia from hypoventilation. Early studies established that continuous administration of oxygen was capable of ameliorating pulmonary hypertension and improving survival in patients with both daytime and nocturnal hypoxemia.[173] More recently, the use of NPPV plus oxygen has been advocated, both in the stable hypercapnic patient as well as during the treatment of acute exacerbations with worsening ventilatory failure. With respect to the former scenario, a meta-analysis of clinical trials with nocturnal NPPV did not support this form of therapy,[174] but a subsequent multicenter trial did demonstrate a reduction in hospitalization and improvement in dyspnea and health-related quality of life[175] as well as a reduction in health care costs.[176] More recently, Dellweg and colleagues[177] used controlled, rather than assisted mode, nocturnal NPPV in 305 COPD patients and found improved diurnal $PaCO_2$, a slight increase in vital capacity, and improved MIP. Budweiser and colleagues[178] found that nocturnal NPPV improved BMI in malnourished COPD patients, presumably a result of reduced caloric expenditure by the respiratory muscles. Most recently, Windisch and colleagues[179,180] have championed the use of nocturnal NPPV aimed at achieving eucapnia, which they term "high-intensity" therapy. Seventy-three patients received bilevel PAP at settings that averaged $28 \pm 5/5 \pm 1$ cm H_2O in their most recent trial, and after 2 months of therapy a significant reduction in $PaCO_2$ and increases in FVC and FEV_1 were achieved.[179] Few data have appeared with respect to the regular use of NPPV during wakefulness in stable hypercapnic COPD patients. However, many groups have examined the use of NPPV during exercise in these individuals and, when examined by meta-analysis, improvements in dyspnea and exercise tolerance seem to be consistently demonstrated.[181] One limitation with respect to using NPPV during exercise relates to the additional effort required by the patient in carrying the necessary equipment, which negated any benefit

in one recent study.[182] Finally, lung reduction surgery (LVRS), in those individuals deemed suitable candidates, has also been shown to ameliorate hypercapnia, with patients having the highest preoperative levels of $PaCO_2$ seeming to benefit the most at 3 to 6 months of follow-up.[183] However, few data concerning long-term effects of LVRS on hypercapnia have appeared, apparently because most studies (including the largest, the National Emphysema Treatment Trial, NETT) excluded patients with the most severe degrees of hypoventilation. For instance, despite original entrance criteria that accepted $PaCO_2$ up to 60 mm Hg, $PaCO_2$ averaged only 43 mm Hg in the NETT after the Data Safety Monitoring Board discontinued enrollment of the most severe candidates (those with FEV_1 <20% of predicted) at an early stage due to unacceptable surgical mortality.[184,185] One study has reported mortality in a small cohort of 6 patients with preoperative $PaCO_2$ greater than 60 mm Hg. At 3 to 6 months, $PaCO_2$ improved from 70.4 ± 9.4 mm Hg to 46.9 ± 3.4 mm Hg, and 5 of 6 patients were alive and "well" after an average of 55 months (range 43–69 months) of follow-up.[186]

The management of acute exacerbations of COPD is somewhat beyond the scope of this review. However, it should be mentioned that NPPV now has assumed a role in the standard treatment of this condition when accompanied by acute ventilatory failure, and this practice has been substantiated by a large volume of clinical investigations and multiple systematic meta-analyses.[187,188] Of note, patients with the most severe exacerbations seem to benefit the most.[189]

Bronchial Asthma

Conventional definitions of bronchial asthma have held that airways obstruction in this disorder is fully reversible, and that this reversibility is the hallmark of the disease. However, more recent analyses have recognized various asthma phenotypes, including those in which full reversibility does not occur.[190] Consequently, the modern definition of asthma encompasses some degree of reversible obstructive impairment as well as the presence of airway inflammation.

Chronic hypoventilation in the asthmatic is virtually never seen unless accompanied by other conditions such as severe obesity, OSAS, COPD, or other comorbidities, but acute ventilatory failure is a known complication of asthmatic exacerbations. The usual course of action when acute ventilatory failure accompanies status asthmaticus has been intubation and mechanical ventilation, but the availability of NPPV has led some investigators to apply this modality in such situations. A few retrospective reports suggest that NPPV in this situation is well tolerated, and has utility in preventing the need for intubation in adults[191,192] and children.[193,194] Only 2 small randomized controlled studies have been reported. In children, Soroksky and colleagues[195] compared 15 patients presenting with status asthmaticus treated with NPPV and conventional medical therapy with 15 receiving only medical therapy. Those patients receiving NPPV exhibited shorter emergency department stays and reduced need for hospitalization. Soma and colleagues[196] studied 44 adults presenting with asthma exacerbations, all of whom received intravenous corticosteroids (5 mg/kg) and were randomized into 3 groups. Fourteen were treated with bilevel PAP at 6/4 cm H_2O and 16 with bilevel PAP at 8/6 cm H_2O, while the remaining 14 did not receive bilevel PAP. Forty subjects completed the study, with 2 in each NPPV group dropping out (1 in each group for clinical deterioration, 1 in each group for inability to perform spirometry). Baseline FEV_1 averaged about 30% to 40% of predicted in each group, indicating fairly severe asthma exacerbations. At 40 minutes and thereafter, FEV_1 improved more in the 8/6 cm H_2O group compared with controls, while Borg scale dyspnea, wheezing, and accessory muscle use were improved in both bilevel PAP groups compared with controls. The weaknesses evident in the latter study include the somewhat unconventional medical treatment (corticosteroids only) and the fairly low values of PAP employed, including only a 2 cm H_2O spread between inspiratory and expiratory pressures. In view of the paucity of data, 2 separate meta-analyses of the efficacy of NPPV for treatment of status asthmaticus have judged this modality to be as yet unproven.[197,198]

SLEEP-RELATED HYPOVENTILATION/ HYPOXEMIA DUE TO PULMONARY PARENCHYMAL OR VASCULAR PATHOLOGY

Any respiratory system disorder that increases the absolute value of dead space or elevates V_d/V_t by reducing tidal volume may potentially lead to hypoventilation. The former category of diseases consist mainly of those that attenuate the pulmonary vasculature, such as primary pulmonary hypertension, chronic pulmonary thromboembolic disease, and pulmonary hypertension secondary to collagen-vascular diseases[199]; interstitial lung diseases such as usual interstitial pneumonia[200–202]; and causes of secondary pulmonary hypertension such as human immunodeficiency virus infection or end-stage liver disease with portal hypertension. Pulmonary parenchymal diseases that reduce

tidal volume due to restrictive ventilatory impairment include interstitial lung disorders such as sarcoidosis, interstitial disease (either primary or associated with collagen-vascular disorders), or cystic fibrosis.[200–202] Compensatory increases in minute ventilation to maintain satisfactory alveolar ventilation may not be sustainable as these conditions reach end stage,[203] or may occur during sleep at an even earlier stage due to the physiologic changes detailed above.[204] Most recently, Lancaster and colleagues[205] reported another possible cause of sleep-related hypoventilation in this population: a surprisingly high prevalence (88%) of OSAS in 50 unselected patients followed for idiopathic pulmonary fibrosis in a university pulmonary clinic. This cohort was a relatively older population (mean age, 64.9 years) of somewhat elevated BMI (mean, 32.3 kg/m^2) but was fairly equally distributed as far as gender (about two-thirds male); therefore, it is unclear whether this was a group in whom demographics alone would suggest a higher than normal prevalence of OSAS. The elevated prevalence of OSAS reported by this group is possibly of great importance but must be corroborated by further studies. With respect to treatment of hypoventilation from pulmonary parenchymal and vascular disease, the key strategy must clearly be effective management (when available) of the primary disorder. The few reports of NPPV treatment for acute exacerbations have not demonstrated any significant effect on outcome, but may help ameliorate patient dyspnea to a modest extent.[200,206] Koschel and colleagues[207] recently reported a trial of NPPV treatment in 10 patients with stable hypercapnic respiratory failure from a variety of interstitial lung diseases. These investigators were able to demonstrate an acute improvement in $PaCO_2$ (from a mean of 57.7 ± 5.1 to 52.3 ± 5.9 mm Hg) while patients were breathing spontaneously, with maximally tolerated values of NPPV (mean pressures were 28.2 ± 2.5/4.2 ± 0.4 cm H_2O). Measures were taken to improve ventilatory performance and patient comfort, including the use of a nonrebreathing circuit with an expiratory valve and a heat and moisture exchanger. However, it must be noted that this was a report of an acute short-term effect, with no long-term follow-up reported.

Of all of the pulmonary parenchymal and vascular disorders, cystic fibrosis (CF) has been studied most extensively with respect to hypoventilation and its management. Cystic fibrosis is a chronic progressive disorder encompassing mucus hypersecretion, impaired clearance of secretions, chronic and/or recurrent respiratory infections, lower airways obstruction, bronchiectasis, and pulmonary parenchymal destruction. As such, it is neither a purely parenchymal nor an exclusively airway disorder, but rather has elements of both restrictive and obstructive ventilatory impairment. Mutations in the cystic fibrosis transmembrane conductance regulator (CFTR) gene lead to defective chloride transport in the respiratory epithelium, causing abnormalities in mucous rheology and consequent defective clearance of airway secretions.[208] This in turn leads to recurrent respiratory tract infections and eventually to chronic infection and/or colonization with resistant bacteria,[209] and then destruction of the airway wall (bronchiectasis), mucous plugging and changes in airway epithelial morphology (airways obstruction), and destruction of lung parenchyma (pulmonary fibrosis). Additional morbidity affecting ventilatory capacity also occurs as a consequence of the pancreatic insufficiency that is caused by many CFTR mutations. Malabsorption and subsequent malnutrition lead to a higher prevalence of osteopenia, osteoporosis, and the development of progressive kyphosis with chest wall restriction that also impairs breathing.[210] Finally, chronic pain is a well-described complication of advanced CF and is often treated with opiates, leading to depressed ventilatory drive.[211] Hypoventilation in CF is therefore the result of a combination of the various mechanical, gas exchange, and ventilatory drive derangements already discussed in detail. As in other respiratory disorders, hypoventilation during sleep may be the earliest manifestation of disease progression.[212] It has been suggested that nocturnal hypoxemia contributes to *cor pulmonale* and progressive functional decline in these patients.[213] Death in CF almost exclusively occurs from respiratory failure.[209]

General management of the patient with CF has been thoroughly covered in recent reviews and is well beyond the scope of this article.[214–217] Lung transplantation similarly has become a standard consideration for the treatment of end-stage disease, and is also discussed elsewhere.[218] As is the case in other disorders of hypoventilation, although oxygen therapy does not treat the primary cause of hypoxemia, it is still widely used in patients with oxyhemoglobin desaturation from CF with or without hypercapnia.[219] There are few rigorous studies of oxygen supplementation in CF, and although symptomatic improvement may be expected, it is unclear whether disease progression or mortality are improved.[220] As is the case with other chronic progressive lung diseases, several groups have reported their

experience in treating small numbers of CF patients with respiratory failure using NPPV,[221,222] but few data have been published with respect to long-term, prospective, randomized controlled trials. Young and colleagues[223] published such a study but incorporated only 8 subjects, demonstrating improved nocturnal ventilation, symptoms, and exercise tolerance when patients received NPPV. Fauroux and colleagues[224] reported a retrospective analysis of the French CF registry, comparing patient data for the year before initiation of NPPV with that from the year after NPPV was started; they also compared prior year data from patients started on NPPV with contemporaneous data from a group of matched controls who did not receive NPPV. For the year prior to starting NPPV, NPPV patients exhibited greater declines in pulmonary function than the matched controls, but the rate of decline became similar to controls after NPPV was started. A recent meta-analysis of this issue did not find enough data to conclude that NPPV had any impact on exacerbations or progression of CF, although it should be noted that the Fauroux study was not included in this review.[225]

CONGENITAL CENTRAL ALVEOLAR HYPOVENTILATION SYNDROME

Congenital central hypoventilation syndrome (CCHS) is a rare condition characterized by abnormal automatic control of breathing, first described by Mellins and colleagues[226] in 1970. In view of the marked worsening of hypoventilation in these patients during sleep, Mellins suggested that the eponym "Ondine's curse" (a reference to a story in Greek mythology, and an eponym originally coined by Severinghaus and Mitchell[227]) be applied to this disorder. Despite the delightful literary panache that this term bestows on the disease, there has been considerable controversy as to whether it is truly applicable and consequently, and perhaps unfortunately, its use has fallen out of favor.[228] The disorder has an estimated incidence that varies widely in different reports, from 1 in 10,000 to 1 in 200,000 live births.[229] In addition to the respiratory control abnormality, the most common clinical manifestations have been aganglionic megacolon (Hirschsprung disease) and the development of neural crest tumors such as neuroblastoma, ganglioneuroblastoma, and ganglioneuroma, a fact that has led to the designation of this disorder as a neurocristopathy.[230] Amiel and colleagues[231] implicated mutations in the *PHOX2B* gene as responsible for CCHS in 2003, and subsequent work has shown that most CCHS patients have mutations leading to polyalanine expansions in this gene.[232] The severity of CCHS manifestations varies, and has been explained by the identification of multiple alleles[233] with different mutations that greatly increase the likelihood of Hirschsprung disease and the development of neural crest tumors.[234] Although most studies implicate the de novo occurrence of mutations, cases of siblings and twins with CCHS suggest that transmission could occur in an autosomal dominant pattern with variable penetration.[235,236]

Although mainly a disorder identified in the pediatric population (and usually shortly after birth), genetic analysis of CCHS family members has demonstrated a small population of adults with mild, previously undetected CCHS.[237] Indeed, CCHS severity can vary over a wide spectrum. Onset of symptoms typically is in the first year of life but may present in the neonate.[238–240] Diagnostic criteria generally require persistent evidence of sleep-associated hypoventilation with arterial pCO_2 greater than mm Hg, and primary cardiac, pulmonary, and neuromuscular disease must be absent. The most severe hypoventilation occurs in stage N3 sleep, when automatic control of breathing predominates, while manifestations are more variable in REM sleep, perhaps caused by the projection of some cortical influence on breathing during phasic REM.[241] Ventilation during wakefulness may or may not be abnormal, and most patients can increase ventilation with exercise, although that response is attenuated and hypercapnia may ensue.[242,243] It is interesting that in CCHS the increase in ventilation with exercise appears to be accomplished by elevating the respiratory rate early on, rather than tidal volume as is the case in normal subjects.[243] Due to the inconsistent ventilatory response to exercise, some authorities proscribe exercise in CCHS patients; in addition, these patients may not experience the normal degree of dyspnea with breath holding, and diving underwater or even swimming have been discouraged. Consistent with a neurocristopathy pathogenesis, patients with CCHS may demonstrate a wide variety of autonomic nervous system abnormalities including those associated with control of heart rate, impaired swallowing, gastroesophageal dysmotility and reflux, pupillary abnormalities, hypotonia, profuse sweating, and absence of fever with infection.[244,245]

The treatment of CCHS in large part revolves around providing ventilatory support tailored to the patient's needs. Some individuals require treatment only during sleep, whereas others must receive mechanical ventilation throughout wakefulness as well.[246] While ventilatory support has in the past required tracheotomy and mechanical ventilation, NPPV is increasingly being employed,[247–251] and as these patients have intact phrenic nerves, diaphragmatic pacing can also be considered.[252] Concerns about the possible occurrence of facial deformities in infants and young children induced by the interfaces required for delivering NPPV have probably inhibited more widespread use of this modality.[253] Outcome over the long term hinges on impeccable attention to ventilatory support and its complications.[229]

SUMMARY

A wide variety of mechanisms can lead to the hypoventilation associated with various medical disorders, which include derangements in central ventilatory control, mechanical impediments to breathing, and abnormalities in gas exchange leading to increased dead space ventilation. The pathogenesis of hypercapnia in OHS remains somewhat obscure, although in many patients comorbid obstructive sleep apnea appears to play an important role. Hypoventilation in neurologic or neuromuscular disorders is primarily explained by weakness of respiratory muscles, although some CNS diseases may affect control of breathing. In other chest wall disorders, obstructive airways disease, and CF, much of the pathogenesis is explained by mechanical impediments to breathing, but an element of increased dead space ventilation often occurs. Central alveolar hypoventilation syndrome involves a genetically determined defect in central respiratory control. Treatment in all of these disorders involves coordinated management of the primary disorder (when possible) and, increasingly, the use of NPPV.

REFERENCES

1. Diem K, Lentner C, editors. Scientific tables. 7th edition. Basel: Ciba-Geigy Limited; 1970. p. 545–70
2. Covelli HD, Black JW, Olsen MS, et al. Respiratory failure precipitated by high carbohydrate loads. Ann Intern Med 1981;95:579–81.
3. Talpers SS, Romberger DJ, Bunce SB, et al. Nutritionally associated increased carbon dioxide production. Excess total calories vs high proportion of carbohydrate calories. Chest 1992;102:551–5.
4. Caruso AL, Bouillon TW, Schumacher PM, et al. Drug-induced respiratory depression: an integrated model of drug effects on the hypercapnic and hypoxic drive. Conf Proc IEEE Eng Med Biol Soc 2007;2007:4259–63.

5. Polkey MI, Lyall RA, Moxham J, et al. Respiratory aspects of neurological disease. J Neurol Neurosurg Psychiatr 1999;66:5–15.

6. Glenn WW, Haak B, Sasaki C, et al. Characteristics and surgical management of respiratory complications accompanying pathologic lesions of the brain stem. Ann Surg 1980;191:655–63.

7. Frankel H, Kazemi H. Regulation of CSF composition- blocking chloride-bicarbonate exchange. J Appl Phys 1983;55:177–82.

8. Norman RG, Goldring RM, Clain JM, et al. Transition from acute to chronic hypercapnia in patients with periodic breathing: predictions from a computer model. J Appl Physiol 2006;100:1733–41.

9. Jennings DB, Chen CC. Ventilation in conscious dogs during acute and chronic hypercapnia. J Appl Phys 1976;41:839–47.

10. Campo A, Frühbeck G, Zulueta JJ, et al. Hyperleptinemia, respiratory drive and hypercapnic response in obese patients. Eur Respir J 2007;30:223–31.

11. D'Alessandro V, Mason T 2nd, Pallone MN, et al. Late-onset hypoventilation without PHOX2B mutation or hypothalamic abnormalities. J Clin Sleep Med 2005;1:169–72.

12. Katz ES, McGrath S, Marcus CL. Late-onset central hypoventilation with hypothalamic dysfunction: a distinct clinical syndrome. Pediatr Pulmonol 2000;29:62–8.

13. Dillard TA, Hnatiuk OW, McCumber TR. Maximum voluntary ventilation. Spirometric determinants in chronic obstructive pulmonary disease patients and normal subjects. Am Rev Respir Dis 1993; 147:870–5.

14. Bergofsky EH. Respiratory failure in disorders of the thoracic cage. Am Rev Respir Dis 1979;119: 643–69.

15. Javaheri S, Sicilian L. Lung function, breathing pattern, and gas exchange in interstitial lung disease. Thorax 1992;47:93–7.

16. Toussaint M, Steens M, Soudon P. Lung function accurately predicts hypercapnia in patients with Duchenne muscular dystrophy. Chest 2007;131: 368–75.

17. Sivak ED, Shefner JM, Sexton J. Neuromuscular disease and hypoventilation. Curr Opin Pulm Med 1999;5:355–62.

18. Misuri G, Lanini B, Gigliotti F, et al. Mechanism of CO_2 retention in patients with neuromuscular disease. Chest 2000;117:447–53.

19. Nunes S, Valta P, Takala J. Changes in respiratory mechanics and gas exchange during the acute respiratory distress syndrome. Acta Anaesthesiol Scand 2006;50:80–91.

20. Burwell CS, Robin ED, Whaley RD, et al. Extreme obesity associated with alveolar hypoventilation - A Pickwickian syndrome. Am J Med 1956;21: 811–8.

21. Dickens C. The posthumous papers of the Pickwick club. London: Chapman & Hall; 1837.

22. Olson AL, Zwillich C. The obesity hypoventilation syndrome. Am J Med 2005;11:948–56.

23. Centers for Disease Control and Prevention. U.S. obesity trends. Available at: http://www.cdc.gov/obesity/data/trends.html. Accessed November 10, 2009.

24. Raebel MA, Malone DC, Conner DA, et al. Health services use and health care costs of obese and nonobese individuals. Arch Intern Med 2004;164: 2135–40.

25. Berg G, Delaive K, Manfreda J, et al. The use of health-care resources in obesity-hypoventilation syndrome. Chest 2001;120:377–83.

26. Strumpf DA, Millman RP, Hill NS. The management of chronic hypoventilation. Chest 1990;98: 474–80.

27. Ganesh S, Alapat P. The prevalence of obesity hypoventilation syndrome in an inner city population. Chest 2007;132(Suppl):651S.

28. Nowbar S, Burkart KM, Gonzales R, et al. Obesity-associated hypoventilation in hospitalized patients: prevalence, effects, and outcome. Am J Med 2004; 116:1–7.

29. Laaban JP, Chailleux E. Daytime hypercapnia in adult patients with obstructive sleep apnea syndrome in France, before initiating nocturnal nasal continuous positive airway pressure therapy. Chest 2005;127:710–5.

30. Mokhlesi B, Tulaimat A, Faibussowitsch I, et al. Obesity hypoventilation syndrome: prevalence and predictors in patients with obstructive sleep apnea. Sleep Breath 2007;11:117–24.

31. Kaw R, Hernandex AV, Walker E, et al. Determinants of hypercapnia in obese patients with obstructive sleep apnea. Chest 2009;136:787–96.

32. Young T, Palta M, Dempsey J, et al. The occurrence of sleep-disordered breathing among middle-aged adults. N Engl J Med 1993;328: 1230–5.

33. Sharp JT, Henry JP, Sweany SK, et al. Total respiratory system inertance and its gas and tissue components in normal and obese men. J Clin Invest 1964;43:503–9.

34. Lopata M, Onal E. Mass loading, sleep apnea, and the pathogenesis of obesity hypoventilation. Am Rev Respir Dis 1982;126:640–5.

35. Waltemath CL, Bergman NA. Respiratory compliance in obese patients. Anesthesiology 1974;41: 84–5.

36. Lazarus R, Sparrow D, Weiss ST. Effects of obesity and fat distribution on ventilatory function. The normative aging study. Chest 1997;111:891–8.

37. Rubinstein I, Zamel N, DuBarry L, et al. Airflow limitation in morbidly obese, nonsmoking men. Ann Intern Med 1990;112:828–32.

38. King GG, Brown NJ, Diba C, et al. The effects of body weight on airway caliber. Eur Respir J 2005; 25:896–901.

39. McLachlan CR, Poulton R, Car G, et al. Adiposity, asthma, and airway inflammation. J Allergy Clin Immunol 2007;119:634–9.

40. Beuther DA, Sutherland ER. Overweight, obesity, and incident asthma. A meta-analysis of prospective epidemiologic studies. Am J Respir Crit Care Med 2007;175:661–6.

41. Sampson MG, Grassino AE. Load compensation in obese patients during quiet tidal breathing. J Appl Phys 1983;55:1269–76.

42. Rapoport DM, Garay SM, Epstein H, et al. Hypercapnia in the obstructive sleep apnea syndrome. A reevaluation of the "Pickwickian syndrome.". Chest 1986;89:627–35.

43. Lin CC. Effect of nasal CPAP on ventilatory drive in normocapnic and hypercapnic patients with obstructive sleep apnoea syndrome. Eur Respir J 1994;7:2005–10.

44. Rapoport DM, Norman RG, Goldring RM. CO_2 homeostasis during periodic breathing: predictions from a computer model. J Appl Phys 1993;75:2302–9.

45. Berger KI, Ayappa I, Sorkin IB, et al. CO_2 homeostasis during periodic breathing in obstructive sleep apnea. J Appl Phys 2000;88:257–64.

46. Berger KI, Ayappa I, Sorkin IB, et al. Postevent ventilation as a function of CO_2 load during respiratory events in obstructive sleep apnea. J Appl Phys 2002;93:917–24.

47. Ayappa I, Berger KI, Norman RG, et al. Hypercapnia and ventilatory periodicity in obstructive sleep apnea syndrome. Am J Respir Crit Care Med 2002;166:1112–5.

48. Berger KI, Norman RG, Ayappa I, et al. Potential mechanism for transition between acute hypercapnia during sleep to chronic hypercapnia during wakefulness in obstructive sleep apnea. Adv Exp Med Biol 2008;605:431–6.

49. Kessler R, Chaouat A, Schinkewitch P, et al. The obesity-hypoventilation syndrome revisited. A prospective study of 34 consecutive cases. Chest 2001;120:369–76.

50. Berger KI, Ayappa I, Chatr-Amontri B, et al. Obesity hypoventilation syndrome as a spectrum of respiratory disturbances during sleep. Chest 2001;120:1231–8.

51. Klein S, Coppack SW, Mohamed-Ali V, et al. Adipose tissue leptin production and plasma Leptin kinetics in humans. Diabetes 1996;45:984–7.

52. O'Donnell CP, Schaub CD, Haines AS, et al. Leptin prevents respiratory depression in obesity. Am J Respir Crit Care Med 1999;159:1477–84.

53. Phipps PR, Starritt E, Caterson I, et al. Association of serum leptin with hypoventilation in human obesity. Thorax 2001;57:75–6.

54. Shimura R, Tatsumi K, Nakamura A, et al. Fat accumulation, leptin, and hypercapnia in obstructive sleep apnea-hypopnea syndrome. Chest 2005; 127:543–9.

55. Makinodan K, Yoshikawa M, Fukuoka A, et al. Effect of serum leptin levels on hypercapnic ventilatory response in obstructive sleep apnea. Respiration 2008;75:257–64.

56. Yee B, Cheung J, Phipps P, et al. Treatment of obesity hypoventilation syndrome and serum leptin. Respiration 2006;73:209–12.

57. Redolfi S, La Piana G, Spandrio S, et al. Long-term non-invasive ventilation increases chemosensitivity and leptin in obesity-hypoventilation syndrome. Respir Med 2007;101:1191–5.

58. Tirlapur VG, Mir MA. Effect of low calorie intake on abnormal pulmonary physiology in patients with chronic hypercapneic respiratory failure. Am J Med 1984;77:987–94.

59. Sugerman HJ, Fairman RP, Sood RK, et al. Long-term effects of gastric surgery for treating respiratory insufficiency of obesity. Am J Clin Nutr 1992; 55:597S–601S.

60. Boone KA, Cullen JJ, Mason EE, et al. Impact of vertical banded gastroplasty on respiratory insufficiency of severe obesity. Obes Surg 1996;6: 454–8.

61. Martí-Valeri C, Sabaté A, Masdevall C, et al. Improvement of associated respiratory problems in morbidly obese patients after open Roux-en-Y gastric bypass. Obes Surg 2007;17:1102–10.

62. The Longitudinal Assessment of Bariatric Surgery (LABS) Consortium. Perioperative safety in the longitudinal assessment of bariatric surgery. N Engl J Med 2009;361:445–54.

63. Tice JA, Karliner L, Walsh J, et al. Gastric banding or bypass? A systematic review comparing the two most popular bariatric procedures. Am J Med 2008;121:885–93.

64. Sullivan CE, Berthon-Jones M, Issa FG. Remission of severe obesity-hypoventilation syndrome after short-term treatment during sleep with nasal continuous positive airway pressure. Am Rev Respir Dis 1983;128:177–81.

65. Berthon-Jones M, Sullivan CE. Time course of change in ventilatory response to CO_2 with long-term CPAP therapy for obstructive sleep apnea. Am Rev Respir Dis 1987;135:144–7.

66. Shivaram U, Cash ME, Beal A. Nasal continuous positive airway pressure in decompensated hypercapnic respiratory failure as a complication of sleep apnea. Chest 1993;104:770–4.

67. Piper AJ, Wang D, Yee BJ, et al. Randomized trial of CPAP vs. bilevel support in the treatment of obesity hypoventilation syndrome without severe nocturnal desaturation. Thorax 2008;63: 395–401.

68. Pérez de Llano LA, Golpe R, Ortiz Piquer M, et al. Short-term and long-term effects of nasal intermittent positive pressure ventilation in patients with obesity-hypoventilation syndrome. Chest 2005; 128:587–94.

69. Pérez de Llano LA, Golpe R, Ortiz Piquer M, et al. Clinical heterogeneity among patients with obesity hypoventilation syndrome: therapeutic implications. Respiration 2008;75:34–9.

70. Masa JF, Celli BR, Riesco JA, et al. The obesity hypoventilation syndrome can be treated with noninvasive mechanical ventilation. Chest 2001; 119:1102–7.

71. de Lucas-Ramos P, de Miguel-Diez J, Santacruz-Siminiani A, et al. Benefits at 1 year of nocturnal intermittent positive pressure ventilation in patients with obesity-hypoventilation syndrome. Respir Med 2004;98:961–7.

72. Chouri-Pontarollo N, Borel JC, Tamisier R, et al. Impaired objective daytime vigilance in obesity-hypoventilation syndrome. Impact of noninvasive ventilation. Chest 2007;131:148–55.

73. Budweiser S, Riedl SG, Jörres RA, et al. Mortality and prognostic factors in patients with obesity-hypoventilation syndrome undergoing noninvasive ventilation. J Intern Med 2007;261:375–83.

74. Piper AJ, Sullivan CE. Effects of short-term NIPPV in the treatment of patients with severe obstructive sleep apnea and hypercapnia. Chest 1994;105: 434–40.

75. Janssens J-P, Metzger M, Sforza E. Impact of volume targeting on efficacy of bi-level non-invasive ventilation and sleep in obesity-hypoventilation. Respir Med 2009;103:165–72.

76. Storre JH, Seuthe B, Fiechter R, et al. Average volume-assured pressure support in obesity hypoventilation. A randomized crossover trial. Chest 2006;130:815–21.

77. Brown LK. Filling in the gaps: the role of non-invasive adaptive servo-ventilation for heart failure-related central sleep apnea. Chest 2008;134:4–7.

78. Zwillich CW, Natalino MR, Sutton FD, et al. Effects of progesterone on chemosensitivity in normal men. J Lab Clin Med 1978;92:262–9.

79. Sutton FD, Zwillich CW, Creagh CE, et al. Progesterone for outpatient treatment of Pickwickian syndrome. Ann Intern Med 1975;83:476–9.

80. Zavorsky GS, Murias JM, Kim DJ, et al. Waist-to-hip ratio is associated with pulmonary gas exchange in the morbidly obese. Chest 2007;131:362–7.

81. Gilchrist JM. Overview of neuromuscular disorders affecting respiratory function. Semin Respir Crit Care Med 2002;23:191–200.

82. Brown LK. Sleep disordered breathing in neurologic disease. Clin Pulm Med 1996;3:22–35.

83. Mehta S. Neuromuscular disease causing acute respiratory failure. Respir Care 2006;51:1016–23.

84. Braun NM, Arora NS, Rochester DF. Respiratory muscle and pulmonary function in polymyositis and other proximal myopathies. Thorax 1983;38: 616–23.

85. Hukins CA, Hillman DR. Daytime predictors of sleep hypoventilation in Duchenne muscular dystrophy. Am J Respir Crit Care Med 2000;161: 166–70.

86. Fallat RJ, Jewitt B, Bass M, et al. Spirometry in amyotrophic lateral sclerosis. Arch Neurol 1979; 36:74–80.

87. Fromageot C, Lofaso F, Annane D, et al. Supine fall in lung volumes in the assessment of diaphragmatic weakness in neuromuscular disease. Arch Phys Med Rehabil 2001;82:123–8.

88. Lechtzin N, Wiener CM, Shade DM, et al. Spirometry in the supine position improves the detection of diaphragmatic weakness in patients with amyotrophic lateral sclerosis. Chest 2002;121:436–42.

89. Black LF, Hyatt RE. Maximum respiratory pressures: normal values and relationship to age and sex. Am Rev Respir Dis 1969;99:696–702.

90. Wilson SH, Cooke NT, Edwards RHT, et al. Predicted normal values for maximal respiratory pressures in Caucasian adults and children. Thorax 1984;39:535–8.

91. Rochester DF, Esau SA. Assessment of ventilatory function in patients with neuromuscular disease. Clin Chest Med 1994;15:751–63.

92. Lawn ND, Fletcher DD, Henderson RD, et al. Anticipating mechanical ventilation in Guillain-Barré syndrome. Arch Neurol 2001;58:893–8.

93. Shiffman PL, Belsh JM. Pulmonary function at diagnosis of amyotrophic lateral sclerosis: rate of deterioration. Chest 1993;103:508–13.

94. Szeinberg A, Tabachnik E, Rashed N, et al. Cough capacity in patients with muscular dystrophy. Chest 1988;94:1232–5.

95. Polkey MI, Green M, Moxham J. Measurement of respiratory muscle strength. Thorax 1995;50: 1131–5.

96. Fitting JW, Paillex R, Hirt L, et al. Sniff nasal pressure: a sensitive respiratory test to assess progression of amyotrophic lateral sclerosis. Ann Neurol 1999;46:887–93.

97. Stefanutti D, Benoist MR, Scheinmann P, et al. Usefulness of sniff nasal pressure in patients with neuromuscular or skeletal disorders. Am J Respir Crit Care Med 2000;162:1507–11.

98. Terzi N, Orlikowski D, Fermanian C, et al. Measuring inspiratory muscle strength in neuromuscular disease: one test or two? Eur Respir J 2008;31:93–8.

99. Koulouris N, Mulvey DA, Laroche CM, et al. The measurement of inspiratory muscle strength by sniff esophageal, nasopharyngeal, and mouth pressure. Am Rev Respir Dis 1989;139:641–6.

100. Miller RG, Jackson CE, Kasarskis EJ, et al. Practice parameter update: the care of the patient with amyotrophic lateral sclerosis: drug, nutritional, and respiratory therapies (an evidence-based review). Neurology 2009;73:1218–26.

101. Similowski T, Mehiri S, Duguet A, et al. Comparison of magnetic and electrical phrenic nerve stimulation in assessment of phrenic nerve conduction time. J Appl Phys 1997;82:1190–9.

102. Pinto S, Turkman A, Pinto A, et al. Predicting respiratory insufficiency in amyotrophic lateral sclerosis: the role of phrenic nerve studies. Clin Neurophysiol 2009;120:941–6.

103. Black LF, Hyatt RE. Maximal static respiratory pressures in generalized neuromuscular disease. Am Rev Respir Dis 1971;103:641–50.

104. Vincken W, Elleker MG, Cosio MG. Determinants of respiratory muscle weakness in stable neuromuscular disorders. Am J Med 1987;82:53–8.

105. Annane D, Orlikowski D, Chevret S, et al. Nocturnal mechanical ventilation for chronic hypoventilation in patients with neuromuscular and chest wall disorders. Cochrane Database Syst Rev 2007;(4):CD001941.

106. Finsterer J. Cardiopulmonary support in Duchenne muscular dystrophy. Lung 2006;184:205–15.

107. Piepers S, van den Berg JP, Kalmijn S, et al. Effect of non-invasive ventilation on survival, quality of life, respiratory function and cognition: a review of the literature. Amyotroph Lateral Scler 2006;7:195–200.

108. Seneviratne J, Mandrekar J, Wijdicks EF, et al. Noninvasive ventilation in myasthenic crisis. Arch Neurol 2008;65:54–8.

109. Wijdicks EF, Roy TK. BiPAP in early Guillain-Barré syndrome may fail. Can J Neurol Sci 2006;33:105–6.

110. Nogués MA, Benarroch E. Abnormalities of respiratory control and the respiratory motor unit. Neurologist 2008;14:273–88.

111. Nogués MA, Roncoroni AJ, Benarroch E. Breathing control in neurological diseases. Clin Auton Res 2002;12:440–9.

112. Boor JW, Johnson RJ, Canales L, et al. Reversible paralysis of automatic respiration in multiple sclerosis. Arch Neurol 1977;34:686–9.

113. Rizvi SS, Ishikawa S, Faling LJ, et al. Defect in automatic respiration in a case of multiple sclerosis. Am J Med 1974;56:433–6.

114. Devereaux MW, Keane JR, Davis RL. Automatic respiratory failure associated with infarction of the medulla. Arch Neurol 1973;29:46–52.

115. Beal MF, Richardson EP Jr, Brandstetter R, et al. Localized brainstem ischemic damage and Ondine's curse after near-drowning. Neurology 1983;33:717–21.

116. Levin BE, Margolis G. Acute failure of automatic respirations secondary to a unilateral brainstem infarct. Ann Neurol 1977;1:583–6.

117. Tsara V, Serasli E, Kimiskidis V, et al. Acute respiratory failure and sleep-disordered breathing in Arnold-Chiari malformation. Clin Neurol Neurosurg 2005;107:521–4.

118. Rabec C, Laurent G, Baudouin N, et al. Central sleep apnoea in Arnold-Chiari malformation: evidence of pathophysiological heterogeneity. Eur Respir J 1998;12:1482–5.

119. Pollack IF, Kinnunen D, Albright AL. The effect of early craniocervical decompression on functional outcome in neonates and young infants with myelodysplasia and symptomatic Chiari II malformations: results from a prospective series. Neurosurgery 1996;38:703–10.

120. Swaminathan S, Paton JY, Ward SL, et al. Abnormal control of ventilation in adolescents with myelodysplasia. J Pediatr 1989;115:898–903.

121. Weese-Mayer DE, Brouillette RT, Naidich TP, et al. Magnetic resonance imaging and computerized tomography in central hypoventilation. Am Rev Respir Dis 1988;137:393–8.

122. Chung HD, DeMello DE, D'Souza N, et al. Infantile hypoventilation syndrome, neurenteric cyst, and syringobulbia. Neurology 1982;32:441–4.

123. Glass GA, Josephs KA, Ahlskog JE. Respiratory insufficiency as the primary presenting symptom of multiple-system atrophy. Arch Neurol 2006;63:978–81.

124. Cormican LJ, Higgins S, Davidson AC, et al. Multiple system atrophy presenting as central sleep apnea. Eur Respir J 2004;24:323–5.

125. Dalmau J. Limbic encephalitis and variants related to neuronal cell membrane autoantigens. Rinsho Shinkeigaku 2008;48:871–4.

126. Russell-Jones DL, Treacher DF, Lenicker HM, et al. Central hypoventilation in a seven year old child following pertussis treated with negative pressure ventilation. Postgrad Med J 1989;65:768–70.

127. White DP, Miller F, Erickson RW. Sleep apnea and nocturnal hypoventilation after western equine encephalitis. Am Rev Respir Dis 1983;127:132–3.

128. Reid AH, McCall S, Henry JM, et al. Experimenting on the past: the enigma of von Economo's encephalitis lethargica. J Neuropathol Exp Neurol 2001;60:663–70.

129. Casals J, Elizan TS, Yahr MD. Postencephalitic parkinsonism- a review. J Neural Transm 1998;105:645–76.

130. Strieder DJ, Baker WG, Baringer JR, et al. Chronic hypoventilation of central origin. A case with encephalitis lethargica and Parkinson's syndrome. Am Rev Respir Dis 1967;96:501–7.

131. Muirhead A, Conner A. The assessment of lung function in children with scoliosis. J Bone Joint Surg Br 1985;67:699–702.

132. Conti G, Rocco M, Antonelli M, et al. Respiratory system mechanics in the early phase of acute respiratory failure due to severe kyphoscoliosis. Intensive Care Med 1997;23:539–44.

133. Phillips MS, Kinnear WJ, Shneerson JM. Late sequelae of pulmonary tuberculosis treated by thoracoplasty. Thorax 1987;42:445–51.

134. Sahin G, Guler H, Calikoglu M, et al. [A comparison of respiratory muscle strength, pulmonary function tests and endurance in patients with early and late stage ankylosing spondylitis]. Z Rheumatol 2006; 65:535–8, 540 [in German].

135. Camiciottoli G, Trapani S, Ermini M, et al. Pulmonary function in children affected by juvenile spondyloarthropathy. J Rheumatol 1999;26: 1382–6.

136. Miles SE, Sandrini A, Johnson AR, et al. Clinical consequences of asbestos-related diffuse pleural thickening: a review. J Occup Med Toxicol 2008;3:20.

137. Miller A, Teirstein AS, Selikoff IJ. Ventilatory failure due to asbestos pleurisy. Am J Med 1983;75:911–9.

138. Lisboa C, Moreno R, Fava M, et al. Inspiratory muscle function in patients with severe kyphoscoliosis. Am Rev Respir Dis 1985;132:48–52.

139. Giordano A, Fuso L, Galli M, et al. Evaluation of pulmonary ventilation and diaphragmatic movement in idiopathic scoliosis using radioaerosol ventilation scintigraphy. Nucl Med Commun 1997; 18:105–11.

140. Chu WC, Li AM, Ng BK, et al. Dynamic magnetic resonance imaging in assessing lung volumes, chest wall, and diaphragm motions in adolescent idiopathic scoliosis versus normal controls. Spine (Phila Pa) 1976;31:2243–9.

141. Kotani T, Minami S, Takahashi K, et al. An analysis of chest wall and diaphragm motions in patients with idiopathic scoliosis using dynamic breathing MRI. Spine (Phila Pa 1976) 2004;29:298–302.

142. Phillips MS, Miller MR, Kinnear WJ, et al. Importance of airflow obstruction after thoracoplasty. Thorax 1987;42:348–52.

143. Clinical indications for noninvasive positive pressure ventilation in chronic respiratory failure due to restrictive lung disease, COPD, and nocturnal hypoventilation—a consensus conference report. Chest 1999;116:521–34.

144. Hill NS, Eveloff SE, Carlisle CC, et al. Efficacy of nocturnal nasal ventilation in patients with restrictive thoracic disease. Am Rev Respir Dis 1992; 145:365–71.

145. Gonzales C, Ferris G, Diaz J, et al. Kyphoscoliotic ventilatory insufficiency: effects of long-term intermittent positive-pressure ventilation. Chest 2003; 124:857–62.

146. Buyse B, Meersseman W, Demedts M. Treatment of chronic respiratory failure in kyphoscoliosis: oxygen or ventilation? Eur Respir J 2003;22:525–8.

147. Jackson M, Smith I, King M, et al. Long term non-invasive domiciliary assisted ventilation for respiratory failure following thoracoplasty. Thorax 1994;49: 915–9.

148. Shneerson JM, Simonds AK. Noninvasive ventilation for chest wall and neuromuscular disorders. Eur Respir J 2002;20:480–7.

149. Schönhofer B, Barchfeld T, Wenzel M, et al. Long term effects of non-invasive mechanical ventilation on pulmonary haemodynamics in patients with chronic respiratory failure. Thorax 2001;56:524–8.

150. Hogg JC. Lung structure and function in COPD. Int J Tuberc Lung Dis 2008;12:467–79.

151. Hogg JC. Pathophysiology of airflow limitation in chronic obstructive pulmonary disease. Lancet 2004;364:709–21.

152. Pistolesi M, Camiciottoli G, Paoletti M, et al. Identification of a predominant COPD phenotype in clinical practice. Respir Med 2008;102:367–76.

153. Friedlander AL, Lynch D, Dyar LA, et al. Phenotypes of chronic obstructive pulmonary disease. COPD 2007;4:355–84.

154. Makita H, Nasuhara Y, Nagai K, et al. Characterization of phenotypes based on severity of emphysema in chronic obstructive pulmonary disease. Thorax 2007;62:932–7.

155. Filley GF, Beckwitt HJ, Reeves JT, et al. Chronic obstructive bronchopulmonary disease. II. Oxygen transport in two clinical types. Am J Med 1968;44: 26–38.

156. Calverley PM. Respiratory failure in chronic obstructive pulmonary disease. Eur Respir J 2003;47(Suppl):26s–30s.

157. Koulouris NG, Latsi P, Dimitroulis J, et al. Noninvasive measurement of mean alveolar carbon dioxide tension and Bohr's dead space during tidal breathing. Eur Respir J 2001;17:1167–74.

158. Fernandes M, Cukier A, Ambrosino N, et al. Respiratory pattern, thoracoabdominal motion and ventilation in chronic airway obstruction. Monaldi Arch Chest Dis 2007;67:209–16.

159. Baldwin ED, Cournand A, Richards DW Jr. Pulmonary insufficiency; physiological classification, clinical methods of analysis, standard values in normal subjects. Medicine (Baltimore) 1948;27:243–78.

160. Bégin P, Grassino A. Inspiratory muscle dysfunction and chronic hypercapnia in chronic obstructive pulmonary disease. Am Rev Respir Dis 1991;143: 905–12.

161. Montes de Oca M, Celli BR. Mouth occlusion pressure, CO_2 response and hypercapnia in severe chronic obstructive pulmonary disease. Eur Respir J 1998;12:666–71.

162. Gorini M, Misuri G, Corrado A, et al. Breathing pattern and carbon dioxide retention in severe chronic obstructive pulmonary disease. Thorax 1996;51:677–83.

163. Tobin MJ, Laghi F, Brochard L. Role of the respiratory muscles in acute respiratory failure of COPD: lessons from weaning failure. J Appl Phys 2009; 107:962–70.

164. De Troyer A, Wilson TA. Effect of acute inflation on the mechanics of the inspiratory muscles. J Appl Phys 2009;107:315–23.

165. King DA, Cordova F, Scharf SM. Nutritional aspects of chronic obstructive pulmonary disease. Proc Am Thorac Soc 2008;5:519–23.

166. Ferreira IM, Brooks D, Lacasse Y, et al. Nutritional supplementation for stable chronic obstructive pulmonary disease. Cochrane Database Syst Rev 2005;(2):CD000998.

167. van Balkom RH, van der Heijden HF, van Herwaarden CL, et al. Corticosteroid-induced myopathy of the respiratory muscles. Neth J Med 1994;45:114–22.

168. Robinson TD, Freiberg DB, Regnis JA, et al. The role of hypoventilation and ventilation-perfusion redistribution in oxygen-induced hypercapnia during acute exacerbations of chronic obstructive pulmonary disease. Am J Respir Crit Care Med 2000;161:1524–9.

169. Flenley DC. Sleep in chronic obstructive lung disease. Clin Chest Med 1985;6:651–61.

170. Bednarek M, Plywaczewski R, Jonczak L, et al. There is no relationship between chronic obstructive pulmonary disease and obstructive sleep apnea syndrome: a population study. Respiration 2005;72:142–9.

171. Bradley TD, Rutherford R, Lue F, et al. Role of diffuse airway obstruction in the hypercapnia of obstructive sleep apnea. Am Rev Respir Dis 1986;134:920–4.

172. Fletcher EC, Shah A, Qian W, et al. "Near miss" death in obstructive sleep apnea: a critical care syndrome. Crit Care Med 1991;19:1158–64.

173. Report of the Medical Research Council Working Party. Long term domiciliary oxygen therapy in chronic hypoxic cor pulmonale complicating chronic bronchitis and emphysema. Lancet 1981;1:681–6.

174. Wijkstra PJ, Lacasse Y, Guyatt GH. A meta-analysis of nocturnal noninvasive positive pressure ventilation in patients with stable COPD. Chest 2003; 124:337–43.

175. Clini E, Sturani C, Rossi A, et al. The Italian multicentre study on noninvasive ventilation in chronic obstructive pulmonary disease patients. Eur Respir J 2002; 20:529–38.

176. Clini EM, Magni G, Crisafulli E, et al. Home noninvasive mechanical ventilation and long-term oxygen therapy in stable hypercapnic chronic obstructive pulmonary disease patients: comparison of costs. Respiration 2009;77:44–50.

177. Dellweg D, Schonhofer B, Haidl PM, et al. Short-term effect of controlled instead of assisted noninvasive ventilation in chronic respiratory failure due to chronic obstructive pulmonary disease. Respir Care 2007;52:1734–40.

178. Budweiser S, Heinemann F, Meyer K, et al. Weight gain in cachectic COPD patients receiving noninvasive positive-pressure ventilation. Respir Care 2006;51:126–32.

179. Windisch W, Haenel M, Storre JH, et al. High-intensity non-invasive positive pressure ventilation for stable hypercapnic COPD. Int J Med Sci 2009;6: 72–6.

180. Windisch W, Kostić S, Dreher M, et al. Outcome of patients with stable COPD receiving controlled noninvasive positive pressure ventilation aimed at a maximal reduction of $Pa(CO_2)$. Chest 2005;128: 657–62.

181. van 't Hul PT, Kwakkel G, Gosselink R. The acute effects of noninvasive ventilatory support during exercise on exercise endurance and dyspnea in patients with chronic obstructive pulmonary disease. A systematic review. J Cardiopulm Rehabil 2002;22:290–7.

182. Dreher M, Doncheva E, Schwoerer A, et al. Preserving oxygenation during walking in severe chronic obstructive pulmonary disease: noninvasive ventilation versus oxygen therapy. Respiration 2009;78:154–60.

183. Shade D Jr, Cordova F, Lando Y, et al. Relationship between resting hypercapnia and physiologic parameters before and after lung volume reduction surgery in severe chronic obstructive pulmonary disease. Am J Respir Crit Care Med 1999;159: 1405–11.

184. Tiong LU, Davies R, Gibson PG, et al. Lung volume reduction surgery for diffuse emphysema. Cochrane Database Syst Rev 2006;(4):CD001001.

185. Criner GJ, Sternberg AL. National emphysema treatment trial. The major outcomes of lung volume reduction surgery in severe emphysema. Proc Am Thorac Soc 2008;5:393–405.

186. Mitsui K, Kurokawa Y, Kaiwa Y, et al. Thoracoscopic lung volume reduction surgery for pulmonary emphysema patients with severe hypercapnia. Jpn J Thorac Cardiovasc Surg 2001;49:481–8.

187. Quon BS, Gan WQ, Sin DD. Contemporary management of acute exacerbations of COPD: a systematic review and metaanalysis. Chest 2008;133:756–66.

188. Ram FS, Picot J, Lightowler J, et al. Non-invasive positive pressure ventilation for treatment of respiratory failure due to exacerbations of chronic obstructive pulmonary disease. Cochrane Database Syst Rev 2004;(3):CD004104.

189. Keenan SP, Sinuff T, Cook DJ, et al. Which patients with acute exacerbation of chronic obstructive pulmonary disease benefit from noninvasive positive-pressure ventilation? A systematic review of the literature. Ann Intern Med 2003;138:861–70.

190. Moore WC, Meyers DA, Wenzel SE, et al. Identification of asthma phenotypes using cluster analysis in the severe asthma research program. Am J Respir Crit Care Med 2010;181:315–23.

191. Meduri GU, Cook TR, Turner RE, et al. Noninvasive positive pressure ventilation in status asthmaticus. Chest 1996;110:767–74.

192. Fernández MM, Villagrá A, Blanch L, et al. Noninvasive mechanical ventilation in status asthmaticus. Intensive Care Med 2001;27:486–92.

193. Carroll CL, Schramm CM. Noninvasive positive pressure ventilation for the treatment of status asthmaticus in children. Ann Allergy Asthma Immunol 2006;96:454–9.

194. Beers SL, Abramo TJ, Bracken A, et al. Bilevel positive airway pressure in the treatment of status asthmaticus in pediatrics. Am J Emerg Med 2007;25:6–9.

195. Soroksky A, Stav D, Shpirer I. A pilot prospective, randomized, placebo-controlled trial of bilevel positive airway pressure in acute asthmatic attack. Chest 2003;123:1018–25.

196. Soma T, Hino M, Kida K, et al. A prospective and randomized study for improvement of acute asthma by non-invasive positive pressure ventilation (NPPV). Intern Med 2008;47:493–501.

197. Keenan SP, Mehta S. Noninvasive ventilation for patients presenting with acute respiratory failure: the randomized controlled trials. Respir Care 2009;54:116–26.

198. Ram FS, Wellington S, Rowe B, et al. Non-invasive positive pressure ventilation for treatment of respiratory failure due to severe acute exacerbations of asthma. Cochrane Database Syst Rev 2005;(3): CD004360.

199. Ting H, Sun XG, Chuang ML, et al. A noninvasive assessment of pulmonary perfusion abnormality in patients with primary pulmonary hypertension. Chest 2001;119:824–32.

200. Nava S, Rubini F. Lung and chest wall mechanics in ventilated patients with end stage idiopathic pulmonary fibrosis. Thorax 1999;54:390–5.

201. Strickland NH, Hughes JM, Hart DA, et al. Cause of regional ventilation-perfusion mismatching in patients with idiopathic pulmonary fibrosis: a combined CT and scintigraphic study. AJR Am J Roentgenol 1993;161:719–25.

202. Renzi G, Milic-Emili J, Grassino AE. Breathing pattern in sarcoidosis and idiopathic pulmonary fibrosis. Ann N Y Acad Sci 1986;465:482–90.

203. Saydain G, Islam A, Afessa B, et al. Outcome of patients with idiopathic pulmonary fibrosis admitted to the intensive care unit. Am J Respir Crit Care Med 2002;166:839–42.

204. McNicholas WT, Coffey M, Fitzgerald MX. Ventilation and gas exchange during sleep in patients with interstitial lung disease. Thorax 1986;41: 777–82.

205. Lancaster LH, Mason WR, Parnell JA, et al. Obstructive sleep apnea is common in idiopathic pulmonary fibrosis. Chest 2009;136:772–8.

206. Al-Hameed FM, Sharma S. Outcome of patients admitted to the intensive care unit for acute exacerbation of idiopathic pulmonary fibrosis. Can Respir J 2004;11:117–22.

207. Koschel D, Handzhiev S, Wiedemann B, et al. Acute effects of NPPV in interstitial lung disease with chronic hypercapnic respiratory failure. Respir Med 2010;104:291–5.

208. Knowles MR, Boucher RC. Mucus clearance as a primary innate defense mechanism for mammalian airways. J Clin Invest 2002;109: 571–7.

209. Gibson RL, Burns JL, Ramsey BW. Pathophysiology and management of pulmonary infections in cystic fibrosis. Am J Respir Crit Care Med 2003; 168:919–51.

210. Aris RM, Renner JB, Winders AD, et al. Increased rate of fractures and severe kyphosis: sequelae of living into adulthood with cystic fibrosis. J Clin Endocrinol Metab 2005;90:1888–986.

211. Ravilly S, Robinson W, Suresh S, et al. Chronic pain in cystic fibrosis. Pediatrics 1996;98:741–7.

212. Milross MA, Piper AJ, Dobbin CJ, et al. Sleep disordered breathing in cystic fibrosis. Sleep Med Rev 2004;8:295–308.

213. Fraser KL, Tullis DE, Sasson Z, et al. Pulmonary hypertension and cardiac function in adult cystic fibrosis. Chest 1999;115:1321–8.

214. Flume PA, Mogayzel PJ Jr, Robinson KA, et al. Cystic fibrosis pulmonary guidelines: treatment of pulmonary exacerbations. Am J Respir Crit Care Med 2009;180:802–8.

215. Flume PA, Robinson KA, O'Sullivan BP, et al. Cystic fibrosis pulmonary guidelines: airway clearance therapies. Respir Care 2009;54:522–37.

216. Stallings VA, Stark LJ, Robinson KA, et al. Evidence-based practice recommendations for nutrition-related management of children and adults with cystic fibrosis and pancreatic insufficiency: results of a systematic review. J Am Diet Assoc 2008;108:832–9.

217. Flume PA, O'Sullivan BP, Robinson KA, et al. Cystic fibrosis pulmonary guidelines: chronic medications for maintenance of lung health. Am J Respir Crit Care Med 2007;176:957–69.

218. Nathan SD. Lung transplantation: disease-specific considerations for referral. Chest 2005; 127:1006–16.

219. Yankaskas JR, Marshall BC, Sufian B, et al. Cystic fibrosis adult care: consensus conference report. Chest 2004;125(Suppl):1S–39S.

220. Zinman R, Corey M, Coates AL, et al. Nocturnal home oxygen in the treatment of hypoxemic cystic fibrosis patients. J Pediatr 1989;114:368–77.

221. Serra A, Polese G, Braggion C, et al. Non-invasive proportional assist and pressure support ventilation in patients with cystic fibrosis and chronic respiratory failure. Thorax 2002;57:50–4.

222. Gozal D. Nocturnal ventilatory support in patients with cystic fibrosis: comparison with supplemental oxygen. Eur Respir J 1997;10:1999–2003.

223. Young AC, Wilson JW, Kotsimbos TC, et al. Randomized placebo controlled trial of non-invasive ventilation for hypercapnia in cystic fibrosis. Thorax 2008;63:72–7.

224. Fauroux B, Le Roux E, Ravilly S, et al. Long-term noninvasive ventilation in patients with cystic fibrosis. Respiration 2008;76:168–74.

225. Moran F, Bradley JM, Piper AJ. Non-invasive ventilation for cystic fibrosis. Cochrane Database Syst Rev 2009;(1):CD002769.

226. Mellins RB, Balfour HH Jr, Turino GM, et al. Failure of autonomic control of ventilation (Ondine's curse). Medicine (Baltimore) 1970;49:487–526.

227. Severinghaus JW, Mitchell RA. Ondine's curse: failure of respiratory center automaticity while awake. J Clin Res 1962;10:122.

228. Nannapaneni R, Behari S, Todd NV, et al. Retracing "Ondine's Curse". Neurosurgery 2005;57:354–63.

229. Trang H, Dehan M, Beaufils F, et al. The French congenital central hypoventilation syndrome registry: general data, phenotype, and genotype. Chest 2005;127:72–9.

230. Bolande RP. The neurocristopathies: a unifying concept of disease arising in neural crest maldevelopment. Hum Pathol 1974;5:409–29.

231. Amiel J, Laudier B, Attié-Bitach T, et al. Polyalanine expansion and frameshift mutations of the paired-like homeobox gene PHOX2B in congenital central hypoventilation syndrome. Nat Genet 2003;33:459–61.

232. Weese-Mayer DE, Berry-Kravis EM. Genetics of congenital central hypoventilation syndrome: lessons from a seemingly orphan disease. Am J Respir Crit Care Med 2004;170:16–21.

233. Berry-Kravis EM, Zhou L, Rand CM, et al. Congenital central hypoventilation syndrome PHOX2B mutations and phenotype. Am J Respir Crit Care Med 2006;174:1139–44.

234. Hamilton J, Bodurtha JN. Congenital central hypoventilation syndrome and Hirschsprung's disease in half-sibs. J Med Genet 1989;26:272–4.

235. Gaultier C, Amiel J, Dauger S, et al. Genetics and early disturbances of breathing control. Pediatr Res 2004;55:729–33.

236. Trochet D, O'Brien LM, Gozal D. PHOX2B genotype allows for prediction of tumor risk in congenital central hypoventilation syndrome. Am J Hum Genet 2005;76:421–6.

237. Antic NA, Malow BA, Lange N, et al. PHOX2B mutation-confirmed congenital central hypoventilation syndrome: presentation in adulthood. Am J Respir Crit Care Med 2006;174:923–7.

238. Weese-Mayer DE, Shannon DC, Keens TG, et al. Idiopathic congenital central hypoventilation syndrome: diagnosis and management. Am J Respir Crit Care Med 1999;160:368–73.

239. Gozal D, Gaultier C. Proceedings from the first international symposium on the congenital central hypoventilation syndrome. Pediatr Pulmonol 1997;23:133–68.

240. Dejhalla M, Parton P, Golombek SG. Case report of Haddad syndrome in a newborn: congenital central hypoventilation syndrome and Hirschsprung's disease. J Perinatol 2006;26:259–60.

241. Gaultier C, Trang-Pham H, Praud JP, et al. Cardiorespiratory control during sleep in the congenital central hypoventilation syndrome. Pediatr Pulmonol 1997;23:140–2.

242. Paton J, Swaminathan S, Sargent C, et al. Hypoxic and hypercapnic ventilatory responses in awake children with congenital central hypoventilation syndrome. Am Rev Respir Dis 1989;140:368–72.

243. Paton J, Swaminathan S, Sargent C, et al. Ventilatory response to exercise in children with congenital central hypoventilation syndrome. Am Rev Respir Dis 1993;147:1185–91.

244. Weese-Mayer DE, Silvestri JM, Huffman AD, et al. Case/control family study of autonomic nervous system dysfunction in idiopathic congenital central hypoventilation syndrome. Am J Med Genet 2001;100:237–45.

245. Chen ML, Keens TG. Congenital central hypoventilation syndrome: not just another rare disorder. Paediatr Respir Rev 2004;5:182–9.

246. Vanderlaan M, Holbrook CR, Wang M, et al. Epidemiologic survey of 196 patients with congenital central hypoventilation syndrome. Pediatr Pulmonol 2004;37:217–29.

247. Windisch W, Hennings E, Storre JH, et al. Long-term survival of a patient with congenital central hypoventilation syndrome despite the lack of continuous ventilatory support. Respiration 2004;71:195–8.

248. Lee P, Su YN, Yu CJ, et al. PHOX2B mutation-confirmed congenital central hypoventilation syndrome in a Chinese family: presentation from newborn to adulthood. Chest 2009;135:537–44.

249. Migliori C, Cavazza A, Motta M, et al. Early use of Nasal-BiPAP in two infants with congenital central hypoventilation syndrome. Acta Paediatr 2003;92:823–6.

250. Villa MP, Dotta A, Castello D, et al. Bi-level positive airway pressure (BiPAP) ventilation in an infant with central hypoventilation syndrome. Pediatr Pulmonol 1997;24:66–9.

251. Tibballs J, Henning RD. Noninvasive ventilatory strategies in the management of a newborn infant and three children with congenital central hypoventilation syndrome. Pediatr Pulmonol 2003;36:544–8.

252. Weese-Mayer DE, Silvestri JM, Kenny AS, et al. Diaphragm pacing with a quadripolar phrenic nerve electrode: an international study. Pacing Clin Electrophysiol 1996;19:1311–9.

253. Fauroux B, Lavis JF, Nicot F, et al. Facial side effects during noninvasive positive pressure ventilation in children. Intensive Care Med 2005;31:965–9.

Disorders of Glucose Metabolism in Sleep-disordered Breathing

Macy M.S. Lui, MRCP, Mary S.M. Ip, MD*

KEYWORDS
- Sleep-disordered breathing
- Disorders in glucose metabolism • Diabetes mellitus
- Insulin resistance • Obesity

Maintenance of plasma glucose concentration within narrow bounds is essential for health. Glucose originates from 3 sources: intestinal absorption of food, glycogenolysis from body storage, and gluconeogenesis chiefly from the liver. Insulin plays a pivotal role in glucose metabolism by inhibiting glycogenolysis and gluconeogenesis, increasing glucose disposal by peripheral tissues, and stimulating glycogen synthesis. Insulin surge comprises the major homeostatic mechanism of the body in the face of acute glucose load, in addition to basal maintenance of glucose supply to various organs. Diabetes mellitus (DM) consists of 2 major forms. Type 1 DM is caused by pancreatic β cell destruction resulting in insulin deficiency. Type 2 DM, which is the more common form in adults, is associated with obesity and characterized by insulin resistance with relatively deficient insulin secretion. The prevalence of type 2 DM is escalating globally alongside the sweeping pandemic of obesity.[1,2]

Type 2 DM develops in stages, with subclinical and clinically manifest phases. Impaired fasting glucose or glucose tolerance forms the intermediate stages between normal glucose tolerance and frank diabetes. Insulin resistance is a state in which a given concentration of insulin is associated with a subnormal glucose response and is present in most patients with type 2 diabetes.

DM is an established major risk factor for atherosclerosis. Deranged states of glucose metabolism, including insulin resistance, glucose intolerance, and type 2 DM, also form the key components of the metabolic syndrome, which is a constellation of cardiometabolic risk factors comprising hypertension, dyslipidemia, and central obesity.

Obstructive sleep apnea (OSA) is characterized by repetitive upper airway obstruction during sleep resulting in intermittent hypoxia and sleep fragmentation. OSA and disorders of glucose metabolism, both strongly associated with obesity and central obesity, not unexpectedly often occur concomitantly in the same individual. Given that recurrent events of sleep-disordered breathing (SDB) are followed by a cascade of pathophysiologic mechanisms that are also established or potential players in the cardiometabolic network, it is worthwhile to explore in depth the relationship between OSA and glucose homeostasis, beyond that of simple coexistence.

There are many tools for assessing glucose metabolism.[3–5] In the clinical setting, simple tests such as measurement of the blood levels of glycosylated hemoglobin (HbA1c), fasting or other spot glucose, fructosamine, and oral glucose tolerance test (OGTT) are used for diagnosis and monitoring of glucose intolerance or diabetic status. A continuous glucose monitoring system (CGMS) involves the use of a subcutaneous sensor to monitor 24-hour interstitial glucose fluctuations.

The quantification of insulin sensitivity/resistance is mainly used in research settings. The tools

Division of Respiratory Medicine and Critical Care Medicine, Department of Medicine, Queen Mary Hospital, The University of Hong Kong, Pokfulam Road, Hong Kong Special Administrative Region, Hong Kong, People's Republic of China
* Corresponding author.
E-mail address: msmip@hkucc.hku.hk

Clin Chest Med 31 (2010) 271–285
doi:10.1016/j.ccm.2010.02.001

range from simple measurements of fasting insulin and glucose levels, their mathematically derived indices such as homeostatic model assessment (HOMA), and other tests of a range of complexity, including intravenous glucose tolerance test, short insulin tolerance test, and hyperglycemic euglycemic clamps.[4] In the hyperinsulinemic euglycemic clamp study, considered the gold standard for assessing insulin sensitivity, insulin-induced glucose uptake is measured while the blood glucose concentration is maintained at a steady concentration via a glucose infusion, to avoid the confounding effects of counter-regulatory hormones such as epinephrine and glucagon.

EPIDEMIOLOGIC AND CLINICAL STUDIES ON OSA AND ALTERATIONS IN GLUCOSE METABOLISM

Despite heterogeneity in study design and protocol, most of the more recent cross-sectional population-based or clinic-based studies found an independent link between OSA and disorders of glucose metabolism (Table 1).

OSA and Insulin Resistance/Glucose Intolerance

The Sleep Heart Health Study on 2656 community-dwelling subjects not on any antidiabetic medications found that the severity of SDB was associated with the degree of insulin resistance and glucose intolerance, independent of age, gender, body mass index (BMI, calculated as weight in kilograms divided by the square of height in meters) and waist circumference.[6] In a case-control study, McArdle and colleagues[7] reported a higher insulin resistance (estimated by HOMA) in OSA compared with age- and weight-matched control white subjects (mean BMI 27 kg/m^2). Similarly, in Japanese men who were lean by preestablished criteria, Kono and colleagues[8] reported higher fasting glucose and insulin resistance in those with OSA, compared with control subjects matched for visceral obesity documented by abdominal computerized tomography. Excessive daytime sleepiness has been suggested to be a phenotypic marker for blood pressure increase and its response in OSA.[9] Barceló and colleagues[10] reported that despite similar BMI and severity of OSA, only OSA subjects who had excessive daytime sleepiness, but not the non-sleepy subjects matched for BMI, had worse insulin resistance than controls without OSA. This was supported by the recent report from Tsai and colleagues,[11] who observed that severe OSA was associated with DM after adjustment for demographics, weight, and neck circumference,

exclusively in sleepy patients on stratified analyses.

Although many of the positive studies only included male subjects, the link between adverse glucose metabolism and OSA may also apply to women, in light of the supportive findings from an epidemiologic study in Sweden which included 400 women.[12] Theorell-Haglöw and colleagues[12] reported a gradual decrease in insulin sensitivity with increasing apnea-hypopnea index (AHI) independent of confounders in women.

Most studies have focused on the effect of SDB on insulin sensitivity/resistance, which reflects tissue response to the effect of insulin on glucose utilization. However, like any other tissue in the body, pancreatic β cells, the source of insulin, are also exposed to the detrimental effects of sleep apnea. Punjabi and Beamer[13] used the frequently sampled intravenous glucose tolerance test to evaluate the dynamic relationship between insulin sensitivity and insulin secretion in 118 subjects with a range of SDB severity. Compared with normal subjects, there was a progressive reduction in insulin sensitivity with increasing severity of SDB, independent of age, sex, race, and percent body fat. The disposition index, a measure of pancreatic β cell function, was also reduced in those with moderate to severe OSA.

The pediatric population has not escaped the sweeping epidemic of obesity, and the prevalence of type 2 DM, previously a disease almost exclusively seen in adults, has now surpassed that of type 1 DM in children and adolescents.[14] Conventionally, OSA in children is related to enlarged tonsils rather than obesity, but there is increasing data to support the growing importance of obesity as a causative factor.[15] Pediatric subjects with SDB have been regarded as a unique nidus for research into the cardiometabolic effects of OSA as they were mostly nonobese. Although the picture is rapidly changing in terms of body habitus, children still have much less preexisting cardiometabolic diseases compared with their adult counterparts. There is increasing data that support an independent association between OSA and adverse glucose metabolism in children and adolescents.[16–18] In the Cleveland Cohort, Redline and colleagues[18] found that after adjusting for age, sex, ethnicity, and preterm status, children with SDB had a 6.49 increased odds of metabolic syndrome compared with those without SDB. However, these findings were challenged by others. In a cohort of 135 children, about half of whom were obese, Tauman and colleagues[19] found that insulin resistance and dyslipidemia were determined primarily by the degree of body adiposity rather than by the severity of SDB among children with OSA. In another study involving non-obese children, severity of OSA was not a significant determinant of insulin resistance.[20]

OSA and DM

In clinical practice, type 2 DM is not uncommonly seen in those who present for suspected SDB. Tamura and colleagues[21] reported a prevalence of DM as high as 30% in 129 Japanese middle-aged adults with OSA, half of whom were of moderate/severe degree, and impaired glucose tolerance (IGT) was found in another 30%. Multiple regression analysis identified male sex and AHI as the independent factors relating to impaired glucose metabolism. Despite the caveat of a single-center sample with potential referral bias, the findings highlight the need for high awareness of metabolic disorders in patients presenting with SDB.

The Wisconsin Sleep Cohort study (n = 1387) reported a 2-fold increase in risk of DM in subjects with OSA (defined by AHI $\geq$ 15) after adjustment for confounders.[22] Nevertheless, causal relationship between OSA and incident diabetes was not demonstrated at 4-year follow-up, unlike the findings in relation to hypertension.[23] Four years is a relatively short follow-up duration, given that the spectrum of glucose metabolic disorders run a slow clinical course, and longer follow-up will hopefully provide more definitive information.

On the other hand, OSA is increasingly recognized among diabetic subjects. West and colleagues[24] recruited male subjects with type 2 DM from a tertiary hospital center and 5 primary care centers in Oxford, UK. With the use of overnight oximetry, the prevalence of OSA (defined as >10/h oxygen saturation dips of $\geq$4%) was estimated to be about 23% in this diabetic population with average BMI of 28.8 kg/m^2 (interquartile range 22.5–39.4). This prevalence estimate of OSA in diabetic men was significantly higher than that reported from a general population in the United Kingdom.[24] These findings were supported by a population-based study in Sweden,[25] which found a much higher prevalence of severe OSA, defined as AHI $\geq$20/h, in diabetic patients than in normoglycemic subjects after adjustment for confounding factors. Recently, the Sleep Ahead Study from the United States reported an alarming prevalence of OSA of more than 86% among obese type 2 diabetic adults[26] and waist circumference was the only predictor for OSA. Although the sample is skewed toward several OSA risk factors, including obesity (mean BMI 36 kg/m^2), age (mean 61 years), and menopause in female subjects (90%), such high prevalence figures

intensify the alarm signal for the magnitude of the health care problem that we are facing.

Several studies have shown supportive evidence for a dose-dependent relationship between the severity of OSA and glucose dysmetabolism,[21,24] although reliable analysis among those on antidiabetic medications may be intrinsically limited by the prevailing clinical practice of adjusting treatment according to the level of HbA1c.

EFFECT OF TREATMENT OF OSA ON GLUCOSE METABOLISM

The effect of treatment of OSA on glucose metabolism may provide clues to the directionality of their association. In adult studies, the intervention was almost exclusively continuous positive airway pressure (CPAP), whereas in children, mostly adenotonsillectomy. Most studies to date have been observational. The treatment periods with CPAP were also variable, ranging from 1 night to 6 months.

Treatment of OSA and Insulin-glucose Metabolism in Nondiabetic Subjects

Many early studies were unable to detect any significant alteration in insulin resistance or their surrogate measures after CPAP treatment of OSA.[3] **Table 2** focuses on published studies in the past decade. Harsch and colleagues[27] used the hyperinsulinemic euglycemic clamp and reported that CPAP treatment of OSA for 2 days promptly improved insulin sensitivity in nondiabetic men. The beneficial effects persisted at 3 months of CPAP treatment, and were apparently more prominent in the nonobese subjects. The same group of investigators also found similar improvement in insulin sensitivity in diabetic subjects with 3-month usage of CPAP.[28] Barceló and colleagues[10] reported that sleepy OSA subjects, who had higher HOMA index than nonsleepy counterparts, at baseline, showed significant decrease with CPAP treatment; such response was not apparent in the nonsleepy group.

Coughlin and colleagues[29] undertook a randomized, placebo-controlled, crossover trial comparing cardiovascular and metabolic outcomes after 6 weeks of therapeutic and sham CPAP in 34 nondiabetic obese men with moderate to severe OSA. No change in fasting glucose levels or HOMA could be demonstrated, despite a significant decrease in blood pressure.

Recently, our group reported a randomized controlled trial of CPAP treatment on insulin sensitivity, using the short insulin tolerance test, in

Table 1
Selected studies on the association of SDB and glucose metabolism in middle-aged adults

Study/Year	Sample	Average BMI (kg/m^2)	Tools Assessing Glucose Metabolism	Findings
Strohl et al 1994[88]	Clinic-based, 261 men with suspected OSA (mean AHI 20)	30	Fasting glucose, insulin	Fasting insulin levels correlated positively with BMI and AHI. Fasting glucose correlated only with BMI
Elmasry et al 2001[25]	Population-based study 116 hypertensive men 25 with DM 8 with IGT 83 without DM/IGT	27–30	Fasting glucose and insulin, HbA1c	The prevalence of severe OSA was significantly higher in diabetic subjects. Significant relationship between variables of SDB and fasting insulin, glucose and HbA1c
Ip et al 2002[89]	Clinic-based 270 nondiabetic Chinese 85 without OSA 185 with OSA	26	Fasting insulin, HOMA	AHI and minimum oxygen saturation are independent determinants of insulin resistance
Meslier et al 2003[90]	Clinic-based 491 men: 90 without OSA 140 mild OSA 79 moderate OSA 182 severe OSA	27–31	Fasting glucose/insulin ratio, OGTT	Both DM and IGT were more common in OSA subjects (30% and 20%), compared with nonapneic snorers (14% and 14%) Insulin sensitivity decreased with increasing severity of OSA
Punjabi et al 2004[6]	Sleep Heart Health Study, 2656 subjects from United States Mean age 68 y	27.4	OGTT, HOMA	Degree of insulin resistance was independently associated with severity of OSA; AHI and minimum oxygen saturation were associated with fasting and 2-h glucose levels

Study	Subjects		Measure	Findings
Reichmuth et al 2005[22]	Wisconsin Sleep Cohort, 1387 subjects, 4-y follow-up in 987 subjects	29	Fasting glucose	DM was more prevalent in OSA (AHI ≥15), odds ratio 2.3 (95% CI 1.28–4.11) after adjustment for age, gender, and habitus; no independent association between incident DM and OSA at 4-y follow-up
Sulit et al 2006[91]	394 subjects from Cleveland Family Study (US)	32	OGTT	Threshold dose response for measures of hypoxic stress (≥2% time with <90% oxygen saturation) and glucose intolerance; adjusted odds ratio 2.33
Makino et al 2006[92]	Clinic-based 213 OSA subjects 30 mild 98 moderate 85 severe	25–28	Fasting glucose and insulin, HOMA	SDB was associated with insulin resistance independent of visceral obesity
Peled et al 2007[93]	Clinic-based 98 with suspected OSA 9 snorers 9 mild OSA 27 moderate 53 severe	25–31	HOMA	Insulin resistance correlated significantly with AHI
Kono et al 2007[8]	94 Japanese men 42 with OSA 52 men without OSA, matched for age, BMI, and visceral fat measured by computed tomography	23	HOMA	Fasting glucose and HOMA were significantly higher in those with OSA. AHI was a predictor of number of metabolic syndrome parameters

(continued on next page)

Table 1
(continued)

Study/Year	Sample	Average BMI (kg/m²)	Tools Assessing Glucose Metabolism	Findings
Sharma et al 2007[94]	40 Indian obese OSA 40 Indian obese non-OSA 40 Indian nonobese controls	30 29 21	Fasting glucose, fasting insulin, HOMA	OSA has no independent association with insulin resistance
Tamura et al 2008[21]	Clinic-based 129 Japanese with OSA 68 severe 41 moderate 20 mild	24–27	75 g OGTT	DM and IGT were more common in those with severe OSA. AHI was independently associated with DM and IGT
Theorell-Haglöw et al 2008[12]	400 female subjects from a city in Sweden	25–31	75 g OGTT	AHI was associated with increased fasting and 2-h insulin levels after adjusting for confounders. A gradual decrease in insulin sensitivity with increasing AHI
Kapsimalis et al 2008[70]	Clinic-based 67 nondiabetic men 15 non-OSA 26 mild-moderate OSA 26 severe OSA	29–31	HOMA	Insulin resistance was not associated with sleep apnea severity independent of obesity
Punjabi et al 2009[13]	118 nondiabetic subjects 39 without SDB 34 mild 22 moderate 23 severe	26–33	FSIVGTT	SDB is associated with impairments in insulin sensitivity, glucose effectiveness, and pancreatic β cell function

Abbreviations: AHI, apnea-hypopnea index; BMI, body mass index; FSIVGTT, frequently sampled intravenous glucose tolerance test; HOMA, homeostatic model assessment; IGT, impaired glucose tolerance; OGTT, oral glucose tolerance test; OSA, obstructive sleep apnea; SDB, sleep-disordered breathing.

61 nondiabetic Chinese men with OSA.[30] Therapeutic CPAP for 1 week improved insulin sensitivity as indicated by greater glucose disposal in response to intravenous insulin, compared with the sham CPAP group. There was a lack of change in HOMA index despite the improvement seen in the short insulin tolerance test, highlighting the variability of the results in relation to the evaluation tools. In contrast to the findings of Harsch and colleagues,[27] the beneficial effect appeared to be more prominent and sustainable in those who were moderately obese, defined according to Asian criteria, with a mean BMI of 28.3 kg/m^2, compared with the nonobese subjects (BMI <25 kg/m^2). However, the number of nonobese subjects was relatively small, limiting any definitive interpretation.

In pediatric subjects, Gozal and colleagues[31] found a brisk increase in fasting levels of insulin and insulin/glucose ratio in the obese, but not the nonobese, group after adenotonsillectomy. In contrast, 2 other studies reported no major changes in insulin and/or HOMA index before and after adenotonsillectomy.[32,33] Nakra and colleagues[34] investigated 34 children, aged 7 to 19 years, with metabolic syndrome, and found that those with SDB had increased sympathetic nervous system activity and nocturnal leptin levels but not worsening of insulin sensitivity based on OGTT, compared with those without SDB; CPAP treatment for 3 months in 11 subjects reduced norepinephrine and leptin levels without any change in insulin sensitivity index.

Treatment of OSA and Glycemic Control in Diabetic Subjects

Several observational studies have reported beneficial effects on glycemic control when OSA is effectively controlled. Babu and colleagues[35] found a significant reduction in postprandial interstitial glucose after 3 months of CPAP therapy, whereas the beneficial effect on HbA1c was confined to those who had higher initial HbA1c levels of >7%. Two further observational studies reported on the effect of CPAP treatment on nocturnal glucose homeostasis using a similar CGMS. Pallayova and colleagues[36] recruited 14 obese subjects with severe OSA and type 2 DM, and demonstrated reduction of nocturnal glucose variability and improved overnight glucose control during CPAP treatment. Dawson and colleagues[37] substantiated this further by reporting a reduction in mean sleeping glucose after treatment with CPAP for an average of 41 days, although there was no change in HbA1c. Dorkova and colleagues[38] also showed that CPAP therapy for

2 months reduced the HOMA index in OSA subjects with metabolic syndrome. Nevertheless, in the only randomized controlled study of CPAP treatment in diabetic subjects published to date, West and colleagues[39] did not find any change in either HbA1c or insulin sensitivity using the hyperinsulinemic euglycemic clamp and HOMA in the group using therapeutic CPAP compared with the group given sham CPAP for 3 months. A limitation of the study was the suboptimal use of CPAP at just less than 4 hours per night even in the therapeutic intervention group, although the treatment did result in reduction of daytime sleepiness and blood pressure.

POTENTIAL MECHANISTIC LINKS BETWEEN OSA AND ADVERSE GLUCOSE METABOLISM
Intermittent Hypoxia

Adipose tissue hypoxia and oxidative stress are potentially important mechanisms in disturbance of glucose homeostasis.[40] In OSA, the pattern of hypoxia is unique in that it is usually not sustained, but one of recurrent intermittent hypoxia with reoxygenation in rapid cycles. The mechanistic role of intermittent hypoxia in the various pathophysiologic sequelae of OSA has been investigated using experimental animal or cell studies exposed to intermittent hypoxic conditions. In leptin-deficient obese mice, Polotsky and colleagues[41] found that the exposure to chronic intermittent hypoxia (30-s hypoxia alternating with 30-s normoxia for 12 h/d) for 12 weeks led to a time-dependent increase in fasting insulin level and deterioration in glucose tolerance and insulin resistance. Iiyori and colleagues[42] applied intermittent hypoxia to lean mice and showed that insulin sensitivity, as assessed by hyperinsulinemic euglycemic clamp, was reduced, although the impairment was independent of autonomic nervous system activity, contradictory to the anticipated role of sympathetic nervous activation as a stress trigger for adverse glucose homeostasis.

Studies of human models of intermittent hypoxia have also been reported recently. Oltmanns and colleagues[43] performed hyperinsulinemic euglycemic clamps in 14 healthy men during normoxia and after 30 min of hypoxia at an oxygen concentration of 75%. Such acute but relatively sustained hypoxia led to worsening of glucose tolerance, increase in heart rate, and increased plasma epinephrine levels. In another study, Louis and Punjabi[44] applied intermittent hypoxia (5% O_2 at 25 cycles/h for 8 hours) on 13 healthy volunteers, using the intravenous glucose tolerance test to assess insulin-dependent and insulin-independent measures of glucose disposal. Compared with

Table 2
Selected clinical studies examining the effect of CPAP on glucose metabolism in adults

Study/Year	Sample	Average BMI (kg/m²)	Tools Assessing Glucose Metabolism	Findings
Brooks et al 1994[95]	10 male subjects with moderate-severe OSA and DM	42	Hyperinsulinemic euglycemic clamp	Insulin sensitivity improved after CPAP for 4 mo
Harsch et al 2004[27]	40 nondiabetic OSA subjects	33	Hyperinsulinemic euglycemic clamp	Insulin sensitivity improved after 2 d of CPAP in nonobese subjects, and after 3 mo in obese subjects
Babu et al 2005[35]	24 subjects with DM and OSA (half being noncompliant)	43	CGMS, HbA1c	CPAP for 3 mo improved postprandial glucose and HbA1c in 17 subjects with baseline HbA1c >7%
Hassaballa et al 2005[96]	38 subjects with DM and OSA (retrospective review)	42	HbA1c	Slightly decreased after about 4 mo of CPAP
Trenell et al 2007[97]	29 OSA subjects: 19 regular CPAP, 10 irregular CPAP	34	Fasting glucose, fasting insulin, HOMA	No change in insulin resistance after CPAP for 12 wk
Coughlin et al 2007[29]	RCT (crossover, CPAP/sham CPAP): 34 nondiabetic OSA subjects	37	Fasting glucose, HOMA	No change after CPAP for 6 wk
West et al 2007[39]	RCT: 42 men with DM and OSA (20 CPAP, 22 sham CPAP)	37	HOMA, HbA1c, euglycemic clamp	No change after CPAP for 3 mo
Barceló et al 2008[10]	44 nondiabetic subjects with OSA (22 with and 22 without EDS matched for age, BMI, and severity of OSA), 23 healthy controls	OSA: 31 Healthy controls: 25	HOMA	CPAP for 3 mo reduced insulin and the HOMA index in patients with EDS, but not in those without EDS
Pallayova et al 2008[36]	14 subjects with severe OSA and DM	37.4	CGMS	Reduction of nocturnal glucose variability and improved overnight glucose control on CPAP

Study	Subjects	BMI	Method	Results
Dawson et al 2008[37]	20 subjects with DM and OSA	39.6	CGMS	Mean sleeping glucose decreased after treatment with CPAP for an average of 41 days (26–96 days). No change in HbA1c
Dorkova et al 2008[38]	32 subjects with severe OSA and metabolic syndrome (16 compliant with CPAP, 16 noncompliant)	35	HOMA	Compliant with treatment with CPAP for 8 wk led to improved HOMA and global CVD risk
Schahin et al 2008[98]	9 nondiabetic OSA subjects	31	Hyperinsulinemic euglycemic clamp	Improvement in insulin sensitivity maintained after 2.9 y of CPAP treatment
Vgontzas et al 2008[99]	16 with OSA; 15 obese controls; 13 nonobese controls	37 35 27	Fasting glucose, insulin, HOMA	No change after CPAP for 3 mo
Cuhadaroğlu et al 2009[100]	44 nondiabetic OSA subjects (31 compliant with CPAP)	32	HOMA	CPAP for 8 wk reduced leptin levels and increased insulin secretion capacity, but not insulin resistance
Lam et al 2009[30]	RCT: 61 OSA subjects without comorbidities (31 CPAP, 30 sham CPAP)	27.5	Short insulin tolerance test, HOMA	Therapeutic nasal CPAP for 1 week improved glucose disappearance rate, and the improvement was maintained after 12 wk of treatment in those with moderate obesity. No change in HOMA

Abbreviations: BMI, body mass index; CGMS, continuous glucose monitoring system; CPAP, continuous positive airway pressure; CVD, cardiovascular disease; EDS, excessive daytime sleepiness; HOMA, homeostatic model assessment; OSA, obstructive sleep apnea; RCT, randomized controlled trial.

normoxia, intermittent hypoxia was associated with a decrease in insulin sensitivity, although no change in pancreatic insulin secretion or cortisol level was found.

Increased oxidative stress has been shown to be a key mechanism for insulin resistance and diabetes.[40] The cyclical hypoxia-reoxygenation that occurs in OSA may be a trigger for formation of reactive oxygen species, the culprit of oxidative stress, although studies on oxidative stress in OSA have shown conflicting results.[3,45] Pialoux and colleagues[46] subjected 10 young healthy men to intermittent hypoxia (cycling between 2 minutes at end-tidal $Po_2 = 45$ Torr and 2 minutes at $P_{ETO_2} = 88$ Torr) of 6 hours per day for 4 days, and found increased production of reactive oxygen species without a compensatory increase in antioxidant activity. Xu and colleagues[47] investigated the effect of intermittent hypoxia on β cells in vitro, and showed that it led to increased β-cell proliferation and cell death, and the cell death response appeared to be caused by oxidative stress.

Sleep Fragmentation, Sleep Loss, Altered Sleep Architecture

Sleep fragmentation and reduced total sleep time commonly take place in OSA. There is abundant data from epidemiologic and laboratory studies to indicate that sleep loss or poor sleep quality, in the absence of SDB, may adversely affect glucose metabolism.[48–52] Yaggi and colleagues[51] studied a cohort of men without diabetes at baseline from the Massachusetts Male Aging Study, and found a 2- and 3-fold increase in the risk of developing diabetes for short and long sleep duration respectively, after about 10 to 15 years of follow-up. In the Sleep Heart Health Study, sleep durations of 6 hours or less or 9 hours or more in 1486 men and women, with adjustment for diabetic risk factors and symptoms of insomnia, were associated with higher prevalence of IGT and diabetes events.[48] Several prospective studies lasting from 7 to 32 years in various ethnic populations have consistently demonstrated a higher risk of glucose intolerance and diabetes for shorter sleep duration and/or poorer sleep quality.[53–56]

Most epidemiologic studies were limited by subjective reporting of sleep duration and quality. In the sleep laboratory, Spiegel and colleagues[57] showed that 2 days of sleep curtailment led to adverse glucose profile and increase in appetite for high caloric density carbohydrates compared with extended sleep. This was accompanied by a decrease in the anorexigenic hormone leptin

and increase in ghrelin, an appetite-stimulating peptide, suggesting that sleep loss may thus predispose to consequent weight gain and dysregulation of glucose metabolism.[58]

In a population-based study using objective assessment of sleep duration with in-laboratory monitoring, the risk of diabetes was 3-fold higher in individuals with insomnia and sleep of 5 hours duration or less, compared with the groups with normal sleep duration and 6 hours sleep or more.[59] Reduction in deep slow-wave sleep, which is common in OSA, might adversely affect the glucose metabolism. Tasali and colleagues[60] found that all-night suppression of slow-wave sleep, without a change in sleep duration, resulted in marked worsening of insulin sensitivity in young healthy adults.

Alterations in Cytokine/Adipokine Release and Inflammation

Many cytokines, in particular adipocytokines, act as mediators of low-grade systemic inflammation, vasculopathy, and adverse glucose metabolism.[61,62] It has been suggested that OSA may act as a trigger for the expression of mediators, such as tumor necrosis factor, that play intermediary pathogenetic roles in adverse glucose metabolism.[63]

The levels of C-reactive marker, a systemic marker of inflammation, correlated positively with HOMA index in a general population followed up for 5 years.[64] In OSA, the levels of C-reactive protein (CRP) has been investigated with conflicting results, mostly relating to the potential confounding effect from obesity. Recently, the authors demonstrated an independent association between severe OSA and increased CRP level in men free of comorbidities, in spite of careful consideration of abdominal obesity measured by computed tomography.[65]

Leptin is an adipokine which plays a key role in the feedback mechanism for suppressing appetite and food intake, and it also has peripheral actions on glucose regulation.[66] Human obesity is characterized by increased rather than low leptin level, reflecting the relative leptin resistance.[67] Despite the tenable hypothesis that OSA may further increase leptin resistance, the data of the relationship between OSA and circulating leptin levels in human studies have been conflicting.[68–72] The secretion of leptin, like many other hormones, may have variation by the time clock, limiting the interpretation of spot level measurements. Nakara and colleagues[34] demonstrated increased leptin levels in OSA with multiple sampling, which decreased with CPAP treatment. In animal experiments, exogenous leptin in genetically leptin-deficient obese mice prevented the emergence of insulin resistance induced by intermittent hypoxia.[41]

Adiponectin is predominantly produced by adipose tissue, and low plasma levels of adiponectin are found to be associated with obesity, metabolic syndrome, diabetes, and other diseases.[73,74] Animal experiments and human studies have shown that adiponectin is a key regulator of insulin sensitivity.[75] There is supporting evidence that OSA is associated with hypoadiponectinemia, independent of obesity, although again, similar to the leptin story, results have not been consistent in different studies.[76,77]

Adipocyte fatty acid–binding protein (A-FABP) is another protein, abundantly expressed by adipocytes, that is important in mediating intracellular fatty acid trafficking and glucose homeostasis.[78] Positive associations between serum A-FABP levels and parameters of adiposity, hyperglycemia, insulin resistance, and the metabolic syndrome have been reported in cross-sectional and longitudinal studies.[79] Our group demonstrated that serum A-FABP levels were significantly higher in those with severe OSA compared with those with milder or no OSA, independent of obesity, suggesting that it may be one of the mediators in the SDB-metabolic link.[80]

Alterations of the Neuroendocrine and Autonomic System

Neuroendocrine and autonomic factors are important in glucose regulation.[81] Epinephrine and cortisol are counter-regulatory hormones with adverse effects on glucose homeostasis. Enhanced sympathetic activity has been convincingly demonstrated in OSA, and the degree of sympathetic activation was found to be correlated with the severity of hypoxia in OSA,[82] whereas studies of cortisol secretion in OSA have shown inconsistent results.[3] In the laboratory, Spiegel and colleagues[57] showed that acute sleep fragmentation, using auditory and mechanical stimulation, decreased insulin sensitivity and glucose effectiveness (the ability of glucose to mobilize itself independent of insulin) the next morning, associated with an increase in the morning levels of cortisol and sympathetic nervous system activity, although not that of systemic inflammation or adipokines. That mechanically induced sleep fragmentation can produce acute adverse effects on glucose homeostasis in healthy subjects was further confirmed recently by the work of Stamatakis and Punjabi.[83]

In the context of glucose metabolism, a lower level of growth hormone would be favorable, whereas a decrease in insulin growth factor (IGF)-1 predicts type 2 diabetes. Several studies investigated the influence of OSA on the somatotropic axis, with evidence showing a reduction of growth hormone and IGF-1 in OSA,[84,85] although these observations were discrepant from the change in growth hormone secretion found in experimental sleep restriction.[86,87]

SUMMARY

Despite proliferating literature, the exact relationship between OSA and alterations in glucose metabolism is still controversial. There is growing evidence to suggest that OSA imposes adverse effects on glucose metabolism, but the translation into clinical effect is not well delineated. Many potential mechanisms are being explored, mostly relating to peripheral tissue response to insulin and more recently regarding pancreatic β cell function of insulin secretion. The effect of OSA on glucose metabolism is likely to be influenced by many personal characteristics. Age, degree of adiposity, lifestyle, comorbidities, and even the stage of glucose disorder itself may modify the relationship between OSA and glucose metabolism. In the biologic system of the human body, all these interact to culminate in clinically relevant outcomes.

REFERENCES

1. Chan JC, Malik V, Jia W, et al. Diabetes in Asia: epidemiology, risk factors, and pathophysiology [review]. JAMA 2009;301(20):2129–40.
2. Janus ED, Watt NM, Lam KS, et al. The prevalence of diabetes, association with cardiovascular risk factors and implications of diagnostic criteria (ADA 1997 and WHO 1998) in a 1996 community-based population study in Hong Kong Chinese. Hong Kong Cardiovascular Risk Factor Steering Committee. American Diabetes Association. Diabet Med 2000;17(10):741–5.
3. Tasali E, Ip MS. Obstructive sleep apnea and metabolic syndrome: alterations in glucose metabolism and inflammation [review]. Proc Am Thorac Soc 2008;5(2):207–17.
4. Muniyappa R, Lee S, Chen H, et al. Current approaches for assessing insulin sensitivity and resistance in vivo: advantages, limitations, and appropriate usage. Am J Physiol Endocrinol Metab 2008;294(1):E15–26.
5. Radikova Z. Assessment of insulin sensitivity/resistance in epidemiological studies. Endocr Regul 2003;37(3):189–94.

6. Punjabi NM, Shahar E, Redline S, et al. Sleep-disordered breathing, glucose intolerance, and insulin resistance: the Sleep Heart Health Study. Am J Epidemiol 2004;160(6):521–30.

7. McArdle N, Hillman D, Beilin L, et al. Metabolic risk factors for vascular disease in obstructive sleep apnea: a matched controlled study. Am J Respir Crit Care Med 2007;175(2):190–5.

8. Kono M, Tatsumi K, Saibara T, et al. Obstructive sleep apnea syndrome is associated with some components of metabolic syndrome. Chest 2007; 131(5):1387–92.

9. Kapur VK, Resnick HE, Gottlieb DJ, et al. Sleep disordered breathing and hypertension: does self-reported sleepiness modify the association? Sleep 2008;31(8):1127–32.

10. Barceló A, Barbé F, de la Peña M, et al. Insulin resistance and daytime sleepiness in patients with sleep apnoea. Thorax 2008;63(11):946–50.

11. Ronksley PE, Hemmelgarn B, Heitman SJ, et al. Obstructive sleep apnea is associated with diabetes in sleepy subjects. Thorax 2009;64(10): 834–9.

12. Theorell-Haglöw J, Berne C, Janson C, et al. Obstructive sleep apnoea is associated with decreased insulin sensitivity in females. Eur Respir J 2008;31(5):1054–60.

13. Punjabi NM, Beamer BA. Alterations in glucose disposal in sleep-disordered breathing. Am J Respir Crit Care Med 2009;179(3):235–40.

14. Vivian EM. Type 2 diabetes in children and adolescents – the next epidemic? Curr Med Res Opin 2006;22:297–306.

15. Bixler EO, Vgontzas AN, Lin HM, et al. Sleep disordered breathing in children in a general population sample: prevalence and risk factors. Sleep 2009; 32(6):731–6.

16. de la Eva RC, Baur LA, Donaghue KC, et al. Metabolic correlates with obstructive sleep apnea in obese subjects. J Pediatr 2002;140(6): 654–9.

17. Li AM, Chan MH, Chan DF, et al. Insulin and obstructive sleep apnea in obese Chinese children. Pediatr Pulmonol 2006;41(12):1175–81.

18. Redline S, Storfer-Isser A, Rosen CL, et al. Association between metabolic syndrome and sleep-disordered breathing in adolescents. Am J Respir Crit Care Med 2007;176:401–8.

19. Tauman R, O'Brien LM, Ivanenko A, et al. Obesity rather than severity of sleep-disordered breathing as the major determinant of insulin resistance and altered lipidemia in snoring children. Pediatrics 2005;116(1):e66–73.

20. Kaditis AG, Alexopoulos EI, Damani E, et al. Obstructive sleep-disordered breathing and fasting insulin levels in nonobese children. Pediatr Pulmonol 2005;40(6):515–23.

21. Tamura A, Kawano Y, Watanabe T, et al. Relationship between the severity of obstructive sleep apnea and impaired glucose metabolism in patients with obstructive sleep apnea. Respir Med 2008;102(10):1412–6.

22. Reichmuth KJ, Austin D, Skatrud JB, et al. Association of sleep apnea and type II diabetes: a population-based study. Am J Respir Crit Care Med 2005; 172(12):1590–5.

23. Peppard PE, Young T, Palta M, et al. Prospective study of the association between sleep-disordered breathing and hypertension. N Engl J Med 2000; 342(19):1378–84.

24. West SD, Nicoll DJ, Stradling JR. Prevalence of obstructive sleep apnoea in men with type 2 diabetes. Thorax 2006;61(11):945–50.

25. Elmasry A, Lindberg E, Berne C, et al. Sleep-disordered breathing and glucose metabolism in hypertensive men: a population-based study. J Intern Med 2001;249(2):153–61.

26. Foster GD, Sanders MH, Millman R, et al. Obstructive sleep apnea among obese patients with type 2 diabetes. Diabetes Care 2009;32(6):1017–9.

27. Harsch IA, Schahin SP, Radespiel-Tröger M, et al. Continuous positive airway pressure treatment rapidly improves insulin sensitivity in patients with obstructive sleep apnea syndrome. Am J Respir Crit Care Med 2004;169(2):156–62.

28. Harsch IA, Schahin SP, Brückner K, et al. The effect of continuous positive airway pressure treatment on insulin sensitivity in patients with obstructive sleep apnoea syndrome and type 2 diabetes. Respiration 2004;71(3):252–9.

29. Coughlin SR, Mawdsley L, Mugarza JA, et al. Cardiovascular and metabolic effects of CPAP in obese males with OSA. Eur Respir J 2007;29(4): 720–7.

30. Lam JC, Lam B, Yao TJ, et al. A randomized controlled trial of nCPAP on insulin sensitivity in obstructive sleep apnoea. Eur Respir J 2010; 35(1):138–45.

31. Gozal D, Capdevila OS, Kheirandish-Gozal L. Metabolic alterations and systemic inflammation in obstructive sleep apnea among nonobese and obese prepubertal children. Am J Respir Crit Care Med 2008;177(10):1142–9.

32. Waters KA, Mast BT, Vella S, et al. Structural equation modeling of sleep apnea, inflammation, and metabolic dysfunction in children. J Sleep Res 2007;16(4):388–95.

33. Apostolidou MT, Alexopoulos EI, Damani E, et al. Absence of blood pressure, metabolic, and inflammatory marker changes after adenotonsillectomy for sleep apnea in Greek children. Pediatr Pulmonol 2008;43(6):550–60.

34. Nakra N, Bhargava S, Dzuira J, et al. Sleep-disordered breathing in children with metabolic

syndrome: the role of leptin and sympathetic nervous system activity and the effect of continuous positive airway pressure. Pediatrics 2008; 122(3):e634–42.

35. Babu AR, Herdegen J, Fogelfeld L, et al. Type 2 diabetes, glycemic control, and continuous positive airway pressure in obstructive sleep apnea. Arch Intern Med 2005;165(4):447–52.

36. Pallayova M, Donic V, Tomori Z. Beneficial effects of severe sleep apnea therapy on nocturnal glucose control in persons with type 2 diabetes mellitus. Diabetes Res Clin Pract 2008;81(1):e8–11.

37. Dawson A, Abel SL, Loving RT, et al. CPAP therapy of obstructive sleep apnea in type 2 diabetics improves glycemic control during sleep. J Clin Sleep Med 2008;4(6):538–42.

38. Dorkova Z, Petrasova D, Molcanyiova A, et al. Effects of continuous positive airway pressure on cardiovascular risk profile in patients with severe obstructive sleep apnea and metabolic syndrome. Chest 2008;134(4):686–92.

39. West SD, Nicoll DJ, Wallace TM, et al. Effect of CPAP on insulin resistance and HbA1c in men with obstructive sleep apnoea and type 2 diabetes. Thorax 2007;62(11):969–74.

40. Furukawa S, Fujita T, Shimabukuro M, et al. Increased oxidative stress in obesity and its impact on metabolic syndrome. J Clin Invest 2004;114: 1752–61.

41. Polotsky VY, Li J, Punjabi NM, et al. Intermittent hypoxia increases insulin resistance in genetically obese mice. J Physiol 2003;552(Pt 1):253–64.

42. Iiyori N, Alonso LC, Li J, et al. Intermittent hypoxia causes insulin resistance in lean mice independent of autonomic activity. Am J Respir Crit Care Med 2007;175(8):851–7.

43. Oltmanns KM, Gehring H, Rudolf S, et al. Hypoxia causes glucose intolerance in humans. Am J Respir Crit Care Med 2004;169(11):1231–7.

44. Louis M, Punjabi NM. Effects of acute intermittent hypoxia on glucose metabolism in awake healthy volunteers. J Appl Physiol 2009;106(5):1538–44.

45. Lavie L. Oxidative stress–a unifying paradigm in obstructive sleep apnea and comorbidities. Prog Cardiovasc Dis 2009;51(4):303–12.

46. Pialoux V, Hanly PJ, Foster GE, et al. Effects of exposure to intermittent hypoxia on oxidative stress and acute hypoxic ventilatory response in humans. Am J Respir Crit Care Med 2009; 180(10):1002–9.

47. Xu J, Long YS, Gozal D, et al. Beta-cell death and proliferation after intermittent hypoxia: role of oxidative stress. Free Radic Biol Med 2009;46(6):783–90.

48. Gottlieb DJ, Punjabi N, Newman AG, et al. Association of sleep time with diabetes mellitus and impaired glucose tolerance. Arch Intern Med 2005;165:863–7.

49. Chaput JP, Despres JP, Bouchard C, et al. Association of sleep duration with type 2 diabetes and impaired glucose tolerance. Diabetologia 2007; 50:2298–304.

50. Knutson KL, Ryden AM, Mander BA, et al. Role of sleep duration and quality in the risk and severity of type 2 diabetes mellitus. Arch Intern Med 2006;166:1768–74.

51. Yaggi HK, Araujo AB, McKinlay JB. Sleep duration as a risk factor for the development of type 2 diabetes. Diabetes Care 2006;29:657–61.

52. Ip M, Mokhlesi B. Sleep and glucose intolerance/ diabetes mellitus. Sleep Med Clin 2007;2(1):19–29.

53. Ayas NT, White DP, Al-Delaimy WK, et al. A prospective study of self-reported sleep duration and incident diabetes in women. Diabetes Care 2003;26:380–4.

54. Bjorkelund C, Bondyr-Carlsson D, Lapidus L, et al. Sleep disturbances in midlife unrelated to 32-year diabetes incidence: the prospective population study of women in Gothenburg. Diabetes Care 2005;28:2739–44.

55. Meisinger C, Heier M, Loewel H. Sleep disturbance as a predictor of type 2 diabetes mellitus in men and women from the general population. Diabetologia 2005;48:235–41.

56. Gangwisch JE, Heymsfield SB, Boden-Albala B, et al. Sleep duration as a risk factor for diabetes incidence in a large U.S. sample. Sleep 2007;30: 1667–73.

57. Spiegel K, Knutson K, Leproult R, et al. Sleep loss: a novel risk factor for insulin resistance and type 2 diabetes. J Appl Physiol 2005;99: 2008–19.

58. Spiegel K, Tasali E, Penev P, et al. Brief communication. Sleep curtailment in healthy young men is associated with decreased leptin levels, elevated ghrelin levels, and increased hunger and appetite. Ann Intern Med 2004;141(11):846–50.

59. Vgontzas AN, Liao D, Pejovic S, et al. Insomnia with objective short sleep duration is associated with type 2 diabetes: a population-based study. Diabetes Care 2009;32(11):1980–5.

60. Tasali E, Leproult R, Ehrmann DA, et al. Slow-wave sleep and the risk of type 2 diabetes in humans. Proc Natl Acad Sci U S A 2008;105(3):1044–9.

61. Andersson CX, Gustafson B, Hammarstedt A, et al. Inflamed adipose tissue, insulin resistance and vascular injury [review]. Diabetes Metab Res Rev 2008;24(8):595–603.

62. Toni R, Malaguti A, Castorina S, et al. New paradigms in neuroendocrinology: relationships between obesity, systemic inflammation and the neuroendocrine system. J Endocrinol Invest 2004; 27(2):182–6.

63. Calvin AD, Albuquerque FN, Lopez-Jimenez F, et al. Obstructive sleep apnea, inflammation, and

the metabolic syndrome. Metab Syndr Relat Disord 2009;7(4):271–8.

64. Park K, Steffes M, Lee DH, et al. Association of inflammation with worsening HOMA-insulin resistance. Diabetologia 2009;52(11):2337–44.

65. Lui MM, Lam JC, Mak HK, et al. C-reactive protein is associated with obstructive sleep apnea independent of visceral obesity. Chest 2009;135(4):950–6.

66. Dyck DJ. Adipokines as regulators of muscle metabolism and insulin sensitivity [review]. Appl Physiol Nutr Metab 2009;34(3):396–402.

67. Blüher S, Mantzoros CS. Leptin in humans: lessons from translational research. Am J Clin Nutr 2009; 89(3):991S–7S.

68. Ip MS, Lam KS, Ho C, et al. Serum leptin and vascular risk factors in obstructive sleep apnea. Chest 2000;118:580–6.

69. Ozturk L, Unal M, Tamer L, et al. The association of the severity of obstructive sleep apnea with plasma leptin levels. Arch Otolaryngol Head Neck Surg 2003;129:538–40.

70. Kapsimalis F, Varouchakis G, Manousaki A, et al. Association of sleep apnea severity and obesity with insulin resistance, C reactive protein, and leptin levels in male patients with obstructive sleep apnea. Lung 2008;186:209–17.

71. Sanner BM, Kollhosser P, Buechner N, et al. Influence of treatment on leptin levels in patients with obstructive sleep apnoea. Eur Respir J 2004;23: 601–4.

72. Harsch IA, Konturek PC, Koebnick C, et al. Leptin and ghrelin levels in patients with obstructive sleep apnoea: effect of CPAP treatment. Eur Respir J 2003;22:251–7.

73. Galic S, Oakhill JS, Steinberg GR. Adipose tissue as an endocrine organ. Mol Cell Endocrinol 2010; 316(2):129–39.

74. Kawano J, Arora R. The role of adiponectin in obesity, diabetes, and cardiovascular disease [review]. J Cardiometab Syndr 2009;4(1):44–9.

75. Han SH, Sakuma I, Shin EK, et al. Antiatherosclerotic and anti-insulin resistance effects of adiponectin: basic and clinical studies [review]. Prog Cardiovasc Dis 2009;52(2):126–40.

76. Lam JC, Xu A, Tam S, et al. Hypoadiponectinemia is related to sympathetic activation and severity of obstructive sleep apnea. Sleep 2008; 31(12):1721–7.

77. Wolk R, Svatikova A, Nelson CA, et al. Plasma levels of adiponectin, a novel adipocyte-derived hormone, in sleep apnea. Obesity Res 2005;13: 186–90.

78. Tso AW, Xu A, Sham PC, et al. Serum adipocyte fatty acid binding protein as a new biomarker predicting the development of type 2 diabetes: a 10-year prospective study in a Chinese cohort. Diabetes Care 2007;30(10):2667–72.

79. Xu A, Wang Y, Xu JY, et al. Adipocyte fatty acid-binding protein is a plasma biomarker closely associated with obesity and metabolic syndrome. Clin Chem 2006;52:405–13.

80. Lam DC, Xu A, Lam KS, et al. Serum adipocyte-fatty acid binding protein level is elevated in severe OSA and correlates with insulin resistance. Eur Respir J 2009;33(2):346–51.

81. Thorens B. Glucose sensing and the pathogenesis of obesity and type 2 diabetes. Int J Obes (Lond) 2008;32(Suppl 6):S62–71.

82. Imadojemu VA, Mawji Z, Kunselman A, et al. Sympathetic chemoreflex responses in obstructive sleep apnea and effects of continuous positive airway pressure therapy. Chest 2007;131(5): 1406–13.

83. Stamatakis K, Punjabi NM. Effects of sleep fragmentation on glucose metabolism in normal subjects. Chest 2010;137(1):95–101.

84. Cooper BG, White JE, Ashworth LA, et al. Hormonal and metabolic profiles in subjects with obstructive sleep apnea syndrome and the acute effects of nasal continuous positive airway pressure treatment. Sleep 1995;18:172–9.

85. Saini J, Krieger J, Brandenberger G, et al. Continuous positive airway pressure treatment. Effects on growth hormone, insulin and glucose profiles in obstructive sleep apnea patients. Horm Metab Res 1993;25:375–81.

86. Spiegel K, Leproult R, Van Cauter E. Impact of sleep debt on metabolic and endocrine function. Lancet 1999;354:1435–9.

87. Speigel K, Leproult R, Colecchia EF, et al. Adaptation of the 24-h growth hormone profile to a state of sleep debt. Am J Physiol Regul Integr Comp Physiol 2000;279:R874–83.

88. Strohl KP, Novak RD, Singer W, et al. Insulin levels, blood pressure and sleep apnea. Sleep 1994; 17(7):614–8.

89. Ip MS, Lam B, Ng MM, et al. Obstructive sleep apnea is independently associated with insulin resistance. Am J Respir Crit Care Med 2002;165: 670–6.

90. Meslier N, Gagnadoux F, Giraud P, et al. Impaired glucose insulin metabolism in males with obstructive sleep apnea syndrome. Eur Respir J 2003;22: 156–60.

91. Sulit L, Storfer-Isser A, Kirchner HL, et al. Differences in polysomnography predictors for hypertension and impaired glucose tolerance. Sleep 2006;29:777–83.

92. Makino S, Handa H, Suzukawa K, et al. Obstructive sleep apnoea syndrome, plasma adiponectin levels, and insulin resistance. Clin Endocrinol 2006;64:12–9.

93. Peled N, Kassirer M, Shitrit D, et al. The association of OSA with insulin resistance, inflammation and

metabolic syndrome. Respir Med 2007;101(8): 1696–701.

94. Sharma SK, Kumpawat S, Gael A, et al. Obesity, not obstructive sleep apnea, is responsible for metabolic abnormalities in a cohort with sleep disordered breathing. Sleep Med 2007;8:12–7.

95. Brooks B, Cistulli PA, Borkman M, et al. Obstructive sleep apnea in obese noninsulin-dependent diabetic patients: effect of continuous positive airway pressure treatment on insulin responsiveness. Clin Endocrinol Metab 1994;79(6):1681–5.

96. Hassaballa HA, Tulaimat A, Herdegen JJ, et al. The effect of continuous positive airway pressure on glucose control in diabetic patients with severe obstructive sleep apnea. Sleep Breath 2005;9(4): 176–80.

97. Trenell MI, Ward JA, Yee BJ, et al. Influence of constant positive airway pressure therapy on lipid storage, muscle metabolism and insulin action in obese patients with severe obstructive sleep apnoea syndrome. Diabetes Obes Metab 2007;9: 679–87.

98. Schahin SP, Nechanitzki T, Dittel C, et al. Long term improvement of insulin sensitivity during CPAP therapy in the obstructive sleep apnea syndrome. Med Sci Monit 2008;14:CR117–21.

99. Vgontzas AN, Zoumakis E, Bixler EO, et al. Selective effects of CPAP on sleep apnea associated manifestations. Eur J Clin Invest 2008;38:585–95.

100. Cuhadaroğlu C, Utkusavaş A, Oztürk L, et al. Effects of nasal CPAP treatment on insulin resistance, lipid profile, and plasma leptin in sleep apnea. Lung 2009;187(2):75–81.

Polysomnography

Behrouz Jafari, MD[a], Vahid Mohsenin, MD[a,b],*

KEYWORDS

- Polysomnography • Rapid eye movement
- Sleep disorders • Sleep study

The science of sleep and the specialty of sleep medicine have evolved rapidly since the initial attempts in the 1930s to develop a consistent framework to describe the complexity of sleep. The methods initially used to characterize correlates of sleep entailed the recording of brain electrical activity in animals in 1875[1] and the subsequent demonstration of the ability to detect and characterize wakeful activity in humans in 1929.[2] Detection and recording of human heart electrical activity were developing at about the same time[3] with identification of cardiac electrical waveforms by Einthoven[4] in 1895. In 1909, Cajal first delineated a network-intermingled collection of nerves and fibers (reticular formation) extending from the spinal cord to the thalamus.[5] Brainstem lesions high up at the midbrain produce continuous electroencephalogram (EEG) characteristics of sleep. The first continuous overnight EEG sleep recordings in humans were published in 1937.[6] The tracings on miles of paper recorded with an 8-ft–long drum polygraph were summarized using a data reduction scheme called sleep staging (stages A, B, C, D, and E), with stages A and B approximately corresponding to the current stage N1, stage C corresponding to stage N2, and stages D and E corresponding to stage N3. They recognized phenomena, such as the fragmentation and fallout of alpha rhythm sleep spindles and high-amplitude slow waves.

The combination of breathing and brain monitoring in physiologic recordings to identify pathologic conditions during sleep evolved in the mid-twentieth century.[7] Later, additional parameters were added when limb myoclonus was described in 1953.[8] Rapid eye movement (REM)–associated respiratory and cardiac effects were identified in 1953 by Aserinsky and Kleitman[9] and later more formally incorporated into the stages of REM sleep. In 1957, Dement and Kleitman[10] proposed the first classification based on an understanding that REM and non-REM (NREM) sleep alternate in successive cycles during the night. They suggested 4 stages (1–4), with stage 1 corresponding to stage N1 at the start of the night and stage R toward morning, stage 2 corresponding to stage N2, and stages 3 and 4 to stage N3.

Establishing a standard for describing sleep recording technique and sleep stage scoring varied widely from one laboratory to the next. Different terminology was used from one sleep center to the next; for example, REM sleep might be called D sleep, paradoxic sleep, desynchronized sleep, or even unorthodox sleep. In response to this circumstance, a committee was formed by members of the Sleep Research Society to standardize the data acquisition and scoring of sleep.[11] The committee recommended the recording of at least 1 EEG derivation, 2 electrooculogram (EOG) derivations, and 1 submental electromyogram (EMG). The recommendation required that sleep be scored in arbitrary epochs of 20 to 30 seconds with a single stage assigned to each epoch. They divided sleep into 5 stages: stages 1 through 4 of NREM sleep and stage REM sleep. Despite occasional suggestions for modifying the system,[11–16] the Rechtschaffen and Kales (R and K) manual remained the standard staging system for human sleep studies for almost 4 decades until 2004, when the board of directors of the American Academy of Sleep Medicine

---

[a] Section of Pulmonary, Critical Care and Sleep Medicine, Yale Center for Sleep Medicine, Yale University School of Medicine, New Haven, CT, USA
[b] Department of Medicine, Yale University School of Medicine, Yale Center for Sleep Medicine, New Haven, CT, USA
* Corresponding author. The John B. Pierce Laboratory, 290 Congress Avenue, New Haven, CT 06519.
E-mail address: Vahid.mohsenin@yale.edu

Clin Chest Med 31 (2010) 287–297
doi:10.1016/j.ccm.2010.02.005

(AASM) commissioned the development of a new manual for the scoring of sleep, including not only sleep staging but also rules for scoring other parameters (ie, arousals, respiratory, cardiac, and movement events).[17] The *AASM Manual for the Scoring of Sleep and Associated Events*, covering all aspects of sleep scoring, were published in 2007.[18] The AASM requires that the new scoring rules be followed in AASM-accredited sleep centers and laboratories.

TECHNIQUES

The polysomnography (PSG) uses various methods to simultaneously and continuously record neurophysiologic, cardiopulmonary, and other physiologic parameters over the course of several hours, usually during an entire night (overnight PSG). PSG provides information on the physiologic changes occurring in many different organ systems in relation to sleep stages and wakefulness. It allows qualitative and quantitative documentation of abnormalities of sleep and wakefulness, sleep-wake transition, and physiologic function of other organ systems that are influenced by sleep. Many of these, such as sleep apnea, may not be present during wakefulness.

Four types of sleep studies are available, depending on the number of physiologic variables recorded[19]:

- Level I. Standard PSG includes EEG (frontal, central, and occipital derivations), EOG, chin EMG, ECG, and recordings of airflow, respiratory effort, oxygen saturation, and limb EMG.[18] A technician is in constant attendance.
- Level II. Comprehensive portable PSG studies are essentially the same as level I, except that a heart rate monitor can replace the ECG and a technician is not in constant attendance.
- Level III. Modified portable sleep apnea testing is a cardiorespiratory study that includes ventilation (at least 2 channels of respiratory movement or respiratory movement and airflow), heart rate or ECG, and oxygen saturation. Ventilation in this case is measured with at least 2 channels of respiratory movement or of airflow. Personnel are needed for preparation, but the ability to intervene is not required for all studies.
- Level IV. Continuous (single or dual) bioparameter recordings where devices that measure a minimum of 1 parameter, usually oxygen saturation, are used.

Video monitoring, although not required, is extremely valuable, from diagnostic and medicolegal perspectives. Additional variables, such as 16-channel EEG recording for seizures, end-tidal CO_2 monitoring, pulse transit time, and esophageal pressure monitoring, can be added according to the clinical indications. The AASM recommends performing at least 6 hours of overnight recording.[19] The neurophysiologic, ECG, and sound channels are sampled at 100 to 1000 Hz with 12- to 20-bit resolution, respiratory mechanical channels at 50 Hz, and pulse oximetry and body position, at a significantly lower rate. The modern-day computerized PSG systems provide powerful tools for technicians and physicians to customize data acquisition. Reference electrodes, resolution, and sensitivity can be changed and digital filters added or removed to minimize recording artifacts. Many of these functions can be performed even after the data are acquired, which allows interpretation of the studies despite malfunction of certain equipment during the recording.[20]

The application of electrodes and sensors to a patient is the most important part of a sleep study. If done poorly, the quality of the data is compromised and a significant amount of the night is spent troubleshooting and problem solving. Filters should not be used to compensate for poor-quality electrode application, because changing filter settings can significantly alter the data, which affects how the study is analyzed.

Electroencephalography

EEG is the recording of surface electrical activity of the brain. Only limited EEG data are obtained during a PSG recording to help identify stages of sleep and wakefulness.

Reliable EEG recording begins with accurate measurement of the human skull, as dictated by the International Federation of Societies for Electroencephalography and Clinical Neurophysiology 10–20 system of electrode placement (**Fig. 1**).[21] Each of the points on the 10–20 map indicates a possible electrode site. Each electrode site is designated with a letter or letters and a number. The letters FP, F, C, P, and O represent frontal pole, frontal, central, parietal, and occipital, respectively. M represents the mastoid process. Odd numbers are used to denote the left-sided electrode placements; even numbers are used to denote the right-sided electrode placements. Z denotes midline electrode placement sites.

It is well recognized that alpha activity associated with wakefulness usually is most prominent when recorded from the occipital region. Although

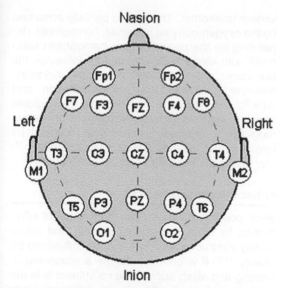

Fig. 1. Schematic representation of the 10–20 electrode placement system.

Williams and coworkers[22] argued as early as 1973 for including a bipolar occipital lead as a matter of routine, it was not adopted as standard technique until 1985 for use on the multiple sleep latency test[23] and 1992 for central nervous system arousal scoring on overnight PSGs.[24] Typically, a monopolar mastoid-referenced derivation from O1, O2, O3, or O4 is suggested.

The recommended derivations are F4-M1, C4-M1, and O2-M1.[18] A minimum of 3 EEG derivations is required to sample activity from the frontal, central, and occipital regions (M1 and M2 refer to the left and right mastoid processes).[18] This recommendation is partly based on K complexes maximally represented with frontal lobe electrodes, sleep spindles maximally seen with central electrodes, and delta activity maximally seen with frontal electrodes.[25] An accepted alternative is to use FZ-CZ, CZ-OZ, and C4-M1 with backup electrodes at FPZ, C3, O1, and M2 for alternative electrode displays in case of primary electrode malfunction.[18]

Electro-oculography

An EOG records changes that occur in the corneoretinal potential with eye movements during sleep and wakefulness. The cornea and retina form a dipole, with the cornea positive in relation to the retina. A movement in the eyes changes the electrical signal in the EOG electrodes, which is recorded as a deflection. The recommended EOG derivations are E1 (left eye)–M2 and E2 (right eye)–M2. E1 is placed 1 cm below the left outer

canthus. E2 is placed 1 cm above the right outer canthus for ease of recognition of REMs.[18]

The EOG is important in the evaluation of sleep and sleep stages. REMs are one of the signs of REM sleep and are essential for the scoring of REM sleep. These movements are seen as sharp bursts of electrical activity. At the time of sleep onset, slow eye movement can be seen.

Electromyogram

Submental and leg (tibialis anterior) EMG recordings are performed routinely during PSG. The submental EMG recordings are essential for scoring sleep stages, especially REM sleep. Three electrodes are placed for submental EMG recordings, to have a backup in case one of them malfunctions during the sleep study. Typically, the submental EMG tone is lowest during REM sleep. It is also helpful in detecting sleep bruxism. Bilateral leg EMG recordings are used to diagnose periodic limb movements of sleep. Additional EMG recordings can be used under special circumstances. For example, both upper and lower extremity EMGs can be recorded for suspected REM behavior disorder, and gastrocnemius muscle EMG could be recorded for diagnosing nocturnal leg cramps.[20]

Air Flow Measurement

The gold standard for measurement of air flow is body plethysmography and pneumotachography; however, they are considered unsuitable for routine PSG.[26] Currently airflow is measured with the help of a thermistor or with a nasal pressure monitor.

The thermistor measures changes in the electrical conductance in response to temperature changes in the probe, which occur with inspiration and expiration. Currently, use of an oronasal thermal sensor is recommended for detection of apnea and is used in conjunction with a nasal pressure transducer to allow the detection of hypopneas.[18] The ability of the nasal pressure transducer to adequately detect respiratory events is comparable to the gold standard approach of the pneumotachometer.[27,28]

Respiratory Effort Measurement

Different monitors have been used in the past to evaluate respiratory effort, including strain gauges, piezoelectric transducers, and impedance pneumography. The current recommendation is esophageal manometry or inductance plethysmography for monitoring and recording respiratory effort.[18] Esophageal manometry involves the passage of a thin flexible tube containing a pressure transducer through the nose or mouth, into the esophagus. Diaphragmatic contraction during inspiration causes a drop in thoracic pressure that is transmitted to the esophagus and detected by the pressure transducer. The reverse occurs during expiration. Esophageal pressure measurements are a sensitive and qualitative index of inspiratory effort. Because esophageal manometry is not well accepted or tolerated by most subjects undergoing PSG, inductance plethysmography has become the method of choice in most sleep laboratories.

Respiratory inductance plethysmography measures respiratory effort from body surface movement. Inductance is the property of a circuit or circuit element that opposes a change in current flow. Bands that contain transducers (which consist of an insulated wire sewn onto an elasticized band in the shape of a horizontally oriented sinusoid) are placed around the rib cage and abdomen.[29] With inspiration and expiration, the changes in the cross-sectional area of the chest and abdomen cause a proportional change in the diameter of the transducer. This change in the diameter of the transducer alters the inductance. These monitors can be calibrated to a known volume, which provides qualitative and quantitative analyses of breath volumes.

Snoring

Snoring is recorded from a snore microphone, and the signal is displayed as a continuous waveform. Technician notes are the most useful way of assessing the severity of snoring. Snoring signal is also prominently reflected in chin EMG and in nasal pressure tracing.

Cardiac Monitoring

Standard recording of cardiac rhythm during PSG is by use of a modified lead II electrograph with 1 lead just inferior to the right clavicle and the other on the left side at the level of the seventh rib. Current recommendations are that several cardiac parameters, such as average heart rate during sleep, highest heart rate during sleep, highest heart rate during recording, bradycardia, and other arrhythmias, be reported in all sleep study interpretations.[18]

Measurement of Oxygenation

The most commonly used noninvasive method for the continuous monitoring of blood oxygen is the use of pulse oximetry, in which the oxygen saturation of arterial blood (SaO_2) is determined by the passage of 2 wavelengths of light (650 nm and 805 nm) through a pulsating vascular bed from 1

sensor to another. The light is partially absorbed by the oxygen-carrying molecule, hemoglobin, depending on the percent of the hemoglobin saturated with oxygen. Several factors influence the accuracy and reliability of pulse oximetry, however, including the sensor location and type[30]; the presence of abnormal hemoglobin species, such as carboxyhemoglobin or methemoglobin[29]; reduced skin perfusion caused by hypothermia; hypotension or vasoconstriction[31]; and change in heart rate and circulation time.[32]

Other Monitoring Devices

Body position is also an important piece of information to monitor, because snoring and upper airway obstruction during sleep are influenced by gravity.[33,34] It is common to see a worsening of snoring and sleep apnea when a subject is in the supine position. Continuous recording of body position is determined by a sensor, which is usually placed on the chest. A common problem with body position sensor is that it may not correlate closely with the actual subject's position and therefore it is important for a technologist to record the subject's body position via camera/video monitoring to confirm accuracy of the body position monitor.

STAGING SLEEP

In 2007, the new *AASM Manual for the Scoring of Sleep and Associated Events* was published, providing a comprehensive reference for the evaluation of PSGs.[18] According to the new criteria, the following staging system was proposed:

- Stage W (wakefulness)
- Stage N1 (NREM stage 1 sleep)
- Stage N2 (NREM stage 2 sleep)
- Stage N3 (NREM stage 3 sleep)
- Stage R (REM sleep).

The change in sleep staging differentiates the scoring rules from those of the R and K manual published in 1968. The basic principle of sleep staging is that the night is divided into 30-second sequential periods, known as epochs. Each epoch is assigned a stage. If 2 or more stages can be identified during a single epoch, the stage comprising the greatest portion of the epoch is assigned. Although an assessment of the overall flow of sleep might be better obtained by relying on identifying the start and end of each stage irrespective of epochs, such a scoring method is cumbersome in the presence of highly fragmented sleep, as may be seen in patients with obstructive sleep apnea syndrome (OSA).

Wakefulness (Stage W)

Wakefulness is defined by the presence of 8 to 13 Hz sinusoidal alpha rhythm in the posterior head regions on the EEG (**Fig. 2**)[18] and greater than 50% of an epoch having this rhythm. Alpha appears with eye closure and attenuates with eye opening. About 10% to 20% of normal subjects have little or no alpha rhythm.[35] When alpha rhythm is not clearly discernable by visual inspection of the EEG, wakefulness can still be scored if the EOG demonstrates any 1 of 3 markers of alertness:

- Eye blinks; blinking results in conjugate vertical eye movements at a frequency of 0.5 to 2 Hz, which are visible on the EOG
- Reading eye movements (which consist of a slow phase followed by a rapid movement in the opposite direction)
- Irregular conjugate eye movements with normal or high chin muscle tone.

Stage N1 Sleep

Although the AASM manual recognizes that many signs of drowsiness are discernable before alpha rhythm is lost, it does specify a single time of sleep onset. This is defined as the start of the first epoch scored as any stage other than stage W, recognizing that in most subjects this is stage N1.[18] This stage is defined by the presence of low-amplitude, mixed-frequency activity of predominantly 4 to 7 Hz (**Fig. 3**).[18] The EOG generally shows slow eye movements and the chin EMG is often lower in amplitude than in stage W. The EEG may show vertex sharp waves, which are sharply contoured waves maximal over the central region, distinguishable from the background EEG and lasting less than 0.5 second. None of these additional features is required for scoring stage N1, although their presence may be helpful in equivocal situations. In subjects who do not have alpha rhythm and show low-amplitude, mixed-frequency activity with the eyes closed even in wakefulness, discerning sleep onset can be problematic. In these circumstances, stage N1 sleep should be scored when slowing of background EEG frequencies by greater than or equal to 1 Hz, vertex sharp wave, or slow eye movements is observed.[36] The onset of slow eye movements usually precedes the other changes and is the criterion most likely to be applied. Because slow eye movements are usually seen when alpha rhythm is still present, the sleep latency is likely to be slightly shorter in subjects who do not show alpha rhythm.[36]

Stage N2 Sleep

Stage N2 sleep is defined by the presence of 1 or more K complexes without associated arousals or 1 or more trains of sleep spindles in the first half of the epoch or in the second half of the prior epoch.[18] A K complex is a well-defined biphasic wave easily discernable from the background EEG with total duration greater than or equal to 0.5 seconds, usually maximal frontally (**Fig. 4**). A sleep spindle is a train of waves with a frequency of 11 to 16 Hz, but usually 12 to 14 Hz, with duration greater than or equal to 0.5 second, usually maximal centrally. There are no defined amplitude criteria for a K complex or a sleep spindle. K complexes can be associated with arousals induced by environmental stimuli or by sleep apnea. In some patients with OSA, sleep can be highly fragmented by repeated apnea-induced arousals with frequent K complexes. K complexes induced by arousals do not represent a deeper level of sleep and so cannot be used to designate stage N2 sleep, unless a spontaneous K complex or sleep spindle is also present in the same epoch. K complexes and sleep spindles are intermittent phenomena and may not always be present in successive epochs. Their absence does not indicate that sleep has reverted to stage N1 unless an arousal occurs or a major body movement followed by slow eye movements is present. Stage N2 sleep terminates when there is a transition to stages W, N3, or R.[36]

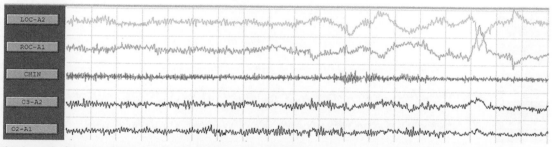

Fig. 2. Wakefulness with presence of alpha waves and REMs.

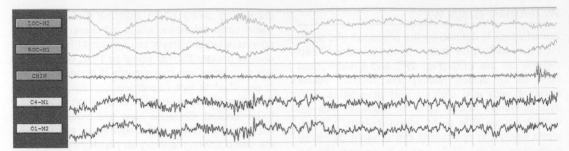

Fig. 3. Stage N1 with mixed-frequency EEG and rolling eye movements.

Stage N3 Sleep

Stage N3 sleep is scored when greater than or equal to 20% of an epoch consists of slow wave activity, defined as waves of frequency of 0.5 to 2 Hz with peak-to-peak amplitude greater than 75 mV recorded over the frontal regions (**Fig. 5**).[18] The frequency band is a subset of the classically defined delta frequency range (<4 Hz) and the term, *delta sleep*, should not be used. Sleep spindles may persist in stage N3 sleep but are not required for scoring.

The neurophysiologic genesis of slow waves differs from that of K complexes,[37] such as growth hormone, is maximally released during slow wave sleep rather than stage N2.[38,39]

Stage R, REM Sleep

REM sleep is scored if an epoch includes low-amplitude, mixed-frequency EEG, REMs, and low chin EMG tone (**Fig. 6**).[18] The EEG is similar to that in stage N1, but some subjects have more prominent alpha frequencies, often at a frequency somewhat slower than that of their alpha rhythm when they are awake. REMs are defined as conjugate, irregular, sharply peaked eye movements with the duration of the initial deflection usually less than 500 milliseconds. Low chin EMG tone implies that the chin EMG amplitude is no higher than in any other stage and is usually at the lowest level of the entire PSG. Certain other phenomena,

if present, may support scoring stage R but are not required. These include saw tooth waves (2–6 Hz sharply contoured or triangular, often serrated waves maximal over the central head regions and frequently preceding bursts of REMs) and transient muscle activity, previously known as phasic muscle twitches (burst of EMG activity lasting <0.25 seconds superimposed on low tone background, which may be present in the chin, anterior tibialis, or EEG-EOG derivations). Detailed rules define when a period of stage R sleep ends.[18] In general, once stage R is scored, subsequent epochs should continue to be scored as stage R until there is a definite change to another stage, an arousal or major body movement is followed by slow eye movements, or K complexes or sleep spindles occur in the absence of REMs, even if chin EMG tone remains low. If an epoch contains REMs and the chin EMG tone is low, stage R should be scored even if K complexes or sleep spindles are present. This latter situation frequently occurs during the first REM period of the night when REM and NREM phenomena intermix. There are also rules concerning the scoring of transition epochs between epochs of definite stage N2 and definite REM sleep. In outline, stage R should be scored if chin EMG tone is low and K complexes and sleep spindles are absent, even if REM has not yet commenced. If K complexes or sleep spindles are present in the transition epochs without REMs, however,

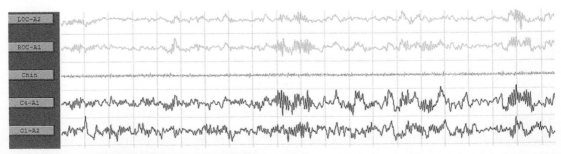

Fig. 4. Stage N2 with K complex and sleep spindles.

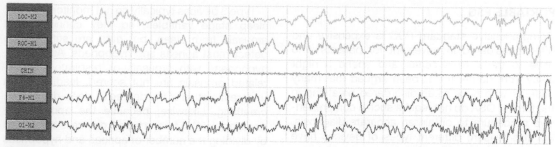

Fig. 5. Stage N3 with delta waves.

these should be scored as stage N2, even if chin muscle tone is low.[18,36]

Major Body Movement

The term, *movement time*, was used in the R and K manual[40] to classify epochs when more than 50% of the EEG was obscured by body movements and muscle artifact. The AASM manual eliminated this term, replacing it with the concept of major body movements. Epochs with major body movements are scored as stage W if any alpha rhythm, even comprising less than half the epoch, is present, or if the preceding or following epoch is scored as stage W. Otherwise, the epoch is given the same stage as the epoch that follows.[18] The logic behind this rule is that major body movements generally result in an arousal or at least a change to a lighter stage of sleep.[36]

Indications for PSG

The Standards of Practice Committee of the AASM reviewed the indications for PSG in 2005 and recommended the following[41]:

- Sleep-related breathing disorders, including OSA, central sleep apnea syndrome (CSA), Cheyne-Stokes respiration (CSR), and alveolar hypoventilation syndrome; upper airway resistance syndrome; the present reference or gold standard for evaluation of sleep and sleep-related breathing is the PSG

- Narcolepsy, parasomnias, sleep-related seizure disorders, restless legs syndrome, periodic limb movement sleep disorder, depression with insomnia
- For continuous positive airway pressure (CPAP) titration in patients with sleep-related breathing disorders; for the assessment of treatment results in some cases; with a multiple sleep latency test in the evaluation of suspected narcolepsy; in evaluating sleep-related behaviors that are violent or otherwise potentially injurious to the patient or others; and in certain atypical or unusual parasomnias. PSG may be indicated in patients with neuromuscular disorders and sleep-related symptoms, to assist in the diagnosis of paroxysmal arousals or other sleep disruptions thought to be seizure related, in a presumed parasomnia or sleep-related seizure disorder that does not respond to conventional therapy, or when there is a strong clinical suspicion of periodic limb movement sleep disorder.

PSG is not routinely indicated to diagnose chronic lung disease; in cases of typical, uncomplicated, and noninjurious parasomnias when the diagnosis is clinically evident; for patients with seizures who have no specific complaints consistent with a sleep disorder; to diagnose or treat restless legs syndrome; for the diagnosis of circadian rhythm sleep disorders; or to establish a diagnosis of depression.

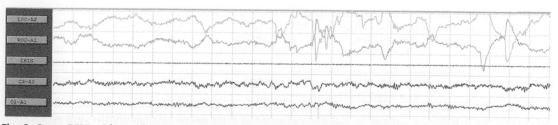

Fig. 6. Stage REM with rapid eye movements and saw tooth waves.

PORTABLE PSG

Comprehensive standard PSG is expensive and often considered inconvenient for patients who have to travel to a center and spend a night away from home. It has been argued that many patients who have sleep-disordered breathing in the form of OSA do not require such a comprehensive procedure to obtain an accurate diagnosis. For this reason, different types of devices have been developed to test for sleep apnea at home or outside the usual environment of a sleep center. Portable monitoring, therefore, in this context means technology that can be performed outside a sleep center and often is unattended. Such devices may be as simple as overnight oximetry or include all the same leads as performed with standard PSG.[42]

In 1994 the AASM noted that the available portable devices had insufficient reliability to allow for widespread usage.[43] In 2005 and 2007, different type of studies emerged, which suggested that in highly selected populations, the outcomes with regards to the use of CPAP were at least equivalent with portable compared with standard PSG.[44,45] Later in 2007, another article was published by the AASM, which set forth some clinical guidelines for use of portable studies.[46] Finally, these devices appeared to have broken through many of the barriers that were preventing it from more widespread usage. AASM divided the technology into different parameters, which may be a more useful way to approach portable devices types (**Tables 1** and **2**).[46] Type 2 devices require experienced technologist to avoid problems with data acquisition that tend to occur with these devices. These types of studies might be best for institutionalized patients who have trouble getting to a sleep center or for hospitalized patients.[42]

Type 3 devices typically do not monitor EEG and sleep stage variables, so they cannot detect arousals from sleep, but data are sufficient to detect most apneas and hypopneas. As a result, hypopneas with arousals or respiratory effort–related arousals are not scored, leading to an underestimation of the degree of sleep-disordered breathing. Likewise, because the apnea-hypopnea index (AHI) from a type 3 device is calculated by dividing the number of apneas and hypopneas (only scored with desaturations) by the entire study duration rather than total sleep time, tends to be underestimated. These calculation changes cause the AHI tends to be derived by a type 3 to be lower than that derived by PSG, which decreases the diagnostic sensitivity.

The information that can be collected from a type 4 device includes frequency of apneas, frequency of hypopneas (with desaturation only), an AHI (as divided by total recording time), baseline Sao_2, mean Sao_2, frequency of desaturation, and nadirs of Sao_2. Therefore, not only do all of the limitations of type 3 devices apply to type 4 devices but also type 4 devices cannot differentiate between obstructive and central/mixed apneas. There are other limitations regarding types 3 and 4 devices. Unlike PSG, in which there are standardized rules for scoring events, there are no published standardized rules for portables. Many devices use proprietary algorithms to score events, and a user cannot alter the scoring.[42] Similarly, the characteristics of overnight pulse oximetry depend on the criteria used to define events. When using a quantitative measure, such as a 4% desaturation, the sensitivity is low for diagnosing OSA; however, the specificity is acceptable.[47–49] When using more qualitative criteria, however, such as analyzing the tracing for frequent desaturations, often known as a saw tooth pattern, the sensitivity improves but the

Table 1
Types of monitoring systems during sleep

	Type 1	Type 2	Type 3	Type 4
Number of leads	≥ 7	≥ 7	≥ 4	1–2
Types of leads	EEG, EOG, EMG, ECG, airflow, effort, oximetry	EEG, EOG, EMG, ECG, airflow, effort, oximetry	Airflow, effort, oximetry, ECG	Oximetry + other (usually airflow)
Setting	Attended usually in a sleep center	Unattended	Unattended	Unattended

Data from Ferber R, Millman R, Coppola M, et al. Portable recording in the assessment of obstructive sleep apnea. ASDA standards of practice. Sleep 1994;17(4):378–92.

Table 2
AASM clinical guidelines: parameters used for portable monitors

Parameter	Examples
Oximetry	
Respiratory monitoring	Effort
	Airflow
	Snoring
	End-tidal CO_2
	Esophageal pressure
Cardiac monitoring	Heart rate
	Heart rate variability
	Arterial tonometry
Measures of sleep/ wake activity	EEG
	Actigraphy
Body position	Accelerometer
Other	

Data from Collop NA, Anderson WM, Boehlecke B, et al. Clinical guidelines for the use of unattended portable monitors in the diagnosis of obstructive sleep apnea in adult patients. Portable Monitoring Task Force of the American Academy of Sleep Medicine. J Clin Sleep Med 2007;3(7):737–47.

specificity falls.[50] A more recent study showed poor consistency between pulmonary physicians interpreting overnight oximetry readings.[51] The low level of consistency suggests there are significant problems with either approach that result in increased false-negative or false -positive tests.

Several studies that have used portable and standard PSG in a highly selected patient population have shown no significant differences in the outcome measures between these two types of monitoring. The absence of difference in the outcomes were, in large part, due to employment of highly trained sleep specialists and the training and education of the patients on the use of these devices.[44,45,52]

Based on the AASM recommendations, portable devices should record airflow, respiratory effort, and blood oxygenation. The most accurate airflow signals would include a thermister and a nasal pressure sensor and the most accurate effort signals would use respiratory inductance plethysmography.

Choosing an appropriate population is important when considering use of portable device to diagnose OSA.[53] As discussed previously, most of the studies showing positive outcomes with portables have been done on patients who had a high likelihood of having OSA. In addition, confounding disorders, such as respiratory disease or cardiac disease, are usually a reason to exclude patients for portables testing. The presence of

other comorbid sleep disorders, such as insomnia, restless legs syndrome, or parasomnias, are also likely to reduce the accuracy of portables, and their use should be avoided.[42]

SUMMARY AND FUTURE

PSG is an essential tool for diagnosis of variety of sleep disorders. The results of PSG should be interpreted in the context of a patient's history and medications and observation in the sleep laboratory. As new technologies evolve, it is expected that the field also will evolve. Further work is needed to determine if computerized scoring, with or without human revision, may one day reliably replace visual scoring in normal and abnormal sleep. Improved techniques to measure and quantify sleep itself will allow for more meaningful assessment of sleep disruption that can lead to the recognition of new disorders and better predictions of the outcomes of these disorders.

REFERENCES

1. Caton R. The electric current of the brain. Br Med J 1875;2:278.
2. Berger H. Uber das elektroenkelphalogramm des Menshcen [About electroencephalogram of Menshcen]. Arch Psychiatr Nervenkr 1929;87: 527–70 [in German].
3. Walter A. A demonstration on man of electromotive changes accompanying the heart beat. J Physiol 1887;8:229–34.
4. Einthoven W. Uber die form des menschlichen electrocardiogramms [About the form of the human electrocardiographic program]. Arch Gesamte Physiol 1895;60:101–23 [in German].
5. Cajal RS. Histologie du systeme nerveux de l'homme et des vertebres. Paris: Norbert Maloine; 1909.
6. Loomis AL, Harvey N, Hobart GA. Cerebral states during sleep, as studied by human brain potentials. J Exp Psychol 1937;21:127–44.
7. Gastaut H, Tassinari CA, Duron B. Polygraphic study of diurnal and nocturnal (hypnic and respiratory) episodal manifestations of Pickwick syndrome. Rev Neurol (Paris) 1965;112:568–79.
8. Symonds CP. Nocturnal myoclonus. J Neurol Neurosurg Psychiatry 1953;16(3):166–71.
9. Aserinsky E, Kleitman N. Regularly occurring periods of eye motility and concomitant phenomena during sleep. Science 1953;118:273–4.
10. Dement W, Kleitman N. Cyclic variations in EEG during sleep and their relation to eye movements, body motility, and dreaming. Electroencephalogr Clin Neurophysiol 1957;9(4):673–90.

11. Hori T, Sugita Y, Koga E, et al. Proposed supplements and amendments to 'a manual of standardized terminology, techniques and scoring system for sleep stages of human subjects', the Rechtschaffen & Kales (1968) standard. Psychiatry Clin Neurosci 2001;55(3):305–10.

12. Himanen SL, Hasan J. Limitations of Rechtschaffen and Kales. Sleep Med Rev 2000;4(2):149–67.

13. Hirshkowitz M. Standing on the shoulders of giants: the standardized sleep manual after 30 years. Sleep Med Rev 2000;4:169–79.

14. McGregor P, Thorpy MJ, Schmidt-Nowara WW, et al. T-sleep: an improved method for scoring breathing-disordered sleep. Sleep 1992;15(4):359–63.

15. Shepard JW. Atlas of sleep medicine Armonk. New York: Futura Publishing Company; 1991.

16. van Sweden B, Kemp B, Kamphuisen HA, et al. Alternative electrode placement in (automatic) sleep scoring (Fpz-Cz/Pz-Oz versus C4-A1). Sleep 1990; 13(3):279–83.

17. Iber C, Ancoli-Israel S, Chambers M, et al. The new sleep scoring manual: the evidence behind the rules. J Clin Sleep Med 2007;3:107.

18. Iber C, Ancoli-Israel S, Chesson A, et al. The AASM manual for the scoring of sleep and associated events—rules, terminology and technical specifications. 1st edition. Westchester (IL): American Academy of Sleep Medicine; 2007.

19. ASDA Standards of Practice. Portable recording in the assessment of sleep. Sleep 1994;17:378–92.

20. Kakkar RK, Hill GK. Interpretation of the adult polysomnogram. Otolaryngol Clin North Am 2007;40:713–43.

21. Jasper HH. The ten twenty electrode system of the International Federation. Electroencephalogr Clin Neurophysiol 1958;10:371–5.

22. Williams RL, Karacan I, Hursch CJ. EEG of human sleep: clinical applications. New York: Wiley; 1974.

23. Carskadon MA, Dement WC, Mitler MM, et al. Guidelines for the multiple sleep latency test (MSLT): a standard measure of sleepiness. Sleep 1986;9(4):519–24.

24. EEG arousals. Scoring rules and examples: a preliminary report from the Sleep Disorders Atlas Task Force of the American Sleep Disorders Association. Sleep 1992;15(2):173–84.

25. Silber MH, Ancoli-Israel S, Bonnet MH, et al. The visual scoring of sleep in adults. J Clin Sleep Med 2007;3(2):121–31.

26. Redline S, Budhiraja R, Kapur V, et al. The scoring of respiratory events in sleep: reliability and validity. J Clin Sleep Med 2007;3(2):169–200.

27. Heitman SJ, Atkar RS, Hajduk EA, et al. Validation of nasal pressure for the identification of apneas/hypopneas during sleep. Am J Respir Crit Care Med 2002;166(3):386–91.

28. Thurnheer R, Bloch KE. Monitoring nasal conductance by bilateral nasal cannula pressure transducers. Physiol Meas 2004;25(2):577–84.

29. Kryger MH, Roth T, Dement WC. Principles and practice of sleep medicine. 3rd edition. Philadelphia: Saunders; 2004.

30. West P, George CF, Kryger MH. Dynamic in vivo response characteristics of three oximeters: Hewlett-Packard 47201A, Biox III, and Nellcor N-100. Sleep 1987;10(3):263–71.

31. Berg S, Haight JS, Yap V, et al. Comparison of direct and indirect measurements of respiratory airflow: implications for hypopneas. Sleep 1997;20(1):60–4.

32. Farre R, Montserrat JM, Ballester E, et al. Importance of the pulse oximeter averaging time when measuring oxygen desaturation in sleep apnea. Sleep 1998;21(4):386–90.

33. McEvoy RD, Sharp DJ, Thornton AT. The effects of posture on obstructive sleep apnea. Am Rev Respir Dis 1986;133(4):662–6.

34. Oksenberg A, Khamaysi I, Silverberg DS, et al. Association of body position with severity of apneic events in patients with severe nonpositional obstructive sleep apnea. Chest 2000;118(4):1018–24.

35. Santamaria J, Chiappa KH. The EEG of drowsiness in normal adults. J Clin Neurophysiol 1987;4(4):327–82.

36. Silber MH. Staging sleep. Sleep Med Clin 2009;4(3):343–52.

37. Steriade M, Amzica F. Slow sleep oscillation, rhythmic K-complexes, and their paroxysmal developments. J Sleep Res 1998;7(Suppl 1):30–5.

38. Holl RW, Hartman ML, Veldhuis JD, et al. Thirty-second sampling of plasma growth hormone in man: correlation with sleep stages. J Clin Endocrinol Metab 1991;72(4):854–61.

39. Van Cautier E, Plat L, Copinschi G. Interrelations between sleep and the somatotrophic axis. Sleep 1998;21:553–66.

40. Rechtschaffen A, Kales A. A manual of standardized terminology, techniques and scoring system for sleep stages of human subjects. Washington, DC: US Government Printing Office NIH publication; 1968.

41. Kushida CA, Littner MR, Morgenthaler T, et al. Practice parameters for the indications for polysomnography and related procedures: an update for 2005. Sleep 2005;28(4):499–521.

42. Collop NA. Portable monitoring. Sleep Med Clin 2009;4:3.

43. Ferber R, Millman R, Coppola M, et al. Portable recording in the assessment of obstructive sleep apnea. ASDA standards of practice. Sleep 1994; 17(4):378–92.

44. Mulgrew AT, Fox N, Ayas NT, et al. Diagnosis and initial management of obstructive sleep apnea

without polysomnography: a randomized validation study. Ann Intern Med 2007;146(3):157–66.

45. Whitelaw WA, Brant RF, Flemons WW. Clinical usefulness of home oximetry compared with polysomnography for assessment of sleep apnea. Am J Respir Crit Care Med 2005;171(2):188–93.

46. Collop NA, Anderson WM, Boehlecke B, et al. Clinical guidelines for the use of unattended portable monitors in the diagnosis of obstructive sleep apnea in adult patients. Portable Monitoring Task Force of the American Academy of Sleep Medicine. J Clin Sleep Med 2007;3(7):737–47.

47. Douglas NJ, Thomas S, Jan MA. Clinical value of polysomnography. Lancet 1992;339(8789):347–50.

48. Gyulay S, Olson LG, Hensley MJ, et al. A comparison of clinical assessment and home oximetry in the diagnosis of obstructive sleep apnea. Am Rev Respir Dis 1993;147(1):50–3.

49. Williams AJ, Yu G, Santiago S, et al. Screening for sleep apnea using pulse oximetry and a clinical score. Chest 1991;100(3):631–5.

50. Series F, Marc I, Cormier Y, et al. Utility of nocturnal home oximetry for case finding in patients with suspected sleep apnea hypopnea syndrome. Ann Intern Med 1993;119(6):449–53.

51. Ramsey R, Mehra R, Strohl KP. Variations in physician interpretation of overnight pulse oximetry monitoring. Chest 2007;132(3):852–9.

52. Berry RB, Hill G, Thompson L, et al. Portable monitoring and autotitration versus polysomnography for the diagnosis and treatment of sleep apnea. Sleep 2008;31(10):1423–31.

53. Epstein LJ, Kristo D, Strollo PJ. Clinical guideline for the evaluation, management and long-term care of obstructive sleep apnea in adults. J Clin Sleep Med 2009;5(3):263–76.

Ambulatory Management of Patients with Sleep Apnea: Is There a Place for Portable Monitor Testing?

Bernie Sunwoo, BSc(Med), MBBS[a],*, Samuel T. Kuna, MD[b,c]

KEYWORDS

- Polysomnogram • Apnea-hypopnea index
- Continuous positive airway pressure
- Cost-effectiveness • Comparative effectiveness

With the increased recognition of sleep apnea, systems for delivering diagnosis and treatment are overwhelmed. There is a need to rethink current strategies.[1]

Obstructive sleep apnea (OSA) is common and, with the increase in obesity in both adults and children, its prevalence is increasing. Substantial evidence shows that OSA is associated with clinically important adverse consequences including daytime hypersomnolence, hypertension, cardiovascular disease, strokes, neurocognitive deficits, diabetes, motor vehicle accidents, decreased quality of life, and increased all-cause mortality.[2–12] Fortunately, effective treatment is available, most commonly in the form of continuous positive airway pressure (CPAP).[13,14] Traditionally, the diagnosis of OSA and titration of CPAP has relied on in-laboratory polysomnography (PSG). This procedure is costly, labor intensive, and limited in availability.[15] Consequently, there has been growing pressure to develop alternative, ambulatory management strategies to diagnose and treat patients with OSA using home, unattended testing with portable monitors.

The role of portable monitoring devices in the diagnosis and management of OSA is rapidly evolving. Several recent reviews and guidelines by government agencies and medical societies have now been published.[16–21] The excellent technology assessment from the Agency for Health Care Research and Quality (AHRQ) highlights the complexities and challenges involved in diagnosing OSA with both in-laboratory PSG and home, unattended, portable monitor testing.[21]

A PROBLEM OF PATIENT ACCESS TO DIAGNOSIS AND TREATMENT

Epidemiologic studies report a high prevalence of OSA worldwide.[12,22,23] Results of the Wisconsin Sleep Cohort Study published in 1993 reported

This work was supported by Grant No. HSR&D 04-021-2.

[a] Division of Pulmonary, Allergy and Critical Care Medicine, Department of Medicine, Hospital of the University of Pennsylvania, University of Pennsylvania, 844 West Gates, Philadelphia, PA 19104, USA
[b] Pulmonary, Critical Care and Sleep Medicine Section, Department of Medicine, Philadelphia VA Medical Center, 3900 Woodland Avenue (111P), Philadelphia, PA 19104, USA
[c] Division of Pulmonary, Allergy and Critical Care Medicine, Department of Medicine, University of Pennsylvania, 844 West Gates, Philadelphia, PA 19104, USA
* Corresponding author.
E-mail address: Bernie.Sunwoo@uphs.upenn.edu

Clin Chest Med 31 (2010) 299–308
doi:10.1016/j.ccm.2010.02.003
0272-5231/10/$ – see front matter © 2010 Elsevier Inc. All rights reserved.

a prevalence of OSA, as defined by an apnea-hypopnea index (AHI) of equal to or greater than five events per hour, in 24% of men and 9% of women aged 30 to 60 years. When the presence of daytime hypersomnolence was included in the definition, the prevalence of OSA in this community-based cohort was 4% of men and 2% of women.[23] The prevalence of OSA in adults increases with age[3,12,23] and it is estimated that 0.7% to 13% of children have OSA.[24] Obesity is one of the most important risk factors for OSA. With the dramatic increase in obesity over the past 25 years, the increasing age of the population, and the growing recognition of the adverse consequences associated with OSA, OSA has exploded into a major public health burden.

Health care systems, especially in developing countries, have not been able to keep up with the increasing patient demand. In the United States, at least 80% of patients with OSA are thought to remain undiagnosed.[25] Whereas the volume of sleep referrals in the USA has increased 12-fold in the last decade, the number of sleep laboratories in the same period has only doubled.[26] In the United Kingdom, the average time from referral to CPAP titration was estimated at 14 months while in Canada it averaged 24 months.[15] In reality, availability is motivated by funding models, with long patient wait times in federal and public healthcare systems. Sleep specialists themselves are in short supply. This has forced many practitioners with little to no training to manage OSA. In some Canadian provinces, primary care physicians order home oximetry to diagnose patients with OSA without referral to a sleep specialist, and in the United Kingdom almost two thirds of all sleep studies are oximetry alone, 20% limited sleep studies, and only 10% full PSG, of which over 50% are performed unattended at home.[15]

PSG IS A FLAWED REFERENCE STANDARD

While the attended, in-laboratory PSG is widely considered the standard in clinical practice for the diagnosis of OSA, it is not a gold standard. The in-laboratory PSG has never been validated and its true sensitivity and specificity in diagnosing OSA is not well documented.[16] The AHI is used by healthcare providers and third-party insurers as a single metric for defining OSA. This emphasis on the centrality of a single number, that is known to vary from night to night, differs from that in other fields where data from physiologic tests are used as just one of many indices to gauge disease severity and to follow treatment responses, but are not used as the sole diagnostic instrument.[27]

Population studies show a unimodal distribution in the AHI and the selection of a particular AHI cut point for the diagnosis of OSA is not based on evidence-based medicine.[28] The recommended AHI cut points of at least 5 events per hour for diagnosis and 5, 15, and 30 events per hour for assessment of mild, moderate, and severe disease severity are recommendations by expert consensus. Indeed, studies have used varying AHI thresholds to define OSA ranging from 5 to 40 events per hour.[21] The known night-to-night variability in AHI on in-laboratory PSG further weakens the clinical utility of this index. Furthermore, the AHI alone correlates weakly with patients' symptoms and treatment outcomes.[20,21,28–31] These weaknesses in the AHI measurement challenge the absolute need for an exact AHI value based on in-laboratory PSG in populations with a high probability for OSA. Comparing portable monitor testing to such a flawed reference standard is clearly problematic.

TYPES OF PORTABLE MONITORS FOR DIAGNOSIS OF OSA

Technological advances have enabled the development of user-friendly portable monitor devices that can diagnose OSA in unattended, out-of-laboratory settings. A wide range of devices are commercially available that vary not only in the number and types of signals recorded, but the sensors used, the methods of scoring, and the criteria used to define respiratory events. Studies using a particular portable monitor cannot be generalized to other monitors—even those in the same class (see later discussion). This lack of standardization limits the ability to perform meta-analyses and evidence-based reviews. Physicians should be aware of the strengths and weaknesses of the specific device chosen for use in their patients.

In 1994, the American Sleep Disorders Association, now the American Academy of Sleep Medicine (AASM), classified sleep testing into four types based on the number and types of signals recorded (**Table 1**).[19] Type 1 testing is full, attended, in-laboratory PSG. Type 2 recordings employ the same signals as in-laboratory PSG and use a minimum of seven channels, but are not attended by trained personnel. Given the patient's inability to self-apply bipolar electrodes, type 2 tests require home set-up by a trained technologist and are not practical for clinical purposes. However, type 2 portable monitors have proven useful in research studies that require full PSG to minimize participant burden, maintain flexibility of scheduling, and standardize recording equipment across sites in multicenter studies.

Table 1
Current classification of the different types of sleep studies

Sleep Test	Description	Personnel	Minimum Signals Required
Type 1	Standard PSG performed in a sleep laboratory	Attended	Minimum of 7 signals, including EEG, EOG, chin EMG, ECG, airflow, respiratory effort, and oxygen saturation
Type 2	Comprehensive portable PSG	Unattended	Same as type 1
Type 3	Portable testing limited to sleep apnea	Attended and unattended	Minimum of 4 signals, including ECG or heart rate, oxygen saturation, and at least 2 channels of respiratory movement, or respiratory movement and airflow
Type 4	Continuous recording of one or two signals	Unattended	Usually pulse oximetry

Abbreviations: EEG, electroencephalogram; EOG, electrooculogram; EMG, electromyogram.
Data from Ferber R, R Millman, M Coppola, et al. Portable recording in the assessment of obstructive sleep apnea. ASDA standards of practice. Sleep 1994;17(4):378–92.

Type 3 monitors record a minimum of four signals, including ECG or heart rate, oxygen saturation, and at least two respiratory channels. Type 3 devices are relatively simple to use. Patients are able to apply the sensors themselves and perform their recordings at home. These monitors do not record signals that discriminate wakefulness from sleep or identify the stages of sleep. Therefore, the severity of OSA on type 3 recordings is usually quantified as the respiratory disturbance index (RDI), the number of apneas and hypopneas per hour of recording instead of per hour of sleep. Type 3 tests in patients who are awake for a significant part of the recording period will underestimate the "true" AHI that would have been obtained on PSG. Type 3 monitors also fail to detect arousals, preventing the scoring of hypopneas associated with arousals (AASM alternative criterion for hypopneas) and respiratory-effort–related arousals. Given the above differences between type 3 monitors and PSG, there is debate as to whether the same AHI cut point used on PSG to diagnose OSA should be selected on portable monitoring testing.[21]

Type 4 monitors record one or two bioparameters with the majority measuring oxygen saturation by pulse oximetry with one or more other signals. Pulse oximetry alone is unable to detect sleep disordered breathing not associated with desaturation, a phenomenon more commonly

seen in children than adults.[19] Recently, the AHRQ broadened the definition of type 4 monitors to include all those that failed to meet criteria for type 3 devices.[21]

A quarter century after its formulation, this classification system is starting to break down. Monitors have been developed that use unconventional signals (eg, peripheral arterial tonometry and wrist actigraphy) and allow selection of different combinations of signals that cross the traditional classification categories.[32,33] Novel technologies are being developed and marketed that outstrip our knowledge about their utility in clinical practice, further challenging the AASM classification. Perhaps the greatest problem however is the lack of standardization of the wide diversity of portable monitors that are commercially available. Over 30 type 2 and type 3 monitors are now marketed and it should not be assumed that the monitors, even those within the same class, are equivalent.[18] No studies to date have compared portable monitoring devices head-to-head and it is currently unknown which combination of signals have the best sensitivity and specificity.[34]

SENSORS USED FOR PORTABLE DIAGNOSTIC MONITORS

Portable monitoring devices differ in not only the numbers and types of signals recorded but in the types of sensors used for these signals. The AASM recommends that portable monitors use the same airflow, effort, and oximetry biosensors conventionally used for in-laboratory PSG. Unfortunately, the lack of standardization of sensors is not unique to portable monitors but also applies to in-laboratory PSG. In standard PSG, an oronasal thermistor and a nasal cannula pressure transducer are now recommended as surrogate markers of airflow.[34] The majority of studies comparing type 3 monitor recordings to PSG were performed with older model monitors that only had the oronasal thermistor signal. Since the nasal pressure signal is a more sensitive indicator of airflow reduction than thermistry, this technical difference may be another reason for the discrepancy between the AHI on in-laboratory PSG and the RDI on home, type 3 testing in direct-comparison studies. For respiratory effort assessment on PSG, the AASM recommends either calibrated or uncalibrated inductance plethysmography, and for oxygenation, pulse oximetry with the appropriate signal averaging time and accommodation for motion artifact is suggested.[34] Depending on the sampling rate, even pulse oximeters can vary substantially in the frequency of artifacts and the accuracy of their signal.[34]

Signal loss is observed more often in home-unattended studies and the success of an ambulatory monitoring program is in large part dependent on minimizing failed recordings. Criteria, such as minimum hours of acceptable oximetry signal, should be set to determine whether a recording is technically acceptable. To minimize failure rate and assure recording quality, it is recommended that the application of sensors or instructions to patients about sensor self-application be performed by experienced sleep technologists under the auspices of an AASM-accredited comprehensive sleep medicine program according to written policies and procedures for portable monitor testing.[34]

SCORING OF PORTABLE DIAGNOSTIC MONITOR STUDIES

Depending on the particular monitor used, scoring the recording may be manual with assistance of computer software, totally automated, or a combination. Overall, manual scoring or manual editing of automated scoring appears to have better agreement with in-laboratory PSG compared with automated scoring.[21,34] The difference between manual and automated scoring may be greater for mild and moderate OSA compared with severe OSA.[21] Moreover, automated scoring algorithms performed by specialized software are

proprietary and can vary across different monitors and even with the specific software version.

Manual scoring of unattended sleep studies is fraught with the same problems encountered in scoring in-laboratory PSGs. The scoring is largely based on pattern recognition of uncalibrated signals. Although the same rules for scoring respiratory events are applied to all four types of sleep testing, there are no uniform scoring criteria for hypopneas.[34,35] This results in interscorer variability in AHI results within a laboratory and wide variability in this measure across laboratories. For this reason, it is critically important for comparative studies to detail the criteria used to score respiratory events on both the PSG and portable monitor recordings.

The 2007 AASM task force on portable monitor testing recommended the review of the recorded signals by board-certified sleep specialists and manual scoring assisted by computer software using scoring criteria consistent with current published AASM standards. It also recommended an ongoing quality improvement program, including interscorer reliability, to assure accuracy and reliability of the testing.[34]

ATTENDED VERSUS UNATTENDED PORTABLE DIAGNOSTIC MONITOR STUDIES

Although intended primarily for unattended recordings, portable monitor testing can be attended, allowing a technologist to intervene if needed. The tests can be performed in various locations from the home to the sleep laboratory. Attended monitoring appears to provide better sensitivity and specificity than unattended recordings with less data loss.[21] These advantages must be balanced against the additional facility-related and personnel costs associated with attended recordings. Unattended sleep studies may have a particularly useful role in the evaluation of patients hospitalized for conditions related to sleep disordered breathing who are too sick to come to the sleep laboratory. There is no direct data on whether and to what extent technologist support and patient education affect the comparison of portable monitors with laboratory-based polysomnography.[21]

AMBULATORY MANAGEMENT OF OSA

Ambulatory management of patients with OSA will only be successful if patients can be diagnosed and initiated on treatment without requiring in-laboratory testing. The initiation and titration of CPAP, the most common treatment for OSA, has traditionally involved an in-laboratory, manual

CPAP titration PSG to determine the optimal pressure setting.[13,14] The reliance on in-laboratory PSG for CPAP titration defeats the ability of home diagnostic portable monitor testing to reduce costs, improve patient access to treatment, and reduce waiting times. The growing demand for in-laboratory testing will only be alleviated by the development of management pathways that are completely ambulatory. Patients diagnosed with OSA on portable monitor testing should be initiated on CPAP treatment without requiring an in-laboratory PSG. This need has encouraged development of alternative approaches to CPAP initiation including home unattended autotitrating CPAP (APAP) devices to determine the optimal fixed CPAP setting, chronic treatment with APAP, CPAP titration based on predicted formulas,[36,37] and even empiric selection of CPAP pressures.[26] Overall, studies comparing these different methods have shown similar improvements in symptoms, ability to eliminate respiratory events in terms of posttreatment AHI, and treatment adherence.[38–40] For example, Masa and colleagues[39] found similar improvements in the AHI and subjective sleepiness in 360 CPAP naïve patients with severe OSA documented by PSG who were randomized to CPAP treatment by either standard full in-laboratory PSG, unattended APAP titration, or setting based on a predicted formula. In the APAP group, optimal CPAP pressures were obtained in 95% of the patients with 82% obtained in just 1 night.[39]

APAP DEVICES

APAP devices automatically and continuously adjust the level of positive airway pressure delivered to the patient based on the presence or absence of snoring, apneas and hypopneas, and inspiratory flow limitation. The algorithms for pressure adjustment are not standardized and vary across manufacturers.[41] The devices record the pressures delivered, air leak from the circuit, and the number of abnormal respiratory events. This information is stored in memory and can be uploaded to a personal computer using computer software. Patients can be loaned APAP devices to use at home, generally for several nights, to determine the fixed CPAP setting needed for treatment. Often the 90th to 95th percentile pressure (ie, the pressure below which the patient spends 90%–95% of the time of use) is generally taken as the optimal fixed-CPAP level.[41,42] APAP-selected fixed-CPAP levels have been shown to reduce AHI to less than 10 events per hour in over 80% of patients.[41–43] Some APAP devices report the average estimated AHI at each pressure

level and permit remote monitoring of their use and performance by either modem or wireless transmission. One could argue that patients with OSA should routinely be treated with APAP rather than fixed CPAP; however, the cost effectiveness of this approach has not been evaluated. While routine treatment with APAP might reduce the amount of required testing, APAP devices are more expensive than CPAP units are and studies do not consistently show that patient adherence to APAP differs from that to CPAP.

APAP units have several disadvantages that need to be addressed when using them in an ambulatory pathway. They do not routinely monitor oxygen saturation, although some offer clip-on oximetry units. Some models are designed to interface with portable monitors to help ensure the adequacy of pressure titration, particularly with regard to oxygen saturation. APAP devices also cannot differentiate central from obstructive apneas.[42] APAP software regulating the pressure changes have therefore been designed not to increase pressure above 10 to 11 cm H_2O in the presence of persistent apneas. All patients being treated with fixed CPAP whether based on an APAP titration or in-laboratory, manual CPAP titration and all patients being treated with APAP should have close clinical follow-up to ensure treatment efficacy and effectiveness.[41] An APAP download showing a persistence of apneas should be followed by an in-laboratory, manual CPAP titration PSG.

VALIDATING HOME, UNATTENDED, PORTABLE MONITOR TESTING

Traditionally, studies have tried to validate portable monitor devices for diagnosis of OSA and APAP devices for CPAP titration by directly comparing the measures obtained by those portable monitoring devices to those obtained on in-laboratory PSG. However, differences in equipment, scoring, testing environment, and the known night-to-night variability in AHI even on PSG make such direct comparisons difficult. The recognition of the deficiencies of this direct comparison have led to comparative effectiveness studies that evaluate clinical outcomes in patients randomized to ambulatory management pathways using portable monitor testing versus traditional in-laboratory management with PSG. Patients randomized to each pathway are then initiated and followed on CPAP or APAP treatment. Clinical outcomes following weeks of treatment in these noninferiority trials have included improvement in symptom scores, self-reported quality of life, adherence to CPAP treatment, and treatment efficacy. Several studies now conclusively demonstrate that, at least in patients with a high probability of OSA, a completely ambulatory approach in terms of diagnosis and CPAP titration is feasible and has equivalent outcomes to in-laboratory management.[28,44,45]

A study by Whitelaw and colleagues[28] compared the ability of physicians to predict which patients with suspected OSA would improve with treatment, as defined by an increase in the Sleep Apnea Quality of Life Index, based on information from a standard PSG or oximeter-based home monitoring. They found physicians' ability to predict treatment outcomes was poor, with correct prediction rates of only 63%, but there was no significant difference between the PSG and home-monitoring group, suggesting that a full-PSG was not necessary for initiation of treatment in a select group.

Mulgrew and colleagues[45] performed a randomized controlled trial comparing an algorithm using a type 4 portable monitor and APAP titration to one using standard in-laboratory PSG in 68 patients with moderate-to-severe OSA. Following 3 months of fixed CPAP treatment, no statistical differences between the two arms were found in AHI on the end-of-study PSG performed on the fixed CPAP setting, change in the Epworth Sleepiness Scale score, or change in Sleep Apnea Quality of Life Index score, but CPAP adherence was greater in participants in the ambulatory arm ($P = .021$).

Using a similar approach, Berry and colleagues[46] randomized 106 veterans with a high likelihood of OSA to either home portable monitor testing for diagnosis followed by APAP titration for those participants with a RDI equal to or greater than five events per hour or to standard in-laboratory PSG for diagnosis and CPAP titration. Following 6 weeks of CPAP treatment, they found no statistical difference in total score on the Epworth Sleepiness Scale, global score on the Functional Outcome of Sleep Questionnaire, CPAP adherence, or patient satisfaction between the two groups.[46]

These studies used comprehensive algorithms, incorporating both portable monitoring to diagnose and initiate treatment of their OSA patients. The protocols were conducted by highly trained and specialized staff, providing thorough education to all patients, with tertiary site backup. It is unclear what impact these factors may have had in determining the outcomes. Antic and colleagues[44] compared a nurse-led model of care using oximetry and home APAP to physician-led care involving standard in-laboratory PSG for diagnosis and CPAP titration in a multicenter randomized controlled trial and, following 3 months of CPAP treatment, showed no significant differences between the two arms in change in the Epworth Sleepiness Scale score, quality of life indices, executive neurocognitive function, CPAP adherence, and total patient satisfaction. However, the nurses in the trial had worked in the field of sleep for a mean of 8.3 years and spent approximately 50 extra minutes with patients than the physician-led group.[44]

SELECTING PATIENTS FOR AMBULATORY MANAGEMENT OF OSA

While the above comparative effectiveness studies provide important new information, their general applicability is limited by their highly restrictive patient selection process. In the study of Antic and colleagues,[44] only 195 (22%) of 1427 potentially eligible patients met all inclusion criteria while in Mulgrew and colleagues[45] study, only 81(4%) of 2216 referred patients were considered eligible after clinical assessment. Selection bias applies to almost all published studies evaluating portable diagnostic monitors and APAP titration units. The studies had strict exclusion criteria, limiting their study population to relatively younger adults without medical comorbidities, such as chronic obstructive pulmonary disease, congestive heart failure, psychiatric disorders, and other sleep disorders. The strict selection criteria of most of these outcomes studies have made it difficult to generalize the results to the population at large. Additional studies are needed on the application of portable monitor testing in special populations: the elderly; patients with comorbid conditions such as chronic heart failure, chronic obstructive pulmonary disease, and neuromuscular disorders; and children. Studies are also needed in patients with milder OSA.

Additional studies are needed to determine whether portable monitor testing should be used to rule in and rule out OSA, or perhaps be restricted to the diagnosis of patients identified with a high pretest likelihood of OSA. Many other questions remain to be answered. Different criteria are used to define high pretest probability and it is unclear exactly how these patients should be identified in clinical practice. Limiting portable monitor testing to patients with a high pretest likelihood of OSA has the advantage of minimizing the number of negative studies and thereby reducing the need for in-laboratory PSG. However, restricting the use of home sleep testing to this subset of patients will hinder attempts to improve access to treatment. Inclusion of a wider range of patients could increase the number of negative studies. However, the additional testing needed to evaluate symptomatic patients with a negative portable monitor test result may decrease the cost effectiveness of the ambulatory management pathway.

CURRENT GUIDELINES FOR USING PORTABLE MONITORS IN AMBULATORY MANAGEMENT OF PATIENTS WITH OSA

The AASM clinical guidelines for use of portable monitor testing was updated in 2007 and recommends the use of portable monitoring devices, recording at a minimum airflow, respiratory effort and blood oxygenation, as an alternative to PSG for the diagnosis of OSA in patients with a high pretest probability for moderate-to-severe OSA, without significant comorbid medical conditions or suspected comorbid sleep disorders.[34] The guidelines emphasize the importance of including a comprehensive clinical evaluation by a trained sleep specialist. The report also states that portable monitoring may be indicated for the diagnosis of OSA in patients for whom in-laboratory PSG is not possible by virtue of immobility, safety, or critical illness. It is also indicated to monitor the response to non-CPAP treatments for sleep apnea.[34] The guidelines do not recommend portable monitoring for general screening of asymptomatic populations.[34] In two recent National Coverage Decisions, the Center for Medicare and Medicaid Services (CMS) in the United States approved coverage for portable monitor testing to diagnose OSA and coverage of CPAP treatment in patients diagnosed with portable monitor testing using type 2, 3, and 4 monitors, the latter requiring the recording of at least three channels.[16] These decisions did not make any specific recommendations about which type of portable monitoring device should be used, nor did they specify the appropriate population to undergo portable monitoring.

The 2007 AASM guidelines state that certain APAP devices may be initiated and used unattended to determine a fixed CPAP treatment pressure for patients with moderate to severe OSA without significant comorbidities.[41] APAP titration is not recommended for patients with significant comorbidities including congestive heart failure and significant lung disease, or those expected to have nocturnal oxyhemoglobin desaturation due to conditions other than OSA.[41] It is not recommended for patients who do not snore and patients with central sleep apnea.[41] APAP devices are also currently not recommended for split-night PSG. In-laboratory PSG is indicated in those patients whose symptoms do not respond to CPAP treatment at a pressure setting selected by APAP titration.[41]

COSTS OF PORTAL MONITOR TESTING

Much of the interest in the ambulatory management of patients with OSA has been driven by the premise that portable monitor testing will be just as effective but less costly than the standard in-laboratory PSG. Assessment of the cost effectiveness of portable monitor testing requires the assessment of both direct and indirect costs for the entire clinical management pathway. These costs include the cost of equipment, laboratory space, personnel including staff training, failed or inconclusive studies ultimately requiring PSG, failure to diagnose concomitant sleep disorders, and the costs arising from complications of undiagnosed and untreated OSA.

Several economic analyses have attempted to address the cost effectiveness of portable monitoring with mixed results.[47–49] One might predict that unattended portable monitor testing would be more cost-effective than in-laboratory testing since the portable monitor recordings do not require a technologist to be in attendance. Supporting this hypothesis, Deutsch and colleagues[49] found home studies and split-night PSG to be cost-effective alternatives to full-night PSG. However, a decision analysis model by Reuven and colleagues[48] challenged the cost advantages of home portable monitor testing, despite demonstrating a 30% lower cost in single, unattended, portable monitoring studies compared with the PSG. Similarly, the decision analysis of Chervin and colleagues[47] suggested greater cost effectiveness with the standard in-laboratory PSG relative to home studies and no testing. These latter studies, however, derived their assumptions for the decision analysis from clinical research studies that may not be applicable to real-world practice. The decreasing cost of portable monitor devices and APAP units along with continued advances in technology improving their sensitivity and specificity since the publication of these studies may invalidate the assumptions used in their decision analyses. More comparative effectiveness studies are needed to provide the evidence required to develop more accurate models. Toward that goal, Antic and colleagues[44] recently published the first prospective study comparing cost effectiveness of ambulatory management of OSA. Their two pathways, nurse-led home testing versus physician-led in-laboratory PSG, had similar improvements in total score on the Epworth Sleepiness Scale but the ambulatory pathway was associated with lower within-study cost per patient.

PREDICTING THE FUTURE

Portable monitor testing for the management of patients with OSA is already well established in many countries. In the United States, it is used extensively by providers in health maintenance organizations and the Veterans Health Administration. The recent decisions by CMS in the United States to approve coverage of portable monitor testing for the diagnosis and initiation of CPAP treatment in patients with OSA is likely to result in a progressively greater role of portable monitor testing in this country's private healthcare sector. Given these recent developments, one can predict that two additional changes will occur in the United States in the near future: coverage by insurers of APAP units for home, unattended titration studies or treatment of OSA, and revision of current reimbursement fees for sleep testing. Coverage of APAP-related services will allow providers to provide this critical component of the ambulatory management pathway. Reimbursement fees are likely to be adjusted to narrow the current large difference in allowable charges between in-laboratory PSG and portable monitor testing. These predictions, if true, will have far-reaching consequences.

The rapid growth of the specialty of sleep medicine over the past 3 decades has been largely driven and structured by the performance of the costly and technologically complex PSG. The availability of less costly and more user friendly devices for management of patients with OSA are likely to lead to the development of clinical management pathways that can be applied by those who are not sleep specialists, including primary care providers. Previous examples of such an evolution of disease management include asthma and diabetes mellitus. Patients with these diseases were originally cared for by allergists, pulmonologists, and endocrinologists. Today, the majority of these patients are managed by primary care providers. OSA is more common than asthma and diabetes and is an acknowledged major public health burden. Nevertheless, the clinical pathways to diagnose and treat patients with OSA using portable monitors still need to be developed and tested. Without well-developed clinical management algorithms, the premature, widespread application of these emerging new technologies by those who are not sleep specialists carries the significant risk of abuse and unacceptable quality of care.

The growing importance of portable monitor testing may be of benefit from the societal and patient perspective, but is viewed by many sleep specialists as a threat to the viability of their specialty. Lower reimbursements for PSG without an increase in fees for portable testing could conceivably dissuade physicians-in-training from specializing in sleep medicine at a time when it is vital that we continue to attract new investigators into this fledgling field. The continuing infusion of new talent into this specialty is vital for the generation of the evidence-based medicine that will guide and justify the use of the emerging technologies. It is to be hoped that any reduction in current reimbursement fees for PSG will be offset by an increase in the relatively low fees for unattended portable monitor testing.

As our knowledge of how to manage patients with OSA evolves, measures taken by insurers and regulatory agencies to promote the ambulatory management of OSA should consider their impact on the quality of patient care and the growth and development of the specialty of sleep medicine. In addition, sleep specialists wedded to the PSG must recognize the inevitability of a prominent role for portable monitor testing in patient care, embrace this new technology as a challenging new opportunity, and not shun it as a threat.

SUMMARY

To date, the diagnosis and treatment of OSA has been dependent on the costly and limited in-laboratory PSG, creating a crisis of access. It has forced stakeholders in healthcare to look increasingly at home portable monitor testing as an alternative strategy. Portable monitors have become technologically sophisticated but vary widely in the numbers and types of signals, sensors, and scoring methods used. As with the development of any other new technology, studies have tried to validate portable monitor testing by comparing these recordings to the current gold standard. However, the PSG has many weaknesses and its position as the reference standard is questioned. Consequently, more recent studies on portable monitor testing have compared clinical outcomes of ambulatory versus in-laboratory management strategies. APAP devices have been incorporated successfully into these ambulatory management pathways, obviating the need for in-laboratory CPAP titration PSG. Initial studies support the use of home-unattended portable monitor testing in the diagnosis of OSA in a select population with a high pretest probability and without comorbidities. Ultimately, the diagnosis and treatment of OSA requires a comprehensive evaluation, and home unattended portable monitoring, like in laboratory PSG, can serve as an objective aid in that process. We need to identify the patients with suspected OSA who should be selected for ambulatory management. We also need to determine whether the ambulatory management algorithms being developed for OSA are cost-effective and address the fundamental issue of access to diagnosis and treatment.

REFERENCES

1. Pack AI. Sleep-disordered breathing: access is the issue. Am J Respir Crit Care Med 2004;169(6): 666–7.
2. Bradley TD, Floras JS. Obstructive sleep apnoea and its cardiovascular consequences. Lancet 2009;373(9657):82–93.
3. Duran J, Esnaola S, Rubio R, et al. Obstructive sleep apnea-hypopnea and related clinical features in a population-based sample of subjects aged 30 to 70 yr. Am J Respir Crit Care Med 2001;163(3 Pt 1): 685–9.
4. Marin JM, Carrizo SJ, Vicente E, et al. Long-term cardiovascular outcomes in men with obstructive sleep apnoea-hypopnoea with or without treatment with continuous positive airway pressure: an observational study. Lancet 2005;365(9464):1046–53.
5. Partinen M, Palomaki H. Snoring and cerebral infarction. Lancet 1985;2(8468):1325–6.
6. Peppard PE, Young T, Palta M, et al. Prospective study of the association between sleep-disordered breathing and hypertension. N Engl J Med 2000; 342(19):1378–84.
7. Punjabi NM, Sorkin JD, Katzel LI, et al. Sleep-disordered breathing and insulin resistance in middle-aged and overweight men. Am J Respir Crit Care Med 2002;165(5):677–82.
8. Shahar E, Whitney CW, Redline S, et al. Sleep-disordered breathing and cardiovascular disease: cross-sectional results of the Sleep Heart Health Study. Am J Respir Crit Care Med 2001;163(1):19–25.
9. Somers VK, White DP, Amin R, et al. Sleep apnea and cardiovascular disease: an American Heart Association/American College Of Cardiology Foundation Scientific Statement from the American Heart Association Council for High Blood Pressure Research Professional Education Committee, Council on Clinical Cardiology, Stroke Council, and Council On Cardiovascular Nursing. In collaboration with the National Heart, Lung, and Blood Institute National Center on Sleep Disorders Research (National Institutes of Health). Circulation 2008; 118(10):1080–111.
10. Teran-Santos J, Jimenez-Gomez A, Cordero-Guevara J. The association between sleep apnea and the risk of traffic accidents. Cooperative Group Burgos-Santander. N Engl J Med 1999; 340(11):847–51.
11. Young T, Finn L, Peppard PE, et al. Sleep disordered breathing and mortality: eighteen-year follow-up of the Wisconsin sleep cohort. Sleep 2008;31(8):1071–8.
12. Young T, Peppard PE, Gottlieb DJ. Epidemiology of obstructive sleep apnea: a population health perspective. Am J Respir Crit Care Med 2002; 165(9):1217–39.
13. American Thoracic Society. Indications and standards for use of nasal continuous positive airway pressure (CPAP) in sleep apnea syndromes. Am J Respir Crit Care Med 1994;150:1738–45.
14. Kushida CA, Littner MR, Hirshkowitz M, et al. Practice parameters for the use of continuous and bilevel positive airway pressure devices to treat adult patients with sleep-related breathing disorders. Sleep 2006;29(3):375–80.
15. Flemons WW, Douglas NJ, Kuna ST, et al. Access to diagnosis and treatment of patients with suspected sleep apnea. Am J Respir Crit Care Med 2004; 169(6):668–72.
16. Centers for Medicare and Medicaid Services. Decision Memo for Continuous Positive Airway Pressure (CPAP) Therapy for Obstructive Sleep Apnea (OSA). (CAG-00093R2). 2008. Available at: http://www.cms.hhs.gov/mcd/viewdecisionmemo.asp?id=204. Accessed February 9, 2010.
17. Chesson AL Jr, Berry RB, Pack A, et al. Practice parameters for the use of portable monitoring devices in the investigation of suspected obstructive sleep apnea in adults. Sleep 2003;26(7):907–13.
18. Collop NA. Portable monitoring for the diagnosis of obstructive sleep apnea. Curr Opin Pulm Med 2008;14(6):525–9.
19. Ferber R, Millman R, Coppola M, et al. Portable recording in the assessment of obstructive sleep apnea. ASDA standards of practice. Sleep 1994; 17(4):378–92.
20. Flemons WW, Littner MR, Rowley JA, et al. Home diagnosis of sleep apnea: a systematic review of the literature. An evidence review cosponsored by the American Academy of Sleep Medicine, the American College of Chest Physicians, and the American Thoracic Society. Chest 2003;124(4):1543–79.
21. Trikalinos TA, Ip S, Raman G, et al. Home diagnosis of obstructive sleep apnea-hypopnea syndrome. Department of Health & Human Services. Agency for Healthcare Research and Quality; 2007. Available at: http://www.ahrq.gov/clinic/techix.htm#competed. Accessed February 9, 2010.
22. Lindberg E, Gislason T. Epidemiology of sleep-related obstructive breathing. Sleep Med Rev 2000;4(5):411–33.
23. Young T, Palta M, Dempsey J, et al. The occurrence of sleep-disordered breathing among middle-aged adults. N Engl J Med 1993;328(17):1230–5.
24. Bixler EO, Vgontzas AN, Lin HM, et al. Sleep disordered breathing in children in a general population

sample: prevalence and risk factors. Sleep 2009;
32(6):731–6.

25. Young T, Evans L, Finn L, et al. Estimation of the
clinically diagnosed proportion of sleep apnea
syndrome in middle-aged men and women. Sleep
1997;20(9):705–6.

26. Patel NP, Ahmed M, Rosen I. Split-night polysomnography. Chest 2007;132(5):1664–71.

27. Colten HR, Altevogt BM, Institute of Medicine (US).
Committee on Sleep Medicine and Research. In:
Sleep Disorders and Sleep Deprivation: an Unmet
Public Health Problem. Washington, DC: The
National Academies Press; 2006.

28. Whitelaw WA, Brant RF, Flemons WW. Clinical usefulness of home oximetry compared with polysomnography for assessment of sleep apnea. Am J Respir
Crit Care Med 2005;171(2):188–93.

29. Bennett LS, Barbour C, Langford B, et al. Health
status in obstructive sleep apnea: relationship with
sleep fragmentation and daytime sleepiness, and
effects of continuous positive airway pressure treatment. Am J Respir Crit Care Med 1999;159(6):
1884–90.

30. Kingshott RN, Engleman HM, Deary IJ, et al. Does
arousal frequency predict daytime function? Eur
Respir J 1998;12(6):1264–70.

31. Lloberes P, Marti S, Sampol G, et al. Predictive
factors of quality-of-life improvement and continuous
positive airway pressure use in patients with sleep
apnea-hypopnea syndrome: study at 1 year. Chest
2004;126(4):1241–7.

32. Morgenthaler T, Alessi C, Friedman L, et al. Practice
parameters for the use of actigraphy in the assessment of sleep and sleep disorders: an update for
2007. Sleep 2007;30(4):519–29.

33. Pittman SD, Ayas NT, MacDonald MM, et al. Using
a wrist-worn device based on peripheral arterial
tonometry to diagnose obstructive sleep apnea: in-
laboratory and ambulatory validation. Sleep 2004;
27(5):923–33.

34. Collop NA, Anderson WM, Boehlecke B, et al. Clinical guidelines for the use of unattended portable
monitors in the diagnosis of obstructive sleep apnea
in adult patients. Portable Monitoring Task Force of
the American Academy of Sleep Medicine. J Clin
Sleep Med 2007;3(7):737–47.

35. Iber C, Ancoli-Israel S, Chesson AL, et al, for the
American Academy of Sleep Medicine. The AASM
manual for the scoring of sleep and associated
events. Rules, terminolgy, and technical specifications. Westchester (IL): American Academy of Sleep
Medicine; 2007.

36. Hoffstein V, Mateika S. Predicting nasal continuous
positive airway pressure. Am J Respir Crit Care
Med 1994;150(2):486–8.

37. Marrone O, Salvaggio A, Romano S, et al. Automatic
titration and calculation by predictive equations for

the determination of therapeutic continuous positive
airway pressure for obstructive sleep apnea. Chest
2008;133(3):670–6.

38. Ayas NT, Patel SR, Malhotra A, et al. Auto-titrating
versus standard continuous positive airway pressure
for the treatment of obstructive sleep apnea: results
of a meta-analysis. Sleep 2004;27(2):249–53.

39. Masa JF, Jimenez A, Duran J, et al. Alternative
methods of titrating continuous positive airway pressure: a large multicenter study. Am J Respir Crit
Care Med 2004;170(11):1218–24.

40. West SD, Jones DR, Stradling JR. Comparison of
three ways to determine and deliver pressure during
nasal CPAP therapy for obstructive sleep apnoea.
Thorax 2006;61(3):226–31.

41. Morgenthaler TI, Aurora RN, Brown T, et al. Practice
parameters for the use of autotitrating continuous
positive airway pressure devices for titrating pressures and treating adult patients with obstructive
sleep apnea syndrome: an update for 2007. An
American Academy of Sleep Medicine report. Sleep
2008;31(1):141–7.

42. Berry RB, Parish JM, Hartse KM. The use of auto-
titrating continuous positive airway pressure for
treatment of adult obstructive sleep apnea. An
American Academy of Sleep Medicine review. Sleep
2002;25(2):148–73.

43. Fletcher EC, Stich J, Yang KL. Unattended home diagnosis and treatment of obstructive sleep apnea without
polysomnography. Arch Fam Med 2000;9(2):168–74.

44. Antic NA, Buchan C, Esterman A, et al. A randomized controlled trial of nurse-led care for symptomatic moderate-severe obstructive sleep apnea. Am
J Respir Crit Care Med 2009;179(6):501–8.

45. Mulgrew AT, Fox N, Ayas NT, et al. Diagnosis and
initial management of obstructive sleep apnea
without polysomnography: a randomized validation
study. Ann Intern Med 2007;146(3):157–66.

46. Berry RB, Hill G, Thompson L, et al. Portable monitoring and autotitration versus polysomnography
for the diagnosis and treatment of sleep apnea.
Sleep 2008;31(10):1423–31.

47. Chervin RD, Murman DL, Malow BA, et al. Cost-
utility of three approaches to the diagnosis of
sleep apnea: polysomnography, home testing,
and empirical therapy. Ann Intern Med 1999;
130(6):496–505.

48. Reuven H, Schweitzer E, Tarasiuk A. A cost-effectiveness analysis of alternative at-home or in-laboratory technologies for the diagnosis of obstructive
sleep apnea syndrome. Med Decis Making 2001;
21(6):451–8.

49. Deutsch PA, Simmons MS, Wallace JM. Cost-effectiveness of split-night polysomnography and home
studies in the evaluation of obstructive sleep
apnea syndrome. J Clin Sleep Med 2006;2(2):
145–53.

Neurobiology of Sleep

Brandon S. Lu, MD, MS[a],*, Phyllis C. Zee, MD, PhD[b]

KEYWORDS

- Sleep neurobiology • Sleep regulation
- Sleep-wake transition • Sleep disorders

Sleep is an evolutionarily conserved process that occupies approximately one-third of a human's life. Although the exact functions of sleep remain elusive, studies of sleep deprivation have shown impairments in cognitive and physical performance,[1,2] and chronic short-sleep duration has been associated with numerous cardiometabolic disturbances, including hypertension,[3] diabetes,[4] and even mortality,[5] emphasizing the importance of sleep for health and performance. Thus, knowledge of the neurobiology of sleep and wake regulation is essential to medicine.

Our understanding of sleep mechanisms has improved drastically in recent years, largely aided by improved methods in molecular and cellular experimental techniques that have allowed direct access to sleep-wake centers in the brain. For example, in vivo microdialysis was used to measure extracellular adenosine concentrations in the basal forebrain of free, living animals to better delineate adenosine's role in sleep.[6] Similarly, lesion of ventrolateral preoptic nucleus (VLPO) cells with direct microinjection of an acid identified distinct cell groups with primary effects on the regulation of rapid eye movement (REM) sleep and non-REM (NREM) sleep.[7]

This article focuses on the how of sleep, not the why of sleep. The authors discuss the wake and sleep centers, the transition between wake and sleep, regulation of REM and NREM sleep, and the homeostatic and circadian regulations of sleep and wakefulness.

WAKE-PROMOTING SYSTEMS

After the initial recording of brain electrical activity by Hans Berger[8] in the 1920s, a major advancement in sleep neurobiology was reached when von Economo[9] described in detail the symptoms and pathology of encephalitis lethargica. He hypothesized that the posterior hypothalamus and rostral midbrain contained centers of wakefulness (lesions in these areas led to excessive sleepiness) and the anterior hypothalamus controlled sleep (lesions led to prolonged insomnia). Moruzzi and Magoun[10] further defined the sleep-wake transition when they demonstrated that stimulation of brainstem reticular formation evoked a generalized desynchronization of electroencephalogram (EEG) activity, simulating arousals from sleep. They hypothesized that a series of reticular relays distributed through the center of the brainstem projects to the basal forebrain and participates in the regulation of wakefulness. Much work has been performed in the last half decade to identify several distinct systems involved in the control of the wake state.

Cholinergic Systems

The "ascending reticular activating system" initially described by Moruzzi and Magoun[10] contains two main branches. The first branch consists of cholinergic neurons originating from the laterodorsal tegmental (LDT) and pedunculopontine nuclei (PPT) of the dorsal midbrain and pons. Dorsal projections from these centers densely innervate the thalamic relay nuclei and

The authors have no financial conflict of interest with the subject discussed in this article.
a Department of Medicine, California Pacific Medical Center, 2351 Clay Street, Suite 501, San Francisco, CA 94115, USA
b Department of Neurology, Northwestern University, 710 North Lake Shore Drive, 11th Floor, Chicago, IL 60611, USA
* Corresponding author.
E-mail address: lubs@sutterhealth.org

the thalamic reticular nuclei, with neurons displaying high firing rates during wakefulness and REM sleep.[11,12] From the thalamus, arousal signal is carried by the thalamocortical tract to activate the cortex, resulting in the desynchronized, low-amplitude EEG signals seen during wakefulness and REM sleep.[13,14]

A ventral projection from the LDT and PPT carries cholinergic neurons to the basal forebrain, where areas such as the substantia innominata and the medial septum and diagonal band of Broca relay the signals to the cerebral cortex.[15] The basal forebrain has high activity during wake and REM sleep, contributing to EEG desynchronization particularly gamma activity (30–60 Hz).[16] Lesions to animal basal forebrain area produced slow delta waves recorded from the cortex during activity and immobility, further suggesting the importance of this area in cortical activation.[17] Aside from its projections to the cerebral cortex, the basal forebrain is also a source of cholinergic activation to the hippocampus and amygdala.[18]

Monoaminergic Pathways

The second branch of the reticular activating system carries mostly monoaminergic neurons to the lateral hypothalamus (LH) and basal forebrain, and ultimately to the cerebral cortex.[19] Monoaminergic nuclei located in the upper brainstem and caudal hypothalamus, which send fibers rostrally, include the locus coeruleus (LC), median and dorsal raphe (DR), tuberomammillary (TMN), substantia nigra (SN), and ventral tegmental area (VTA).

Norepinephrine
The LC is the main source of brain norepinephrine and carries projections to subcortical relay stations (ie, thalamus and hypothalamus) as well as the cortex. In contrast to the cholinergic system, LC neurons discharge highly during wake, less during NREM sleep, and are virtually off during REM sleep.[20,21] Increasing LC neuronal activity in experimental studies promoted wakefulness, whereas LC inactivation led to a shift of EEG from low-amplitude, high-frequency to large-amplitude, slow-wave activity, confirming the role of LC in wakefulness.[22,23]

The LC-norepinephrine system also functions in the regulation of behavioral state. It displays pronounced sensitivity to stressors and has been implicated in stress-related arousal. Consistent with this suggestion, bilateral suppression of LC discharge blocked stressor-induced EEG activation in halothane-anesthetized rats.[24,25]

Serotonin
Serotoninergic—5-hydroxytryptamine (5-HT)—neurons originate in the DR nuclei and, similar to the norepinephrine neurons of the LC, are very active during wake, less active during NREM sleep, and silent during REM sleep.[26] Our understanding of the sleep-wake property of 5-HT has changed over time. Earlier works pointed to 5-HT as a somnogenic agent based on studies which showed that 5-HT increased sleep and inhibition of 5-HT synthesis suppressed NREM and REM sleep.[27] Furthermore, perfusion of a 5-HT$_{1A}$ agonist into the DR-increased REM sleep—a finding consistent with likely activation of presynaptic autoreceptors leading to decreased 5-HT neurotransmission.[28] More recently, however, several studies have shown that 5-HT promotes wakefulness by using various 5-HT receptor agonists/antagonists, 5-HT precursors, or reuptake inhibitors to increase quiet waking and decrease REM sleep.[29–31] Like norepinephrine, 5-HT also regulates behavioral state.

Histamine
The TMN in the posterior hypothalamus is the sole source of histamine (H) in the brain and it sends projections to the entire central nervous system. Active mainly during the waking period, the TMN has little if any activity during sleep, particularly in REM sleep.[32,33] In studies of animals and from clinical experience, drugs that block histamine H$_1$ receptors (eg, diphenhydramine) increase both NREM and REM sleep.[34] Different types of histamine receptor exist, however, providing distinct pharmacologic targets in the same system—H$_1$ and H$_2$ receptors are mostly excitatory in nature, whereas H$_3$ receptors act as inhibitory auto- and heteroreceptors. In fact, H$_3$ receptor antagonists are being developed for the management of narcolepsy.[35]

Dopamine
Dopamine (DA)-containing neurons that are relevant to the sleep-wake cycle are predominantly found in the SN and VTA. These nuclei have interconnections with many nuclei in the brainstem as well as the LH, basal forebrain, and the thalamus. Two subtypes of DA receptors have been cloned—the D1-like and D2-like subfamilies[36]—with the D1 receptor being postsynaptic and its stimulation leading to behavioral arousal, increased wake, and decreased slow-wave sleep (SWS) and REM sleep. The D2 receptors are autoreceptors and postsynaptic receptors that have a biphasic response to agonists—low doses leading to decreased wake and increased SWS and REM sleep, and high doses having the

opposite effect.[37] Distinct from other monoaminergic neurons in the brainstem, DA-containing neurons do not change firing rate across sleep-wake state; rather, the burst activity of DA-containing neurons occurs in a temporal pattern, associated with reward, locomotion, and cognition.[38,39] DA neuronal firing depends upon inputs from the prefrontal cortex, the LH, and cholinergic as well as other monoaminergic nuclei in the brainstem.[40–43]

The wake-promoting effect of DA is readily apparent when one considers that amphetamines promote wakefulness by enhancing DA release and preventing its reuptake by DA transporter.[44] Medications that block DA receptors, such as antipsychotics, often lead to sleepiness, and patients with Parkinson's disease often exhibit excessive daytime sleepiness, which may be partially attributed to DA deficiency.[45] Interestingly, dopamine agonists have been associated with sudden sleep attacks. The mechanism of this phenomenon is possibly due to down-regulation of DA input by the medications binding to presynaptic DA receptors.[46] Taken together, these data clearly support the wake-promoting action of DA.

Orexin/Hypocretin Pathway

In 1998, two groups of scientists independently discovered orexin/hypocretin,[47,48] a neuropeptide synthesized predominantly in the posterior and LH. Orexinergic neurons play an essential role for the stabilization of wakefulness by projecting and binding to its two receptors, Ox1 and Ox2, found diffusely throughout the central nervous system, including the cerebral cortex, forebrain, thalamus, and brainstem arousal nuclei.[49–54] In addition to cortical activation, orexin stimulates somatic motor neurons and the sympathetic nervous system to maintain a waking state.[55,56] It is thus not unexpected to find that orexin neurons discharge exclusively during wake and are off during both SWS and paradoxic sleep.[57]

The clinical importance of orexin emerged when subsequent studies disrupting the orexin/hypocretin pathway using orexin knockout[58] and hypocretin (orexin) receptor 2 gene (*Hcrtr2* or *Ox2*) mutation[59] models produced animals with narcolepsy with cataplexy. About 90% of human narcoleptics with cataplexy are found to have low to undetectable levels of orexin in their cerebrospinal fluid, and human narcoleptics have a 90% reduction in brain orexin neurons, with evidence pointing to a degenerative process as the cause.[60,61]

Of all the arousal systems discussed, the orexin/hypocretin system seems to have the most potent effect on maintaining wakefulness. Even after massive destruction of animal norepinephrine neurons in the LC, neither a comatose state nor a reduction of waking measured by cortical activation was seen. The same can be said for the cholinergic and other monoaminergic brainstem systems—suggesting a redundancy to those arousal systems.[62] The consequence of a defective orexin system is well illustrated in narcolepsy. The orexin/hypocretin system thus performs its critical role of preventing sleep by its excitatory actions on other arousal systems and also providing excitatory input on cortical, motor, and sympathetic systems (**Table 1**).

NREM SLEEP SYSTEMS

The notion that sleep simply results from inactivity of the ascending arousal systems has proven to be erroneous with the discovery of specific brain regions that actively control NREM and REM

Table 1
Activity of wake and sleep centers

	Wake	NREM Sleep	REM Sleep
LDT/PPT (Acetylcholine)	↑↑ [a]	_[b]	↑↑
LC (Norepinephrine) DR (5-HT) TMN (Histamine) SN/VTA (Dopamine)	↑↑	↑[c]	–
Lateral Hypothalamus (Orexin/Hypocretin)	↑↑	–	–
VLPO - cluster (Galanin & GABA)	–	↑↑	–
VLPO - extended (Galanin & GABA)	–	–	↑↑

Abbreviations: GABA, γ-aminobutyric acid; LDT, laterodorsal tegmental; PPT, pedunculopontine tegmental.
[a] high activity.
[b] low or negligible activity.
[c] activity.

sleep. The centers that facilitate sleep include the VLPO and the median preoptic nucleus (MnPN). These areas are active at the transition from waking to sleep and inhibit the firing of arousal centers for sleep initiation and maintenance.

VLPO

The VLPO is located in the anterior hypothalamus and corresponds to the lesioned area in von Economo's patients with encephalitis lethargica who developed profound insomnia.[9] Scientists have discovered that projections from the VLPO reach monoaminergic arousal centers and are active during sleep, using inhibitory neurotransmitters galanin and γ-aminobutyric acid (GABA).[63] These cells form a dense cluster that has heavy innervations to the histaminergic neurons of the TMN, as well as a more diffuse extended part of the nucleus that provides output to the cholinergic LDT/PPT and monoaminergic LC and DR. To further define the function of the VLPO cluster, targeted lesions of the area led to a dramatic decrease in NREM sleep.[7] The extended VLPO (eVLPO), on the other hand, showed activity that correlated with REM sleep (see **Table 1**).[64] The orexin neurons of the LH also receive inhibitory input from the VLPO.[65]

The activity of the VLPO is partially controlled by the same monoaminergic centers that it inhibits. All major monoaminergic nuclei send inhibitory projections to the VLPO so that the sleep and wake systems are reciprocally connected.[66] There are mutual projections between the VLPO and the orexin neurons in the LH. However, the VLPO does not contain orexin receptors such that orexin neurons likely inhibit the VLPO via an indirect mechanism.[67]

MnPN

Similar to the VLPO, the MnPN uses GABA to send inhibitory projections to many of the same arousal targets. The nuclei differ in the temporal pattern of discharge during routine sleep and following sleep deprivation. MnPN neurons tend to display highest activity early in NREM sleep with gradual decline through the sleep period, whereas VLPO neurons demonstrate sustained discharge.[68] In experiments with sleep-deprived rats, it was found that MnPN showed peak activity during sleep deprivation, before the onset of recovery sleep. VLPO, in contrast, showed increased activity only after sleep onset.[69] These data suggest a homeostatic regulatory role for the MnPN.

THE SLEEP-WAKE TRANSITION (FLIP-FLOP SWITCH)

The sleep and wake systems are mutually inhibitory and activity of one system will inhibit activity of the opposing system. Such a circuit is termed a flip-flop switch by engineers who designed such systems to be in one state or another, but never in-between (much like the on-off light switch).[70] Because each state will reinforce its own stability when active (eg, the arousal system will inhibit the sleep system to decrease its own inhibitory feedback, and vice versa), the flip-flop switch is inherently stable and tends to avoid intermediate states (**Fig. 1**).

However, the flip-flop switch may be weakened and state transitions can occur frequently when one side becomes less able to inhibit the other side. An example is the suggested loss of VLPO neurons in the elderly that can lead to sleep

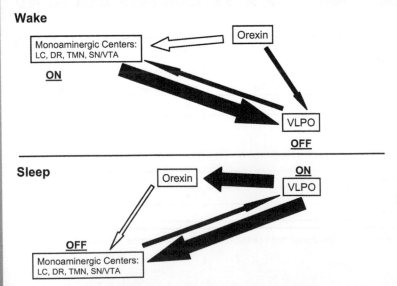

Fig. 1. Regulation of wake and sleep: flip/flop switch. The mutual inhibitory wake and sleep systems each reinforces its own stability when active. The orexin system is a stabilizer by its excitatory action on monoaminergic systems and inhibitory action on the VLPO. Solid arrows represent inhibitory action; open arrows; excitatory action. Thickness of arrows represent strength of relationship.

fragmentation at night and sleepiness or napping during the day, both commonly seen with aging.[19] Orexin has been proposed as a stabilizer of the switch by virtue of its indirect inhibitory action on the VLPO. The orexin neurons actively reinforce the monoaminergic arousal tone by its excitatory activity, thus preventing the rapid and frequent transitions in behavioral states seen in narcoleptics who lack orexin.[70]

REM SLEEP SYSTEMS

REM sleep was previously thought to be controlled by the interplay between the active pontine cholinergic nuclei and inactive monoaminergic nuclei that occurs during REM sleep.[71] Indeed, this concept was supported by evidence that cholinergic stimulation promoted REM sleep and monoamine re-uptake inhibition (eg, antidepressants) reduced REM sleep.[72,73] However, limited change in REM sleep was observed when either set of nuclei was selectively lesioned.[74,75] More recent works have identified distinct REM-on and REM-off regions that also function in a flip-flop switch manner to regulate REM sleep (**Fig. 2**).[76]

REM-off Region

By tracing the projections of the orexin neurons (excitatory and REM-inactive) and eVLPO (inhibitory and REM-active), scientists have identified a REM-off region as a crescent-shaped arc of tissue in the mesopontine tegmentum, consisting of the ventrolateral part of the periaqueductal gray matter (vlPAG) and the lateral pontine tegmentum (LPT). Consistent with an earlier report,[77] lesions at these sites led to increased amounts of REM sleep during both light and dark

periods in rats. In addition, bouts of cataplexy-like state with desynchronized EEG and atonia were also seen.[76]

REM-on Region

The efferent projections of the REM-off region and c-Fos protein expression (an immediate early gene that is upregulated in response to many extracellular signals) were examined during enhanced-REM sleep to determine the site of a REM-on region. It was seen that the REM-off region provided heavy projection to the sublaterodorsal nucleus (SLD; also known as the subcoeruleus area or peri-locus coeruleus alpha) and the periventricular gray matter.[76] This finding was consistent with earlier studies which showed that neurons in the SLD are REM-active and stimulation of the region increased REM-sleep–like behavior.[78,79]

The ventral SLD (vSLD), an area below the periventricular gray matter, has been shown to be responsible for the atonia seen during REM sleep. In fact, animals with lesion of the vSLD were noted to exhibit complex motor behaviors during REM sleep.[80] More extensive studies have demonstrated that the vSLD produces atonia by means of direct glutaminergic spinal projections to interneurons that inhibit spinal motor neurons by glycine and GABA neurotransmitters.[81]

Regulation of REM Sleep

Akin to the transition between wake and sleep, the control of REM sleep is regulated by a system that resembles a flip-flop switch.[76] The REM-on and REM-off neurons of the SLD/subcoeruleus region and vlPAG-LPT, respectively, mutually send

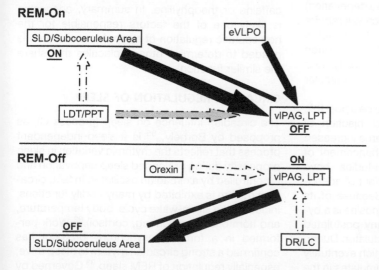

REM-On

SLD/Subcoeruleus Area
ON

LDT/PPT

eVLPO

vlPAG, LPT
OFF

REM-Off

Orexin

ON
vlPAG, LPT

OFF
SLD/Subcoeruleus Area

DR/LC

Fig. 2. Regulation of REM sleep: flip-flop switch. The REM-on and REM-off neurons of the SLD/subcoeruleus region and vlPAG-LPT, respectively, mutually send reciprocal GABAergic inhibitory neurons to the other. The cholinergic LDT/PPT have been proposed to excite the REM-on region and inhibit the REM-off region, while the orexin and monoaminergic systems may both excite the REM-off region. Solid arrows represent inhibitory action; dashed solid arrows, inhibitory (hypothesized) action; dashed open arrows, excitatory (hypothesized) action. Thickness of arrows represents strength of relationship. LPT, lateral pontine; SLD, sublaterodorsal.

reciprocal GABAergic inhibitory neurons to the other. As each side inhibits the other, it also disinhibits and reinforces its own firing, stabilizing the switch.

To integrate the roles of the pontine cholinergic and monoaminergic nuclei (previously thought to be the REM switch) with the recent concept of the REM flip-flop switch, it might be more appropriate to think of the pontine cholinergic and monoaminergic nuclei as REM modulators.[82] For example, the REM-active cholinergic neurons of the LDT/PPT may inhibit the LPT (cholinergic agonists injected into the LPT were shown to cause a REM state[83]) and also directly excite the SLD/subcoeruleus REM-on region. Similarly, 5-HT (DR) and norepinephrine (LC) neurons may actively excite the vlPAG-LPT REM-off neurons to prevent sudden, unexpected transitions into REM sleep. To reinforce the REM-off region, the orexin neurons have also been posited to project excitatory neurons to that area[84] to prevent REM occurring during wake. In narcolepsy with cataplexy, the lack of orexin projection to the REM-off neurons weakens the inhibition of REM-on neurons, allowing for more frequent and inappropriate transitions into REM. Conversely, the eVLPO has known GABAergic projections to the REM-off vlPAG-LPT region, likely to inhibit the area during REM sleep.[64]

HOMEOSTATIC REGULATION OF SLEEP

In 1982, Borbély[85] proposed the classic model of sleep regulation involving both a homeostatic (Process S) and circadian (Process C) process (**Fig. 3**). The sleep-dependent Process S, also known as "sleep propensity," builds during the waking period and is dissipated by sleep. The longer an individual is wake (eg, sleep deprivation) the higher the sleep propensity, which will require extra recovery sleep to dissipate. EEG spectral analysis-measured slow wave activity is often used as the surrogate for sleep propensity, and adenosine has been proposed as its molecular equivalent.[85,86]

Adenosine was initially observed to be a possible somnogen when its injection, and injection of adenosine analogs, to the preoptic area increased total sleep primarily through an enhancement of SWS.[87] Since then, numerous studies have demonstrated the sleep-inducing effect of adenosine, both in cats and dogs.[88,89] Because of its hypnotic effect and the fact that adenosine is a by-product of energy metabolism, many postulated that adenosine is a homeostatic modulator. During wakefulness, the brain uses ATP, which eventually breaks down to adenosine and accumulates in the

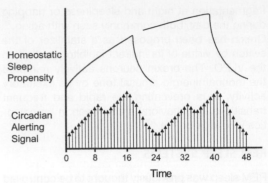

Fig. 3. The two-process model of wake and sleep, as proposed by Borbély85 and Edgar and colleagues94 Top: The homeostatic sleep propensity builds during wake and is dissipated during sleep (*left*). Sleep propensity continues to accumulate with sleep deprivation (*right*), and exponentially declines during the sleep period. Bottom: An independent circadian alerting signal from the suprachiasmatic nucleus (SCN) interacts with the homeostatic sleep propensity to regulate the timing and duration of sleep.

brain, including the basal forebrain. Indeed, basal forebrain adenosine concentration has been shown to progressively increase with each succeeding hour of sleep deprivation and decrease during SWS.[6]

A differential effect of adenosine has been found depending of its site of activity and receptor type. In the basal forebrain, adenosine binds to A1 receptors to decrease wakefulness signals sent to the cortex.[90] Whereas adenosine in the VLPO binds to A2 receptors to induce Fos expression and increase sleep.[91] Most people have had personal experiences with adenosine's role in sleepiness with the use of coffee or tea, beverages which contain the adenosine receptor antagonist caffeine or theophylline. In summary, adenosine is likely one of the factors responsible for the homeostatic regulation of sleep. More research is needed to determine other molecules that share the similar function.

CIRCADIAN REGULATION OF SLEEP

The circadian influence on sleep (process C), as proposed by Borbély, [85] is a sleep-independent process that reflects the rhythmic variation in sleep propensity during prolonged sleep deprivation and is controlled by a circadian oscillator. In fact, circadian rhythm is exhibited by many bodily functions, including the sleep-wake cycle, body temperature, and hormone secretion (eg, cortisol).[92] Work performed in a forced desynchrony protocol has confirmed a strong circadian rhythm to sleep drive, especially regulation of REM sleep.[93] Governed by the anterior hypothalamic suprachiasmatic nucleus (SCN), the master clock of the body, human circadian rhythm cycles in a near-24-hour rhythm driven by rhythmic expressing clock genes. Because the period of the endogenous circadian rhythm is not precisely 24 hours, the master clock must entrain, or be reset, daily to entraining agents, the most powerful of which is light.

Edgar and colleagues[94] expanded upon the model by proposing that the SCN actively initiates and maintains wakefulness and opposes the homeostatic sleep tendency during the subjective day (see **Fig. 3**). Much work has been performed to elucidate the link between the SCN and the sleep system. The SCN has indirect projections to both the VLPO sleep center and wake-promoting orexin neurons in the LH via the adjacent subparaventricular zone (SPZ) and the dorsomedial nucleus of the hypothalamus (DMH).[95,96] The function of the SPZ was identified because, similar to SCN ablation, lesions of the ventral SPZ led to abolishment of sleep-wake circadian rhythm, along with rest–activity and feeding rhythms.[97] The SPZ in turn projects mainly to the DMH, which has an activating effect, as lesions of this region led to more sleep and less locomotor activity.[98] The DMH sends GABAergic neurons to the VLPO (inhibiting sleep and promote wakefulness) and glutaminergic and thyrotropin-releasing hormone neurons to the LH (excitatory to the orexin neurons).[96] The presence of intermediate relay stations between the SCN and the sleep and wake centers of the hypothalamus allow for differential effects of the SCN in diurnal versus nocturnal animals. While the SCN is always active during the light period, its signal is alerting in diurnal organisms (wake promoting) and inhibitory in nocturnal organisms (sleep promoting).[19] The pathways connecting the SCN and the sleep and wake centers thus provide an anatomic basis for the circadian regulation of the sleep-wake cycle.

In Borbély's[85] two-process model of sleep and wake, sleep propensity and duration are determined by the interaction of Processes S and C. The model is able to simulate the variations of sleep duration as a function of sleep onset time, and it describes the cyclic alternation between NREM and REM sleep as a result of reciprocal interaction between the two states. While this model has been pivotal in our conceptualization of sleep and wake, it will undoubtedly be refined as our anatomic and molecular understandings of sleep and circadian regulation evolve (**Fig. 4**).

SUMMARY

There has been significant progress in our knowledge of the mechanisms underlying the regulation

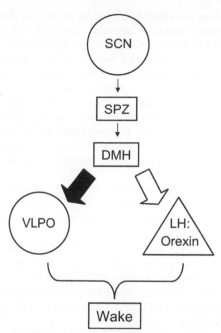

Fig. 4. Circadian regulation of wakefulness. The SCN indirectly inhibits the VLPO and activates the orexin system to promote wakefulness. Solid arrow represents inhibitory action; open arrow, excitatory action.

of sleep and wakefulness. Novel neurotransmitters, pathways, and receptors have been discovered to refine prior theories and define new hypotheses. For example, recent studies have pointed to mutually inhibitory pathways that regulate the switch between wakefulness and sleep, and between NREM and REM sleep, much like flip-flop switches. Similarly, the importance of the wake-promoting orexin pathway has been demonstrated in animal models, as well as in humans with narcolepsy. These new findings have provided novel targets for the development of agents to manage clinical sleep disorders such as insomnia, hypersomnia, and narcolepsy. The concept of interacting circadian and homeostatic systems in regulating sleep and wakefulness has facilitated our understanding of sleep onset and maintenance. This two-process model will undoubtedly be modified as the molecular basis of each system is further elucidated. As we improve our understanding of sleep and wake regulation, novel behavioral and pharmacologic targets for the treatment of sleep disorders will emerge to improve sleep and wake functions and mitigate the negative effects of poor sleep on health.

REFERENCES

1. Durmer JS, Dinges DF. Neurocognitive consequences of sleep deprivation. Semin Neurol 2005; 25:117–29.

2. Oliver SJ, Costa RJ, Laing SJ, et al. One night of sleep deprivation decreases treadmill endurance performance. Eur J Appl Physiol 2009;107:155–61.

3. Gottlieb DJ, Redline S, Nieto FJ, et al. Association of usual sleep duration with hypertension: the Sleep Heart Health Study. Sleep 2006;29:1009–14.

4. Ayas NT, White DP, Al-Delaimy WK, et al. A prospective study of self-reported sleep duration and incident diabetes in women. Diabetes Care 2003;26:380–4.

5. Patel SR, Ayas NT, Malhotra MR, et al. A prospective study of sleep duration and mortality risk in women. Sleep 2004;27:440–4.

6. Porkka-Heiskanen T, Strecker RE, Thakkar M, et al. Adenosine: a mediator of the sleep-inducing effects of prolonged wakefulness. Science 1997; 276:1265–8.

7. Lu J, Greco MA, Shiromani P, et al. Effect of lesions of the ventrolateral preoptic nucleus on NREM and REM sleep. J Neurosci 2000;20:3830–42.

8. Berger H. Ueber das Elektroenkephalogrammdes Menschen. J Psychol Neurol 1930;40:169–79 [in German].

9. von Economo C. Sleep as a problem of localization. J Nerv Ment Dis 1930;71:249–59.

10. Moruzzi G, Magoun HW. Brain stem reticular formation and activation of the EEG. Electroencephalogr Clin Neurophysiol 1949;1:455–73.

11. Armstrong DM, Saper CB, Levey AI, et al. Distribution of cholinergic neurons in rat brain: demonstrated by the immunocytochemical localization of choline acetyltransferase. J Comp Neurol 1983; 216:53–68.

12. Woolf NJ. Cholinergic systems in mammalian brain and spinal cord. Prog Neurobiol 1991;37: 475–524.

13. Jasper HH, Tessier J. Acetylcholine liberation from cerebral cortex during paradoxical (REM) sleep. Science 1971;172:601–2.

14. Steriade M, Datta S, Pare D, et al. Neuronal activities in brain-stem cholinergic nuclei related to tonic activation processes in thalamocortical systems. J Neurosci 1990;10:2541–59.

15. Rye DB, Wainer BH, Mesulam MM, et al. Cortical projections arising from the basal forebrain: a study of cholinergic and noncholinergic components employing combined retrograde tracing and immunohistochemical localization of choline acetyltransferase. Neuroscience 1984;13:627–43.

16. Jones BE. Activity, modulation and role of basal forebrain cholinergic neurons innervating the cerebral cortex. Prog Brain Res 2004;145:157–69.

17. Buzsaki G, Bickford RG, Ponomareff G, et al. Nucleus basalis and thalamic control of neocortical activity in the freely moving rat. J Neurosci 1988;8: 4007–26.

18. Mesulam MM, Mufson EJ, Wainer BH, et al. Central cholinergic pathways in the rat: an overview based on an alternative nomenclature (Ch1-Ch6). Neuroscience 1983;10:1185–201.

19. Saper CB, Scammell TE, Lu J. Hypothalamic regulation of sleep and circadian rhythms. Nature 2005; 437:1257–63.

20. Hobson JA, McCarley RW, Wyzinski PW. Sleep cycle oscillation: reciprocal discharge by two brainstem neuronal groups. Science 1975;189:55–8.

21. Aston-Jones G, Bloom FE. Activity of norepinephrine-containing locus coeruleus neurons in behaving rats anticipates fluctuations in the sleep-waking cycle. J Neurosci 1981;1:876–86.

22. Berridge CW, Foote SL. Effects of locus coeruleus activation on electroencephalographic activity in neocortex and hippocampus. J Neurosci 1991;11: 3135–45.

23. Berridge CW, Page ME, Valentino RJ, et al. Effects of locus coeruleus inactivation on electroencephalographic activity in neocortex and hippocampus. Neuroscience 1993;55:381–93.

24. Berridge CW. Noradrenergic modulation of arousal. Brain Res Rev 2008;58:1–17.

25. Valentino RJ, Page ME, Curtis AL. Activation of noradrenergic locus coeruleus neurons by hemodynamic stress is due to local release of corticotropin-releasing factor. Brain Res 1991;555:25–34.

26. Trulson ME, Jacobs BL. Raphe unit activity in freely moving cats: correlation with level of behavioral arousal. Brain Res 1979;163:135–50.

27. Koella WP. Serotonin and sleep. Exp Med Surg 1969;27:157–68.

28. Bjorvatn B, Fagerland S, Eid T, et al. Sleep/waking effects of a selective 5-HT1A receptor agonist given systemically as well as perfused in the dorsal raphe nucleus in rats. Brain Res 1997;770:81–8.

29. Bjorvatn B, Ursin R. Effects of zimeldine, a selective 5-HT reuptake inhibitor, combined with ritanserin, a selective 5-HT2 antagonist, on waking and sleep stages in rats. Behav Brain Res 1990; 40:239–46.

30. Bjorvatn B, Ursin R. Effects of the selective 5-HT1B agonist, CGS 12066B, on sleep/waking stages and EEG power spectrum in rats. J Sleep Res 1994;3: 97–105.

31. Ursin R. The effects of 5-hydroxytryptophan and L-tryptophan on wakefulness and sleep patterns in the cat. Brain Res 1976;106:105–15.

32. Ko EM, Estabrooke IV, McCarthy M, et al. Wake-related activity of tuberomammillary neurons in rats. Brain Res 2003;992:220–6.

33. Siegel JM, Boehmer LN. Narcolepsy and the hypocretin system—where motion meets emotion. Nat Clin Pract Neurol 2006;2:548–56.

34. Tasaka K, Chung YH, Sawada K, et al. Excitatory effect of histamine on the arousal system and its inhibition by H1 blockers. Brain Res Bull 1989;22: 271–5.

35. Sander K, Kottke T, Stark H. Histamine H3 receptor antagonists go to clinics. Biol Pharm Bull 2008;31: 2163–81.

36. Weiner DM, Levey AI, Sunahara RK, et al. D1 and D2 dopamine receptor mRNA in rat brain. Proc Natl Acad Sci U S A 1991;88:1859–63.

37. Monti JM, Monti D. The involvement of dopamine in the modulation of sleep and waking. Sleep Med Rev 2007;11:113–33.

38. Le Moal M, Simon H. Mesocorticolimbic dopaminergic network: functional and regulatory roles. Physiol Rev 1991;71:155–234.

39. Schultz W. Predictive reward signal of dopamine neurons. J Neurophysiol 1998;80:1–27.

40. Fadel J, Deutch AY. Anatomical substrates of orexin-dopamine interactions: lateral hypothalamic projections to the ventral tegmental area. Neuroscience 2002;111:379–87.

41. Kitai ST, Shepard PD, Callaway JC, et al. Afferent modulation of dopamine neuron firing patterns. Curr Opin Neurobiol 1999;9:690–7.

42. Lokwan SJ, Overton PG, Berry MS, et al. Stimulation of the pedunculopontine tegmental nucleus in the rat produces burst firing in A9 dopaminergic neurons. Neuroscience 1999;92:245–54.

43. White FJ. Synaptic regulation of mesocorticolimbic dopamine neurons. Annu Rev Neurosci 1996;19: 405–36.

44. Wisor JP, Nishino S, Sora I, et al. Dopaminergic role in stimulant-induced wakefulness. J Neurosci 2001; 21:1787–94.

45. Rye DB. Parkinson's disease and RLS: the dopaminergic bridge. Sleep Med 2004;5:317–28.

46. Monti JM, Jantos H, Fernandez M. Effects of the selective dopamine D-2 receptor agonist, quinpirole on sleep and wakefulness in the rat. Eur J Pharmacol 1989;169:61–6.

47. Sakurai T, Amemiya A, Ishii M, et al. Orexins and orexin receptors: a family of hypothalamic neuropeptides and G protein-coupled receptors that regulate feeding behavior. Cell 1998;92:573–85.

48. de Lecea L, Kilduff TS, Peyron C, et al. The hypocretins: hypothalamus-specific peptides with neuroexcitatory activity. Proc Natl Acad Sci U S A 1998;95:322–7.

49. Bayer L, Eggermann E, Saint-Mleux B, et al. Selective action of orexin (hypocretin) on nonspecific thalamocortical projection neurons. J Neurosci 2002; 22:7835–9.

50. Burlet S, Tyler CJ, Leonard CS. Direct and indirect excitation of laterodorsal tegmental neurons by Hypocretin/Orexin peptides: implications for wakefulness and narcolepsy. J Neurosci 2002;22:2862–72.

51. Eggermann E, Serafin M, Bayer L, et al. Orexins/hypocretins excite basal forebrain cholinergic neurones. Neuroscience 2001;108:177–81.

52. Eriksson KS, Sergeeva O, Brown RE, et al. Orexin/hypocretin excites the histaminergic neurons of the tuberomammillary nucleus. J Neurosci 2001;21: 9273–9.

53. Horvath TL, Peyron C, Diano S, et al. Hypocretin (orexin) activation and synaptic innervation of the locus coeruleus noradrenergic system. J Comp Neurol 1999;415:145–59.

54. Liu RJ, van den Pol AN, Aghajanian GK. Hypocretins (orexins) regulate serotonin neurons in the dorsal raphe nucleus by excitatory direct and inhibitory indirect actions. J Neurosci 2002;22: 9453–64.

55. Shirasaka T, Nakazato M, Matsukura S, et al. Sympathetic and cardiovascular actions of orexins in conscious rats. Am J Phys 1999;277:R1780–5.

56. Yamuy J, Fung SJ, Xi M, et al. Hypocretinergic control of spinal cord motoneurons. J Neurosci 2004;24:5336–45.

57. Lee MG, Hassani OK, Jones BE. Discharge of identified orexin/hypocretin neurons across the sleep-waking cycle. J Neurosci 2005;25:6716–20.

58. Chemelli RM, Willie JT, Sinton CM, et al. Narcolepsy in orexin knockout mice: molecular genetics of sleep regulation. Cell 1999;98:437–51.

59. Lin L, Faraco J, Li R, et al. The sleep disorder canine narcolepsy is caused by a mutation in the hypocretin (orexin) receptor 2 gene. Cell 1999;98:365–76.

60. Mignot E, Lammers GJ, Ripley B, et al. The role of cerebrospinal fluid hypocretin measurement in the diagnosis of narcolepsy and other hypersomnias. Arch Neurol 2002;59:1553–62.

61. Thannickal TC, Moore RY, Nienhuis R, et al. Reduced number of hypocretin neurons in human narcolepsy. Neuron 2000;27:469–74.

62. Jones BE. Arousal systems. Front Biosci 2003;8: s438–51.

63. Sherin JE, Shiromani PJ, McCarley RW, et al. Activation of ventrolateral preoptic neurons during sleep. Science 1996;271:216–9.

64. Lu J, Bjorkum AA, Xu M, et al. Selective activation of the extended ventrolateral preoptic nucleus during rapid eye movement sleep. J Neurosci 2002;22: 4568–76.

65. Sakurai T, Nagata R, Yamanaka A, et al. Input of orexin/hypocretin neurons revealed by a genetically encoded tracer in mice. Neuron 2005;46:297–308.

66. Chou TC, Bjorkum AA, Gaus SE, et al. Afferents to the ventrolateral preoptic nucleus. J Neurosci 2002;22:977–90.

67. Marcus JN, Aschkenasi CJ, Lee CE, et al. Differential expression of orexin receptors 1 and 2 in the rat brain. J Comp Neurol 2001;435:6–25.

68. Suntsova N, Szymusiak R, Alam MN, et al. Sleep-waking discharge patterns of median preoptic nucleus neurons in rats. J Physiol 2002;543:665–77.

69. Gvilia I, Xu F, McGinty D, et al. Homeostatic regulation of sleep: a role for preoptic area neurons. J Neurosci 2006;26:9426–33.

70. Saper CB, Chou TC, Scammell TE. The sleep switch: hypothalamic control of sleep and wakefulness. Trends Neurosci 2001;24:726–31.

71. Espana RA, Scammell TE. Sleep neurobiology for the clinician. Sleep 2004;27:811–20.

72. Kubin L. Carbachol models of REM sleep: recent developments and new directions. Arch Ital Biol 2001;139:147–68.

73. Qureshi A, Lee-Chiong T Jr. Medications and their effects on sleep. Med Clin North Am 2004;88: 751–66, x.

74. Jones BE, Harper ST, Halaris AE. Effects of locus coeruleus lesions upon cerebral monoamine content, sleep-wakefulness states and the response to amphetamine in the cat. Brain Res 1977;124:473–96.

75. Shouse MN, Siegel JM. Pontine regulation of REM sleep components in cats: integrity of the pedunculopontine tegmentum (PPT) is important for phasic events but unnecessary for atonia during REM sleep. Brain Res 1992;571:50–63.

76. Lu J, Sherman D, Devor M, et al. A putative flip-flop switch for control of REM sleep. Nature 2006;441: 589–94.

77. Sastre JP, Buda C, Kitahama K, et al. Importance of the ventrolateral region of the periaqueductal gray and adjacent tegmentum in the control of paradoxical sleep as studied by muscimol microinjections in the cat. Neuroscience 1996;74:415–26.

78. Boissard R, Gervasoni D, Schmidt MH, et al. The rat ponto-medullary network responsible for paradoxical sleep onset and maintenance: a combined microinjection and functional neuroanatomical study. Eur J Neurosci 2002;16:1959–73.

79. Sakai K, Crochet S, Onoe H. Pontine structures and mechanisms involved in the generation of paradoxical (REM) sleep. Arch Ital Biol 2001;139:93–107.

80. Sanford LD, Morrison AR, Mann GL, et al. Sleep patterning and behaviour in cats with pontine lesions creating REM without atonia. J Sleep Res 1994;3:233–40.

81. Chase MH, Soja PJ, Morales FR. Evidence that glycine mediates the postsynaptic potentials that inhibit lumbar motoneurons during the atonia of active sleep. J Neurosci 1989;9:743–51.

82. Fuller PM, Saper CB, Lu J. The pontine REM switch: past and present. J Physiol 2007;584: 735–41.

83. Brischoux F, Mainville L, Jones BE. Muscarinic-2 and orexin-2 receptors on GABAergic and other neurons in the rat mesopontine tegmentum and their potential role in sleep-wake state control. J Comp Neurol 2008;510:607–30.

84. Lu J. Neuroanatomical and genetic dissection of brain circuitry regulating REM sleep behavior disorder (RBD) and cataplexy. Sleep Med 2007; 8:S8.

85. Borbély AA. A two process model of sleep regulation. Hum Neurobiol 1982;1:195–204.

86. Benington JH, Heller HC. Restoration of brain energy metabolism as the function of sleep. Prog Neurobiol 1995;45:347–60.

87. Ticho SR, Radulovacki M. Role of adenosine in sleep and temperature regulation in the preoptic area of rats. Pharmacol Biochem Behav 1991;40:33–40.

88. Feldberg W, Sherwood SL. Infections of drugs into the lateral ventricle of the cat. J Physiol 1954;123: 148–67.

89. Haulica I, Ababei L, Branisteanu D, et al. Preliminary data on the possible hypnogenic role of adenosine. Rev Roum Physiol 1973;10:275–9.

90. Strecker RE, Morairty S, Thakkar MM, et al. Adenosinergic modulation of basal forebrain and preoptic/anterior hypothalamic neuronal activity in the control of behavioral state. Behav Brain Res 2000; 115:183–204.

91. Scammell TE, Gerashchenko DY, Mochizuki T, et al. An adenosine A2a agonist increases sleep and induces Fos in ventrolateral preoptic neurons. Neuroscience 2001;107:653–63.

92. Moore RY. A clock for the ages. Science 1999;284: 2102–3.

93. Dijk DJ, Czeisler CA. Contribution of the circadian pacemaker and the sleep homeostat to sleep propensity, sleep structure, electroencephalographic slow waves, and sleep spindle activity in humans. J Neurosci 1995;15:3526–38.

94. Edgar DM, Dement WC, Fuller CA. Effect of SCN lesions on sleep in squirrel monkeys: evidence for opponent processes in sleep-wake regulation. J Neurosci 1993;13:1065–79.

95. Watts AG, Swanson LW, Sanchez-Watts G. Efferent projections of the suprachiasmatic nucleus: I. Studies using anterograde transport of Phaseolus vulgaris leucoagglutinin in the rat. J Comp Neurol 1987;258:204–29.

96. Chou TC, Scammell TE, Gooley JJ, et al. Critical role of dorsomedial hypothalamic nucleus in a wide range of behavioral circadian rhythms. J Neurosci 2003;23:10691–702.

97. Lu J, Zhang YH, Chou TC, et al. Contrasting effects of ibotenate lesions of the paraventricular nucleus and subparaventricular zone on sleep-wake cycle and temperature regulation. J Neurosci 2001;21: 4864–74.

98. Deurveilher S, Semba K. Indirect projections from the suprachiasmatic nucleus to major arousal-promoting cell groups in rat: implications for the circadian control of behavioural state. Neuroscience 2005;130:165–83.

Circadian Rhythm Sleep Disorders

Naveen Kanathur, MD, John Harrington, MD*,
Teofilo Lee-Chiong Jr, MD

KEYWORDS

- Circadian rhythm disorders • Actigraphy
- Melatonin • Bright light

THE CIRCADIAN NEUROBIOME

Because there is insufficient cellular energy for organisms to perform their functions at the same constant rate and at the same time, all biologic processes show rhythmicity, each with its own unique frequency, amplitude, and phase (ie, temporal position of the rhythm in relation to an external factor such as the environmental light-dark cycle). These biologic rhythms are controlled by endogenous rhythm generators that establish the primary rhythm, and external factors called zeitgebers that are able to adjust (entrain) the phase of the intrinsic rhythm. The zeitgebers either cause a phase advance or shift of a period to an earlier time in the 24-hour cycle, or cause a phase delay or shift of a period to a later time.

The term circadian is derived from the Latin word *circa*, which means about, and *die*, which means day. Most intrinsic human circadian rhythms, if allowed to free-run in the absence of zeitgebers, will have a periodicity that is not exactly 24 hours but is slightly longer at about 24.2 hours. To function optimally in a 24-hour world, a rhythm has to undergo entrainment each day to synchronize itself to the external time as well as to other biologic rhythms. As an example, the phase of the sleep-wake cycle can be reset forward or backward with light presented at dawn or dusk, respectively. Similarly, melatonin administration can phase delay the circadian sleep-wake rhythms when taken in the morning, and phase advance them when given in the afternoon or early evening. Light is the predominant zeitgeber of the circadian sleep-wake cycle and

can induce specific phase shifts depending on the timing, intensity, and duration of light exposure, Other external synchronizers include meals or daytime social activities, but these nonphotic stimuli have a weaker influence on the sleep-wake cycle than light.

In mammals, the suprachiasmatic nucleus in the anterior hypothalamus serves as the primary generator of circadian rhythms. Other anatomic sites may also harbor endogenous clocks. The activity of the suprachiasmatic nucleus is independent of the environment, being more active during the daytime than at night. This circadian neurosystem promotes wakefulness during the day and, by doing so, helps to consolidate sleep during the night.

CIRCADIAN RHYTHM SLEEP DISORDERS

Optimal sleep and wakefulness requires proper timing and alignment of desired sleep-wake schedules and circadian rhythm-related periods of alertness. Persistent or recurrent mismatch between endogenous circadian rhythms and the conventional sleep-wake schedules of the environmental day can give rise to several circadian rhythm sleep disorders, with the affected persons presenting with complaints of insomnia, excessive sleepiness, or both.

There are 6 basic disorders of the circadian sleep-wake cycle. The disorders are classified as primary if they are caused by alterations of the endogenous circadian pacemakers (eg, advanced sleep phase syndrome [ASPS], delayed sleep phase syndrome [DSPS], free-running circadian

Division of Sleep Medicine, Department of Medicine, National Jewish Health, 1400 Jackson Street, Denver, CO 80206, USA
* Corresponding author.
E-mail address: harringtonj@njhealth.org

Clin Chest Med 31 (2010) 319–325
doi:10.1016/j.ccm.2010.02.009

rhythm syndrome, and irregular sleep-wake rhythm syndrome) or secondary if they are produced by an inability to adjust promptly to changes in environmental time (eg, shift work sleep disorder [SWSD] and jet lag). Disturbances of circadian sleep-wake rhythms can develop secondary to medical and neurologic disorders, such as encephalopathy from liver cirrhosis or dementia; or from the use of specific drugs or substances.[1] In all these cases, a misalignment between the endogenous sleep-wake cycles and external circadian synchronizing factors are discernible on sleep diaries or actigraphy recorded over several days or weeks.

Advanced Sleep Phase Syndrome

Persons with this syndrome generally report sleep times occurring between 6 PM and 9 PM, and wake-up times between 2 AM and 5 AM. An inability to delay bedtimes is coupled with spontaneous morning awakenings that are several hours earlier than desired. Thus, affected individuals may complain of excessive sleepiness in the late afternoon or early evening or terminal insomnia.[2] This shift in the major sleep period to an earlier time is stable and is often present for many years. Sleep, itself, is normal for age and undisturbed.

ASPS affects approximately 1% of middle-aged adults.[3] The onset of ASPS is typically during middle age, and prevalence increases with aging. Cases of familial ASPS, an autosomal variant, have been reported and are caused by a mutation in a gene located near the telomere of chromosome 2q.[4] Other familial ASPS cases have been associated with a missense mutation in a different casein kinase 1 delta gene.[5]

Although many individuals are able to maintain this altered sleep-wake schedule without distress or impairment, others may experience significant sleep deprivation if later bedtimes are attempted because of the persistence of early morning awakenings. In addition, conditioned insomnia may develop if maladaptive responses to the early morning awakenings occur.

Possible pathogenetic mechanisms for this syndrome include genetic mutations mentioned earlier, enhanced retinal sensitivity to morning light exposure,[6] or very short endogenous circadian period lengths.[7] Bedtime behavior most likely has a contributory role; further phase advances can result from greater morning light exposure after consistently early awakenings as well as limited evening light exposure caused by earlier bedtimes.

Diagnosis of ASPS relies on a thorough sleep history and sleep diaries recorded over several days. Psychiatric evaluation may occasionally be required to exclude mood disorders, because major depression may also present with early morning awakenings. Actigraphy can aid diagnosis in cases with atypical presentations or involving patients who are unable to reliably self-monitor their bedtimes and wake-up times. Actigraphy provides estimates of periods of sleep (or inactivity) and wakefulness (or activity), such as total wake time, total sleep time, frequency of awakenings, and wake time after sleep onset, using accelerometers that are worn on the wrist. Because of its portability, an actigraph allows extended monitoring over several days to weeks, with minimal patient bias or compliance, while the patient maintains customary daytime and nighttime activities.

Polysomnography is not routinely indicated for diagnosis. However, if performed for other reasons it shows normal sleep-onset latency and duration and quality of sleep when monitored over the usual advanced sleep schedule, or shortened sleep-onset latency and decreased total sleep time when recorded during conventional sleep-wake times. In one study, timing of sleep onset and offset was advanced in subjects with familial ASPS compared with controls, whereas sleep duration and quality remained unchanged.[7] Therapy for ASPS involves administering bright light during the early evening to phase delay the circadian sleep-wake rhythms.[8] This therapy should be complemented by minimizing light exposure in the early morning. Chronotherapy, which involves gradually shifting sleep time until the desired bedtime is achieved, may also be tried but seems to be less effective than phototherapy. Supporting evidence for proposed beneficial effects or safety of timed administration of low-dose melatonin in the morning for ASPS remains insufficient.[2]

Delayed Sleep Phase Syndrome

This syndrome involves a chronic inability to sleep during conventional hours, with the major nighttime sleep period occurring later than is desired or socially acceptable. Thus, there is a persistent delay in habitual bedtimes with persons unable to fall asleep until the early morning hours, commonly from 1 AM to 6 AM, and an equally delayed arising time occurring in the late morning or early afternoon from 10 AM to 2 PM.[2]

Persons with this syndrome generally describe feeling relatively more alert in the late evening and sleepier in the morning; thus, they may present with complaints of sleep-onset insomnia and excessive sleepiness in the morning if they try to sleep and awaken at times closer to socially accepted norms. Sleep deprivation may develop if earlier wake-up times are enforced and would, in turn, have a negative impact on academic or job performance. Habitual absence or tardiness for early work or school schedules is not uncommon. Furthermore, secondary-conditioned insomnia may arise because persons attempt to fall asleep at earlier times when the propensity to sleep is reduced. Aside from an inability to voluntarily advance their sleep time, they have no other sleep disturbances; and sleep duration and quality are normal if they go to bed at their preferred schedule and if sleep is allowed to continue until spontaneous awakening.

DSPS has an estimated prevalence of 0.1% to 0.2% in the general population, and accounts for about 5% of cases of chronic insomnia encountered in the sleep clinic. DSPS is probably the most common circadian rhythm sleep disorder. Based on a retrospective case series study of 322 patients with circadian rhythm sleep disorders, the majority (83.5%) had a diagnosis of DSPS.[9] Onset is usually during adolescence or early adulthood, and the course tends to be persistent. A positive family history of the syndrome can be elicited in a significant number of individuals, but a genetic basis for the disorder remains incompletely understood.

This syndrome is postulated to involve alterations in the circadian pacemaker with a phase delay in relation to conventional sleep-wake schedules and an inability to advance the phase to correct the disturbance. This syndrome has also been reported in association with traumatic brain injury.[10] DSPS should be differentiated from other disorders that are associated with sleep-onset insomnia, such as conditioned psychophysiologic insomnia, or mood or anxiety disorders. Altered sleep-wake patterns arising from acquired lifestyle or poor sleep hygiene may also present similarly.

Diagnosis is made from a compatible sleep history, often aided by well-kept sleep diaries. Actigraphy may be considered and shows a consistent delay in habitual sleep times. Polysomnography is not indicated for diagnosis; findings include prolonged sleep-onset latency and decreased total sleep time when performed during desired conventional sleep-wake times, but is generally normal for age when recorded at the habitual delayed sleep periods.

Therapy for DSPS involves phototherapy, pharmacotherapy, and chronotherapy.[8] Phototherapy for DSPS consists of timed early morning exposure and avoidance of bright light in the evening.[11] Neither the optimum duration nor the intensity of

light exposure has been established, and clinicians have used different schedules. Suggested schedules have included 20 minutes of morning light exposure at 10,000 lux, or longer duration of exposures using lesser light intensities. Bright light boxes that generate light at 5000 to 10,000 lux are commercially available. Shorter wavelength light in the blue-green light spectrum (470–525 nm) seems to be more effective in phase-advancing circadian rhythm compared with longer wavelength light.[12] During the summer, outdoor sunlight exposure can be used instead of light box therapy. Timing of light administration after core body temperature has reached a minimum is important because exposure to light before the temperature nadir could further phase delay circadian rhythms. Because identifying an individual's specific temperature nadir, often about 1 to 2 hours after the habitual midsleep time, is difficult and impractical in the clinical setting, bright light therapy may be initiated at the person's habitual awakening time and applied at successively earlier times (eg, 30 minutes to 1 hour every few days) until phase advancement is seen. Light therapy is associated with several adverse effects, including ocular damage, headaches, nausea, and skin dryness and erythema. Phototherapy should not be used in those with retinopathy, photosensitivity, mania, bipolar disorder, and migraine headaches. An ophthalmologic examination is advisable before initiating bright light therapy in patients with suspected retinal and ocular disorders.

Melatonin, when given in the early evening, may help induce a phase advance of the sleep period.[13] The phase-shifting effect of melatonin is opposite to that of bright light and is less potent than the latter; however, it possesses a mild hypnotic effect that may contribute to decreasing sleep-onset latency. Varying doses of melatonin (0.3 mg and 3 mg) have been shown to be effective in phase-advancing circadian rhythms, and the magnitude of the phase advance seems to be better with earlier administration.[14] Persons who choose to take melatonin in the early evening should be instructed to refrain from driving or engaging in potentially dangerous activities for several hours after ingesting melatonin, and informed that it is not approved by the Food and Drug Administration as therapy for circadian rhythm sleep disorders. A combination of appropriately timed afternoon melatonin and morning bright light therapy can produce a larger phase advance than bright light exposure alone.[15] It is tempting to provide immediate relief from sleep-onset insomnia with hypnotic medications. Although these agents may improve sleep-onset latency and sleep efficiency, these changes are transient; and often, partial and hypnotic agents are generally not effective for long-term use.

With chronotherapy, either progressive phase delay or progressive phase advancement of the major sleep episode is used to achieve a more conventional bedtime pattern.[16] Progressive phase delay involves delaying bedtime and wake-up times by about 2 to 3 hours each day on successive days, allowing the major sleep episode to march around the clock until a desired bedtime is reached. Physical activities, meal times, and light exposure are timed to coincide with the progressive delay in wake-up times, and napping is discouraged. Because this approach requires several days to fully complete the cycle, sleep and work may be disrupted when sleep is scheduled during the daytime. The case of a patient with DSPS who developed a free-running circadian rhythm after chronotherapy has been reported.[17] Another technique that has been described involves progressively phase advancing bedtimes, usually by 30 to 60 minutes every 3 to 4 days, until more conventional sleep-wake schedules are attained. It is important to maintain the newly acquired sleep pattern once a desired sleep-wake schedule has been established because the risk of relapse may be high. In addition to proper sleep hygiene, maintaining a regular sleep schedule throughout the week is essential. Ongoing maintenance therapy using periodic timed bright light exposure or melatonin administration may be considered for persons with a history of repeated relapse.

Free-Running Circadian Rhythm Syndrome

This circadian rhythm sleep disorder, also referred to as nonentrained or non–24-hour sleep-wake syndrome, results from lack of synchronization between the endogenous sleep-wake circadian rhythm and the 24-hour environmental light-dark cycle. Rarely encountered in the general population, it is seen most frequently in totally blind individuals who lack photic entrainment.[2] About 70% of blind individuals complain of chronic sleep-wake disturbances, and 40% describe chronic recurring and cyclical insomnia. Prevalence of free-running rhythm in cohorts of blind individuals has been around 5% to 15%; furthermore, more than half of blind individuals without any light perception show this rhythm.[18] In these individuals, sleep-wake patterns freed of exogenous photic entraining influences rely almost entirely on intrinsic biologic rhythms that free-run at a periodicity of slightly over 24 hours. Thus, sleep-onset and wake-up times are delayed by about 1 hour or more each day, resulting in the major sleep period

shifting progressively throughout the day and on to the afternoon and evening before cycling back to the morning. Symptoms reflect the progressive delay in sleep schedules as well as the cyclic variability of sleep disturbance. Affected individuals may complain of periodically recurring problems of excessive sleepiness or insomnia that are separated by periods of complete, albeit brief, disappearance of symptoms. Patients who are allowed to sleep ad libitum may also have minimal symptoms.

Pathogenesis involves lack or weakness of environmental entraining influences or decreased sensitivity to them. Most totally blind persons who do not have retinas have no light stimuli reaching the suprachiasmatic nucleus, and are thus unable to entrain to environmental light. However, certain blind individuals are capable of partially entraining to the environment using either photic cues via an intact and functional retinohypothalamic pathway (ie, melatonin suppression is observed with light exposure) or nonphotic factors such as regular mealtimes or social activities.

Onset can occur at any age, and course tends to be chronic, with many persons unable to maintain the tightly scheduled lifestyle required for schooling or employment. Most affected persons are totally blind. Less commonly, this syndrome can be encountered in sighted individuals with severely schizoid or avoidant personality disorders, mental retardation, or dementia—some of whom may have diminished sensitivity to the phase-shifting effects of light or an extremely lengthy endogenous circadian period that is beyond the range for external 24-hour entrainment.

Diagnosis is made by sleep diaries or actigraphy performed over several days or weeks. Nighttime and 24-hour polysomnography may show highly variable sleep onset and offset times, but sleep efficiency and total sleep time are usually normal. If polysomnography is recorded at a fixed time over several days, sleep-onset latency will be observed to get progressively longer whereas total sleep time may become commensurately shorter. Neurologic and psychiatric evaluations should be entertained in sighted persons to exclude any occult central nervous system or psychiatric pathology.

Therapy is often challenging. Evening administration of melatonin may be tried first.[8,19] Low doses of melatonin (0.5 mg) seem to be as effective as higher doses.[20] Entrainment may take weeks to months after starting melatonin treatment. Persons with intact light perception may benefit from daytime bright light treatment. In all patients, strengthening nonphotic entrainment by strict regulation of the timing of bedtime, arising times, activities, and meals are important but are less consistently effective. Chronic reliance on hypnotic agents to improve sleep and on stimulants to enhance daytime performance should be avoided.

Irregular Sleep-Wake Rhythm Syndrome

Stable circadian sleep-wake rhythms are absent in this syndrome, in which the patient manifests disorganized and highly variable sleep and wake-up times from one day to the next.[2] Bedtimes and wake-up times are inconsistent and unpredictable as is sleep duration. Indeed, the major nocturnal sleep period is fragmented into 3 or more short naps occurring randomly throughout the day and night. Despite this variability in sleep and wake-up times, total sleep duration in a 24-hour period is generally normal or near normal for age.

This disorder is rare in the general population and seems to affect both genders equally. This disorder is most commonly seen in persons with severe brain dysfunction, such as dementia, head injury, or recovery from coma, in persons who have concurrent abnormalities of the circadian neurosystem, or who have severely deficient entrainment by environmental circadian synchronizing factors. Less commonly, it can be seen in cognitively intact individuals who chronically ignore environmental and social time cues by indiscriminate napping or voluntarily spending excessive time in bed during the day (ie, severely poor sleep hygiene). Onset can occur at any age.

Diagnosis is established by compatible sleep history and sleep diaries. Actigraphy is particularly helpful, especially if performed over several days to weeks, and confirms the irregularly irregular patterns of sleep and waking. A polyphasic sleep schedule is evident on 24-hour polysomnography.

Therapy needs to be individualized and centers on proper sleep hygiene (maintenance of regular schedules of sleep and wakefulness as well as daytime activities, such as meals; and limiting time spent in bed to actual sleeping), timed bright light therapy in the morning, and administration of melatonin in the evening.[8] Chronic use of hypnotic agents has unpredictable, but most likely limited long-term efficacy.

Jet Lag

Jet lag refers to the transient sleep disturbance, insomnia, and daytime hypersomnolence that develop after rapid eastward or westward air travel across multiple time zones. Jet lag arises from the traveler's inability to rapidly realign his or her intrinsic circadian rhythm, which remains synchronized to the original home time zone, to the new destination time zone.[21] Thus, persons traveling eastward are phase delayed relative to the new environmental clock time and develop difficulty with falling asleep and awakening the next day. Conversely, westward travelers are phase advanced and, therefore, experience excessive sleepiness in the early evening as well as earlier-than-usual awakenings in the morning. Sleep is frequently disturbed with frequent arousals and diminished sleep efficiency. Total sleep time may be reduced if social commitments do not permit ad libitum sleep to occur. Daytime performance is impaired and many travelers may complain of decreased alertness, nonspecific gastrointestinal disturbances, malaise, fatigue, and decreased mood.

Symptoms generally develop within a day or two of transmeridian air travel, and remit spontaneously within a few days, approximately a day for every time zone change. Sleep disturbance persists longer after eastward travel, which requires advancing the circadian phase, than westward travel. In addition, severity of symptoms is related to the direction of travel (more pronounced sleep disturbance with eastward travel), number of time zone changes, rapidity of travel, and individual differences in susceptibility. Aging also increases the likelihood of sleep disturbance during transmeridian-air travel.[22] It is, nonetheless, important to note that not every east-west traveler develops jet lag, and that north-south travel does not produce jet lag symptoms.

Diagnosis is often readily apparent from the clinical history, and frequent travelers commonly describe similar symptoms after flights in the past. If polysomnography is performed during the first few nights of arrival at the new destination, it will show diminished sleep efficiency and depending on the direction of jet travel, either prolonged-sleep-onset latency or early morning awakenings.

Jet travelers should be advised to immediately adapt their sleep-wake schedules to the new destination time on the day of arrival. Seasoned travelers may choose to begin shifting their sleep-wake schedules in the appropriate direction for several days before travel. Inappropriate timing of light exposure may further delay resynchronization; therefore, it is essential to properly time bright light exposure and light restriction, depending on the direction of travel as well as the number of time zone changes. For instance, westward travel from New York to California would require afternoon light at destination, but travel from New York to Asia would need morning light at destination. Similarly, eastward travelers from California to New York would benefit from morning light exposure at destination, but those flying from California to Europe would need afternoon light at destination. For additional information regarding phototherapy for travel, the reader is advised to consult sleep medicine textbooks or online travel services.

Administration of short-acting hypnotic agents or melatonin at bedtime may lessen jet lag symptoms after eastward jet travel. In a study of 130 eastward (5–9 time zones) traveling subjects, administering 10 mg zolpidem for 3 consecutive nights after travel produced longer total sleep duration, decreased nocturnal awakenings, and improved sleep quality compared with placebo.[23] Melatonin taken at the destination bedtime reduced jet lag symptoms in those traveling through greater than 5 or more time zones.[24] Although not specifically studied for jet lag, newer melatonin receptor agonists may have potential for treatment of this condition.[25] Caffeine may be used to minimize excessive daytime sleepiness.[26]

Shift Work Sleep Disorder

Shift work involves any employment outside of the conventional 8 AM to 5 PM work schedule, and includes rotating shifts, random work assignments, or regular nighttime or early morning shift work. In SWSD, sleep disturbance and work impairment results directly from the disparity in timing between the demands for sleep and the requirements of work in the evening, as well as increases in homeostatic sleep drive and circadian alerting influences in the daytime after night shift work.[21] In addition, many shift workers revert back to traditional daytime activities and nighttime sleep during nonworking days, further disrupting the circadian entraining effects of time cues of sunlight and social activities.

Sleep is frequently reported as unsatisfying or nonrestorative. Sleep-onset latency begun on the morning after night sleep may be prolonged, and sleep may be characterized by frequent arousals. On the other hand, workers starting early schedules, such as between 3 AM and 6 AM, may be compelled to sleep earlier than desired, leading to complaints of sleep-initiation insomnia and difficulty waking up in the early morning. Other features of SWSD include chronic fatigue and malaise, mood disorder, and nonspecific complaints such as dyspepsia. Risk of alcohol and substance dependency may be increased.

There are great individual differences in tolerance to shift work, and not every shift worker develops this disorder. Several factors may increase susceptibility to SWSD, including aging, morningness diurnal preference, presence of other sleep-related disorders, and the extent of daytime activities and commitments. Both genders are affected equally, but women describe worse daytime sleep than do men. The course of sleep disturbance parallels the schedule of the shift work period and generally remits with termination of shift work.

SWSD can pose a significant hazard in the work environment, and increases the risk of physical injuries and work-related accidents because of diminished vigilance secondary to sleep deprivation and circadian changes in levels of alertness.

A thorough sleep history recorded over several days including workdays and nonworkdays, aided by actigraphy, establishes the diagnosis. Therapy should be directed at improving nighttime alertness with the use of evening light exposure; properly timed napping,[27] either before night shift or early during the work hours; and stimulant agents, such as caffeine, modafinil, or armodafinil.[8,28–32] Daytime sleep duration and quality can be enhanced by intermittent use of hypnotic agents or melatonin; however, these agents do not significantly improve nighttime work performance or alertness. Other causes of sleep disturbance or excessive sleepiness, such as environmental sleep disruptors, inadequate sleep hygiene, obstructive sleep apnea, and narcolepsy, must be addressed and managed appropriately.

SUMMARY

Evaluation of suspected circadian rhythm sleep disorders requires proper monitoring of sleep diaries, often over several days to weeks. Actigraphy is useful for diagnosis and monitoring response to therapy. Polysomnography is not routinely indicated. Therapy should be individualized and often includes, in varying combinations, planned napping, phototherapy, and the use of melatonin. Stimulant and hypnotic agents may be considered for SWSD and jet lag.

REFERENCES

1. American Academy of Sleep Medicine. The international classification of sleep disorders: diagnostic and coding manual. 2nd edition. Westchester (IL): American Academy of Sleep Medicine; 2005.
2. Sack R, Auckley D, Auger RR, et al. Circadian rhythm sleep disorders: part II, advanced sleep phase disorder, delayed sleep phase disorder, free-running disorder, and irregular sleep-wake rhythm. Sleep 2007;30(11):1484–501.

3. Ando K, Kripke DF, Ancoli-Israel S. Estimated prevalence of delayed and advanced sleep phase syndromes. Sleep Res 1995;24:509.

4. Toh KL, Jones CR, He Y, et al. An hPer2 phosphorylation site mutation in familial advanced sleep phase syndrome. Science 2001;291:1040–3.

5. Xu Y, Padiath QS, Shapiro RE, et al. Functional consequences of a CKI mutation causing familial advanced sleep phase syndrome. Nature 2005; 434:640–4.

6. Rufiange M, Dumont M, Lachapelle P. Correlating retinal function with melatonin secretion in subjects with an early or late circadian phase. Invest Ophthalmol Vis Sci 2002;43:2491–9.

7. Jones CR, Campbell SS, Zone SE, et al. Familial advanced sleep-phase syndrome: a short-period circadian rhythm variant in humans. Nat Med 1999; 5:1062–5.

8. Morgenthaler TI, Lee-Chiong T, Alessi C, et al. Standards of Practice Committee of the AASM. Practice parameters for the clinical evaluation and treatment of circadian rhythm sleep disorders. An American Academy of Sleep Medicine report. Sleep 2007;30(11):1445–59.

9. Dagan Y, Eisenstein M. Circadian rhythm sleep disorders: toward a more precise definition and diagnosis. Chronobiol Int 1999;16:213–22.

10. Quito C, Gellido C, Chokroverty S, et al. Posttraumatic delayed sleep phase syndrome. Neurology 2000;54:250–2.

11. Rosenthal NE, Joseph-Vanderpool JR, Levendosky AA, et al. Phase-shifting effects of bright morning light as treatment for delayed sleep phase syndrome. Sleep 1990;13:354–61.

12. Wright HR, Lack LC, Kennaway DJ. Differential effects of light wavelength in phase advancing the melatonin rhythm. J Pineal Res 2004;35:1–5.

13. Dagan Y, Yovel I, Hallis D, et al. Evaluating the role of melatonin in the long-term treatment of delayed sleep phase syndrome (DSPS). Chronobiol Int 1998;15(2):181–90.

14. Mundey K, Benloucif S, Harsanyi K, et al. Phase-dependent treatment of delayed sleep phase syndrome with melatonin. Sleep 2005;28:1271–8.

15. Revell VL, Burgess HJ, Gazda CJ, et al. Advancing human circadian rhythms with afternoon melatonin and morning intermittent bright light. J Clin Endocrinol Metab 2006;91:54–9.

16. Czeisler CA, Richardson GS, Coleman RM, et al. Chronotherapy: resetting the circadian clocks of patients with delayed sleep phase insomnia. Sleep 1981;4:1–21.

17. Oren DA, Wehr TA. Hypernyctohemeral syndrome after chronotherapy for delayed sleep phase syndrome. N Engl J Med 1992;327:1762.

18. Sack RL, Lewy AJ, Blood ML, et al. Circadian rhythm abnormalities in totally blind people: incidence and clinical significance. J Clin Endocrinol Metab 1992; 75:127–34.

19. Sack RL, Brandes RW, Kendall AR, et al. Entrainment of free-running circadian rhythms by melatonin in blind people. N Engl J Med 2000; 343(15):1070–7.

20. Hack LM, Lockley SW, Arendt J, et al. The effects of low-dose 0.5-mg melatonin on the free-running circadian rhythms of blind subjects. J Biol Rhythms 2003;18:420–9.

21. Sack RL, Auckley D, Auger RR, et al. Circadian rhythm sleep disorders: part I, basic principles, shift work and jet lag disorders. Sleep 2007; 30(11):1460–83.

22. Monk T. Aging human circadian rhythms: conventional wisdom may not always be right. J Biol Rhythms 2005;20(4):366–74.

23. Jamieson AO, Zammit GK, Rosenberg RS, et al. Zolpidem reduces the sleep disturbance of jet lag. Sleep Med 2001;2:423–30.

24. Herxheimer A, Petrie KJ. Melatonin for the prevention and treatment of jet lag. Cochrane Database Syst Rev 2002;(2):CD001520.

25. Hirai K, Kita M, Ohta H, et al. Ramelteon (TAK-375) accelerates re-entrainment of circadian rhythm after a phase advance of the light-dark cycle in rats. J Biol Rhythms 2005;20:27–37.

26. Beaumont M, Batejat D, Peirard C, et al. Caffeine or melatonin effects on sleep and sleepiness after rapid eastward transmeridian travel. J Appl Phys 2004;96(1):50–8.

27. Purnell MT, Feyer AM, Herbison GP. The impact of a nap opportunity during the night shift on the performance and alertness of 12-h shift workers. J Sleep Res 2002;11:219–27.

28. Walsh JK, Randazzo AC, Stone KL, et al. Modafinil improves alertness, vigilance, and executive function during simulated night shifts. Sleep 2004; 27(3):434–9.

29. Czeisler CD, DF, Walsh JK, et al. Modafinil for the treatment of excessive sleepiness in chronic shift work sleep disorder. Sleep 2003;26:A114.

30. Czeisler C. Absence of detectable effect of modafinil on daytime sleep after a simulated night shift in SWSD patients. Sleep 2003;26:A115.

31. Czeisler CA, Walsh K, Roth T, et al. Modafinil for excessive sleepiness associated with shift-work sleep disorder. N Engl J Med 2005;353(5):478–86.

32. Czeisler CA, Walsh JK, Wesnes KA, et al. Armodafinil for treatment of excessive sleepiness associated with shift work disorder: a randomized controlled study. Mayo Clin Proc 2009;84(11): 958–72.

The Evaluation and Management of Insomnia

Karl Doghramji, MD

KEYWORDS
- Insomnia • Mood disorders • Anxiety disorders
- Chronic obstructive pulmonary disease

Sleep is vital for normal biologic and psychological functioning. Insomnia, which is the inability to obtain adequate sleep quantity or quality, represents the second most commonly expressed complaint in medical practice after pain.[1] It is also expressed by a third of all adults during the course of a year.[2] Insomnia is defined by the complaint alone; there is no objective test for insomnia. It should be distinguished from sleep deprivation or curtailment in that insomnia occurs despite adequate opportunity for sleep, whereas sleep deprivation results from an imposed curtailment of this opportunity.

Nosologic systems add certain qualifiers to this definition such as the presence of daytime consequences, duration, and frequency.

1. The International Classification of Sleep Disorders, Second Version (ICSD-2),[3] defines insomnia as (1) a complaint of difficulty initiating or maintaining sleep or waking up too early or poor sleep quality, (2) occurring despite adequate opportunity and circumstances for sleep, (c) and being associated with daytime impairments such as fatigue, poor attention concentration or memory, poor performance, mood disturbance, daytime sleepiness, reduction in motivation, proneness to errors and accidents, somatic symptoms such as tension headaches and gastrointestinal symptoms, and concerns or worries about sleep.
2. The Diagnostic and Statistical Manual of Mental Disorders (DSM-IV TR)[4] definition is similar to that of the ICSD-2; yet it adds a duration criterion of 1 month.
3. The International Classification of Disorders-10 (ICD-10)[5] introduces a frequency criterion: the sleep disturbance must occur at least 3 nights a week.

Various demographic factors are associated with an increased risk for insomnia.[6–10] These include female gender, especially during pregnancy and peri- and postmenopause; older age; being divorced, widowed, or single; unusual work schedules; sleeping in noisy environments; unemployment and lower socioeconomic status; poor mental and physical health; and the presence of multiple medical and psychiatric disorders.

Insomnia is associated with various impairments, including decreased quality of life, cognitive deficits, occupational difficulties, and an increased risk of future, new, psychiatric disorders.[11–13] The risk of future psychiatric disorders is the greatest when insomnia persists for prolonged periods of time.[14] It is not surprising, therefore, that insomniacs use health care resources at a rate higher than the general population. Insomnia has even been linked to increased mortality.[15,16] Even though many of these impairments have been understood from studies examining insomniacs suffering from a wide variety of comorbid conditions, obscuring cause and effect relationships, recent studies with insomniacs who lack evidence of comorbid conditions reveal an increased risk for psychomotor performance

Department of Psychiatry and Human Behavior, Jefferson Sleep Disorders Center, Thomas Jefferson University, 211 South Ninth Street, Suite 500, Philadelphia, PA 19107, USA
E-mail address: Karl.Doghramji@jefferson.edu

Clin Chest Med 31 (2010) 327–339
doi:10.1016/j.ccm.2010.03.001
0272-5231/10/$ – see front matter © 2010 Elsevier Inc. All rights reserved.

deficits when responding to challenging reaction time tasks in insomniacs.[17]

PATHOPHYSIOLOGY

The pathophysiology of insomnia is poorly understood. Recent studies reveal evidence of heightened arousal, or hyperarousal, not only during sleep but also around the clock. Despite poor sleep quantity and quality at night, insomniacs are less able than normal controls to fall asleep during daytime nap opportunities.[18]

Hyperarousal is evident in cognitive and psychological functions. Insomniacs typically describe speeded thoughts as they lie in bed. They also describe difficulty relaxing, feeling tense and anxious, being overly preoccupied with a myriad of thoughts, and feeling worried and depressed.[19] Hyperarousal in psychological realms is believed to represent a heightened predisposition for exaggerated reactions to environmental stressors, or precipitants, such as job loss and breaches in social relationships; therefore, insomniacs require less activation by external events to achieve high levels of internal arousal, which in turn lead to disturbed sleep. Insomniacs are also known to display cognitive hyperarousal because they carefully monitor mental and body sensations and external cues such as the bedroom clock and environmental noises at bedtime. They also typically have distorted and maladaptive beliefs about sleep itself, including the belief that poor sleep is

inevitable, that the lack of a full night of sleep will invariably lead to disastrous health consequences, and that a minimum of 8 hours of sleep per day is critical to maintain health. Such catastrophizing is encouraged by many nights of poor sleep, which can foment cognitive rumination and worry about not falling asleep and about the potential for disastrous next-day consequences of sleeplessness. This cycle of apprehension and worry can perpetuatee insomnia and make future sleep even less likely. Hyperarousal also becomes a learned response because bedtime rituals and the bedroom environment itself become contextual cues for arousal rather than for sleep. The interaction between predisposing, precipitating, and perpetuating factors in the genesis and progression of insomnia is depicted in **Fig. 1**.

Hyperarousal is also evident in a wide array of biologic functions as evidenced by an increase in high-frequency brain wave activity during sleep,[20] an increase in brain global glucose metabolic rates during wakefulness and sleep,[21] an increase in levels of cortisol and adrenocorticotropic hormone during sleep,[22] an increase in heart rate,[23] and an increase in whole-body metabolic rate.[24]

Genetic vulnerability may play a role in insomnia, as this condition is more likely in monozygotic twins than dizygotic twins.[25] Genetics may also play a role in certain conditions of insomnia, such as delayed sleep phase syndrome and advanced sleep phase syndrome, in which the circadian

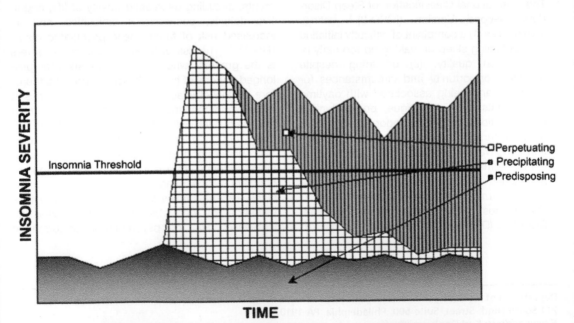

Fig. 1. Factors in the genesis and progression of insomnia (*Data from* Yang CM, Spielman AJ, Glovinsky P. Nonpharmacologic strategies in the management of insomnia. Psychiatr Clin North Am 2006;29(4):895–919.)

system is deranged. A mutation in a human clock gene (*Per2*) was shown to produce advanced sleep phase syndrome, and a functional polymorphism in *Per3* is associated with delayed sleep phase syndrome.[26]

DIFFERENTIAL DIAGNOSIS

When insomnia occurs without an identifiable underlying cause, it is often referred to as primary insomnia or insomnia syndrome.[4,27] Although primary insomnia is presumed to be an independent disorder, other medical, psychiatric, and sleep disorders can coexist with primary insomnia; yet they are presumed not to be causally related to the insomnia complaint. Primary insomnia is thought to have a prevalence of 2% to 4% of the adult population.[28]

Insomnia that is thought to be causally related to coexisting medical or psychiatric conditions has been traditionally referred to as secondary insomnia.[4,27] However, because the direction of causality and the nature of the association between insomnia and coexisting conditions are not always apparent, a recent National Institutes of Health State-of-the-Science Conference noted a preference for the term comorbid insomnia.[27] This category of insomnia represents most insomnias.

Insomnia can be related to maladaptive habits and behaviors.[29] These are listed in **Box 1**.

Almost any psychiatric and medical condition can be associated with insomnia.[14,30,31] Psychiatric disorders, notably depressive and anxiety disorders, are the most prevalent conditions associated with insomnia. Medical conditions, in particular cardiorespiratory conditions, such as mycordial infarction, congestive heart failure, and chronic obstructive pulmonary disease (COPD), are also commonly associated with insomnia.[32] **Table 1** lists selected comorbid insomnia disorders and their hallmark symptoms. Various medications can also cause the complaint of insomnia, including anticholinergics, antihypertensives, antineoplastics, central nervous system stimulants, hormones, antidepressants, antipsychotics, and withdrawal from sedating agents.[29]

SELECTED COMORBID INSOMNIAS
Mood Disorders

About 14% to 20% of insomniacs have major depression.[14] Therefore, one has to maintain a high index of suspicion for depression when encountering patients with insomnia. Conversely, most patients with major depression complain of insomnia, characterized by difficulty falling asleep,

---

Box 1
Habits and behaviors that aggravate insomnia

1. Habits and behaviors related to sleep and the sleep environment that aggravate insomnia

   - Caffeine and alcohol before bedtime
   - Nicotine (smoking and cessation)
   - Large meals or excessive fluid intake within 3 hours of bedtime
   - Exercising within 3 hours of bedtime
   - Using the bed for nonsleep activities (work, telephone, Internet)
   - Staying in bed while awake for extended periods of time
   - Activating behaviors up to the point of bedtime
   - Excessive worrying at bedtime
   - Clock-watching before sleep onset or during nocturnal awakenings
   - Exposure to bright light before bedtime or during awakenings
   - Keeping the bedroom too hot or too cold
   - Noise
   - Behaviors of a bed partner (eg, snoring, leg movements)

2. Daytime habits and behaviors that aggravate insomnia

   - Prolonged bedrest, inactivity, and excessive napping
   - Insufficient light exposure
   - Frequent travel and shift work

---

frequent nocturnal awakenings, early morning awakening, nonrestorative sleep, decreased total sleep, disturbing dreams, and daytime fatigue.[33] In bipolar depression, although insomnia is a common complaint, hypersomnia, or prolonged sleep times, is more frequently reported with daytime fatigue. During manic periods, however, patients usually report significantly reduced sleep times, often with a subjective sense of a decreased need for sleep.

The identification of depression in the context of insomnia is complicated by longitudinal studies indicating that insomnia is commonly seen far before the onset of the full-blown depressive syndrome. In fact, insomnia is more likely to emerge before the onset of the acute phase of a mood disorder than after.[34] Studies also indicate that unremitting insomnia confers an increased risk for the development of new psychiatric disorders, in particular major depression, over the course of the ensuing year, a risk that diminishes if the insomnia resolves.[14] Therefore, chronic insomnia should alert the clinician to the possibility of the future emergence of a mood disorder. In

Table 1
Hallmark symptoms of selected comorbid insomnia disorders

Disorder	Hallmark Symptoms
Psychophysiologic Insomnia	"Trying" to fall asleep Difficulty falling asleep at desired bedtime Frequent nocturnal awakenings Anxiety regarding sleeplessness
Restless Legs Syndrome	Irresistible urge to move the extremities Limb paresthesia Onset of symptoms during periods of rest and in the evening or at bedtime Relief of symptoms with movement
Periodic Limb Movement Disorder	Repetitive involuntary movements of the extremities during sleep or just before falling asleep
Obstructive Sleep Apnea Syndrome	Snoring Breathing pauses during sleep Choking Gasping Morning dry mouth
Chronic Obstructive Pulmonary Disease	Dyspnea
Gastroesophageal Reflux	Epigastric pain or burning Laryngospasm Acid taste in mouth Sudden nocturnal awakenings
Prostatic Hypertrophy	Frequent nocturia
Nocturnal Seizures	Thrashing in bed Loss of bladder or bowel control
Nocturnal Panic Attacks	Sudden surges of anxiety Tachycardia Diaphoresis Choking Laryngospasm
Posttraumatic Stress Disorder	Recurring, vivid dreams and nightmares Anxiety and hypervigilance in sleep environment
Delayed Sleep Phase Syndrome	Inability to fall asleep at desired time Inability to awaken at desired time
Advanced Sleep Phase Syndrome	Inability to stay awake until the desired bedtime Inability to remain asleep until the desired awakening time

Data from Doghramji K, Doghramji P. Clinical management of insomnia. 1st edition. West Islip (NY): Professional Communications, Inc; 2006.

addition, poor response to the treatment of insomnia should alert the clinician to the possibility of an underlying, disguised mood, substance use, or anxiety disorder that may warrant independent management.

The first step in the treatment of disturbed sleep in the context of mood disorders is the management of the underlying disorder. The short-term subjective effects of some of the more commonly used pharmacologic agents are listed in **Table 2**.[35] It should be noted that antidepressant medications are not approved by the US Food and Drug Administration (FDA) for the treatment of insomnia itself.

Effective pharmacologic treatment of the mood disorder does not always dissipate insomnia; in fact, less than 20% of full responders to antidepressant treatment are free of all major depressive disorder symptoms and nearly half the responders have persistent sleep disturbances.[36] In such cases, the addition of hypnotic medications and insomnia-specific cognitive behavioral therapy (CBT) may be helpful, as discussed in a later

Table 2
Primary sleep/wakefulness effects of pharmacologic agents used for the treatment of mood disorders

Medication	Sedation	Insomnia
Heterocyclic Antidepressant		
Amitriptyline	✔	
Imipramine	✔	
Doxepin	✔	
Nortriptyline	✔	
Clomipramine		✔
Desipramine		✔
Protriptyline		✔
Monoamine Oxidase Inhibitors		
Phenelzine		✔
Isocarboxazid		✔
Tranylcypromine		✔
Selective Serotonin Reuptake Inhibitors		
Fluoxetine		✔
Paroxetine	✔	
Sertraline		✔
Other Antidepressants		
Trazodone	✔	
Nefazodone	✔	
Bupropion		✔
Venlafaxine		✔
Mirtazapine	✔	

section. CBTs are also effective for the management of insomnia that occurs in the context of mood disorders.

Anxiety Disorders

Anxiety disorders represent the most frequently encountered psychiatric disorders in individuals with insomnia.[8] The anxiety disorders that are typically associated with insomnia include generalized anxiety disorder (GAD) and posttraumatic stress disorder (PTSD). All phases of sleep are affected, leading to the complaint of difficulties with sleep initiation and maintenance. In PTSD, insomnia is associated with distressing dreams and nightmares, reflections of the reexperiencing of the traumatic event. In panic disorder, insomnia can take the form of sudden awakenings from sleep, with episodes of sleep panic, during which somatic symptoms such as tachycardia and shortness of breath are typical.[37] Insomnia in panic disorder can, therefore, mimic the sudden awakenings of sleep-related breathing disorders and gastroesophageal reflux.

Nonpharmacologic treatments for GAD, such as CBT and relaxation training, can also ameliorate insomnia.[38] In PTSD, for example, imagery rehearsal for the nightmares can diminish nightmares and insomnia.[39] Pharmacologic treatments for insomnia and the underlying anxiety disorder include the benzodiazepine receptor agonists (γ-aminobutyric acid type A [$GABA_A$] receptor agonists), although individual agents may not have a US FDA–approved indication for both conditions. Antidepressants can also ameliorate insomnia in various anxiety disorders as discussed earlier, and if insomnia persists after the management of the underlying anxiety disorder, the addition of hypnotic agents can be helpful.

COPD

Sleep disturbances are the third most commonly reported symptoms, after dyspnea and fatigue, in COPD,[40] and 53% of patients with chronic bronchitis complain of insomnia compared with 36% of subjects without any respiratory disease.[41] Patients with COPD complain of difficulty falling asleep and maintaining sleep. Insomnia can be a result of disease-specific factors,[42] such as

1. Excessive mucus production and cough and the increased work of breathing associated with airflow limitation. These are likely to be exacerbated by the supine position and lead to inspiratory resistance and enhanced ventilatory effort, which in turn increases the frequency of arousals during sleep in normal subjects and is likely to contribute to arousals in patients with COPD
2. Nocturnal dyspnea, also enhanced by the supine position
3. Oxyhemoglobin desaturation during sleep, which is exaggerated during rapid eye movement sleep when postural muscle tone is normally at its lowest point during sleep. The response to hypoxemia or hypercapnia is an increase in ventilation and respiratory effort, which in turn leads to sleep-related arousals.

Secondary causes may also be involved, such as depression and anxiety, which are commonly comorbid with COPD, as well as medications used to treat COPD.

EVALUATION

The primary goal of the evaluation process is to identify comorbid disorders, which in turn can be managed directly. A systematic and comprehensive evaluation is essential.[43,44]

History

Nocturnal and daytime habits and behaviors that can disrupt sleep should be systematically asked for (see **Box 1**). Other aspects of the history are outlined in **Box 2**.

The hallmark symptoms of the various disorders described earlier should be asked for (see **Table 1**). Interviewing a bed partner can be useful in obtaining information regarding snoring, breathing pauses during sleep, limb movements, and the extent and frequency of naps. The history should also include the past medical history, history of medications and substances, social and occupational history for areas that can contribute to irregular sleep/wake habits, and family history, because certain sleep disorders, such as restless legs syndrome and obstructive sleep apnea syndrome (OSAS) and possibly primary insomnia, can have a familial basis.

Physical Examination

A physical examination can yield essential information; for example, a neck circumference of 16 in or greater in women and 17 in or greater in men are associated with an increased risk for sleep-related breathing disorders.

Tests and Inventories

The Insomnia Severity Index is a useful scale for quantifying the severity of insomnia at baseline and after treatment (**Fig. 2**).[45] Sleep logs are useful in defining the nature of the insomnia complaint and following insomnia patterns over time (**Fig. 3**). Their use is essential in all cases of chronic insomnia because insomniacs' recollection of their sleep is obfuscated by their tendency to report only the most problematic nights of sleep. The Fatigue Severity Scale[46] and the Epworth Sleepiness Scale (reproduced elsewhere in this issue)[47] are useful in quantifying daytime consequences. General serum laboratory tests including thyroid function studies can be considered if not current. Polysomnography or a referral to a sleep medicine specialist should be considered if the evaluation raises the suspicion of OSAS or periodic limb movement disorder, if the patient reports violent or potentially injurious nocturnal behaviors, for the evaluation of paroxysmal awakenings or other disturbances in sleep that are thought to be seizure related, if the office-based evaluation is not fruitful, or if the patient does not respond appropriately to treatment of the presumed disorder.

MANAGEMENT

Clinical wisdom suggests that management should optimally be directed toward comorbid conditions, with the anticipation that this strategy will also mitigate insomnia. However, as described earlier, insomnia often persists despite effective management of comorbid conditions. Therefore, direct management of insomnia is often necessary. Other clinical situations may even favor direct management of insomnia at the outset of treatment, as, for example, in the case of a patient in whom sleeplessness causes significant impairment in daytime function and jeopardizes safety and in the case of a patient who has developed an autonomous, self-perpetuating insomnia fueled by anxiety and apprehension regarding the prospect of further sleeplessness.

Nonpharmacologic Methods

Most insomniacs respond to nonpharmacologic methods.[48–51] When compared with pharmacologic methods, nonpharmacologic methods are at least as efficacious and have the advantage of longer duration of benefit. These methods are summarized in **Table 3**.

Box 2
Elements of the sleep/wake history in the evaluation of insomnia

1. Nature of the insomnia
   - Nocturnal pattern (initial, middle, terminal)
   - Duration (acute, long term)
   - Frequency (eg, nightly, weekly, monthly)
   - Precipitants (eg, illnesses, shiftwork, medications, substances)
   - Perpetuating factors (eg, learned/conditioned response, hyperarousal, sleep hygiene habits)

2. Daytime consequences
   - Fatigue
   - Irritability
   - Anergy
   - Memory impairment
   - Mental slowing

3. Patterns of sleep and wakefulness
   - Bedtime
   - Sleep latency (time to fall asleep after lights out)
   - Nocturnal awakenings; number and duration
   - Time of final morning awakening
   - Rising time (ie, time out of bed)
   - Number, time, and duration of daytime naps
   - Daytime symptoms including levels of sleepiness and fatigue over the course of the day

Insomnia Severity Index (ISI)

Subject ID: _____   Date: _____

For each question below, please circle the number corresponding most accurately to your sleep patterns in the **LAST MONTH.**

For the first three questions, please rate the **SEVERITY** of your sleep difficulties.

1. Difficulty falling asleep:

None	Mild	Moderate	Severe	Very Severe
0	1	2	3	4

2. Difficulty staying asleep:

None	Mild	Moderate	Severe	Very Severe
0	1	2	3	4

3. Problem waking up too early in the morning:

None	Mild	Moderate	Severe	Very Severe
0	1	2	3	4

4. How **SATISFIED**/dissatisfied are you with your current sleep pattern?

Very Satisfied	Satisfied	Neutral	Dissatisfied	Very Dissatisfied
0	1	2	3	4

5. To what extent do you consider your sleep problem to **INTERFERE** with your daily functioning (e.g., daytime fatigue, ability to function at work/daily chores, concentration, memory, mood).

Not at all Interfering	A Little Interfering	Somewhat Interfering	Much Interfering	Very Much Interfering
0	1	2	3	4

6. How **NOTICEABLE** to others do you think your sleeping problem is in terms of impairing the quality of your life?

Not at all Noticeable	A little Noticeable	Somewhat Noticeable	Much Noticeable	Very Much
0	1	2	3	4

7. How **WORRIED**/distressed are you about your current sleep problem?

Not at all	A Little	Somewhat	Much	Very Much
0	1	2	3	4

Guidelines for Scoring/Interpretation:

Add scores for all seven items = _____
Total score ranges from 0-28

0-7	= No clinically significant insomnia
8-14	= Subthreshold insomnia
15-21	= Clinical insomnia (moderate severity)
22-28	= Clinical insomnia (severe)

Fig. 2. The Insomnia Severity Index. (*Courtesy of* CM Morin, PhD, Quebec, Canada; with permission.)

Sleep hygiene education is not a stand-alone treatment for insomnia; however, it is regarded as an important foundation on which other therapies can be based. There is considerable variation in the nature of its various elements and how it is practiced. Some of the more commonly described elements are listed in **Box 3**.

Pharmacologic Agents

Hypnotic agents

Bromide, introduced in the mid-1800s, was the first agent specifically used as a sedative hypnotic.

Chloral hydrate, paraldehyde, urethan, and sulfonyl soon followed. Chloral hydrate, although still available and an effective hypnotic, is rarely used because of a wide array of adverse effects, including rapid development of tolerance, seizures and delirium following rapid discontinuation, physical and psychological dependence, and hepatic damage. The ratio of lethal to therapeutic dose is narrow, and overdose can result in severe respiratory depression and death. The barbiturates (eg, phenobarbital, secobarbital, butabarbital, amobarbital, and pentobarbital) were introduced in the early 1900s but are also rarely used as

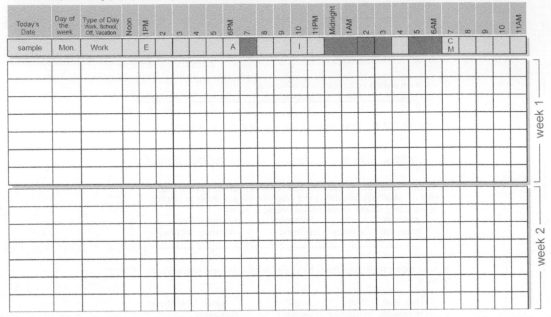

Fig. 3. Sleep log. (*From* http://AASMnet.org, copyright American Academy of Sleep Medicine; with permission.)

hypnotics because of concerns regarding residual sedation (hangover) and psychological dependence. Barbiturate overdose, especially when it involves alcohol, can be fatal.[52]

Agents commonly used for insomnia are listed in **Table 4**. Zolpidem has recently been developed as a sublingual dissolving tablet and as an oral spray. All are benzodiazepine receptor agonists (BzRAs), with the exception of ramelteon, which is a melatonin receptor agonist. The BzRAs bind to the benzodiazepine recognition site of the GABA$_A$ receptor complex and augment the effects of GABA. GABA$_A$ receptors are widely distributed in the central nervous system (CNS), including in the cortex, basal ganglia, and cerebellum. Consequently, these mediate a wide variety of clinical effects, including anxiety, cognition, vigilance, memory, and learning. GABA is also the major neurotransmitter of neurons in brain structures that are believed to be involved in the generation of sleep, such as the ventrolateral preoptic nucleus of the hypothalamus.[53] Ramelteon is a melatonin receptor agonist and acts at the MT1 and MT2 receptors, which are located in the suprachiasmatic nucleus.[54] This structure is also believed to

be important in the control of sleep and wakefulness.[55]

All hypnotics can diminish sleep latency, the time needed to fall asleep after retiring. However, they differ in the extent to which they are effective for sleep maintenance difficulties. In general, the longer half-life hypnotics are better suited for insomniacs who awaken in the middle of the night or early in the morning and have difficulty in getting back to sleep. When considering the nonbenzodiazepine hypnotics, zolpidem ER and eszopiclone have been shown to diminish wake after sleep onset, or the time dedicated to awakening after falling asleep, a measure of sleep continuity. On the other hand, the ability to decrease wake after sleep onset has not been demonstrated for zaleplon and zolpidem.[56]

The main adverse effects of the BzRAs are daytime sedation and psychomotor and cognitive impairment, the likelihood of which is greater with the longer half-life hypnotics and in the case of hypnotics with active metabolites. Therefore, the clinical challenge in using this class of compounds is the identification of a particular medication along the half-life continuum that produces maximum

Table 3
Nonpharmacologic therapies of insomnia

Technique	Goal	Method
Stimulus Control Therapy[a]	Strengthen bed and bedroom as sleep stimuli	If unable to fall asleep within 20 min, get out of bed and repeat as necessary
Relaxation Therapies[a]	Reduce arousal and decrease anxiety	Biofeedback, progressive muscle relaxation
Restriction of Time in Bed (Sleep Restriction)	Improve sleep continuity by limiting time spent in bed	Decrease time in bed to equal time actually asleep and increase as sleep efficiency improves
Cognitive Therapy	Dispel faulty beliefs that may perpetuate insomnia	Talk therapy to dispel unrealistic and exaggerated notions about sleep
Paradoxic Intention	Relieve performance anxiety	Try to stay awake
Sleep Hygiene Education	Promote habits that help sleep; eliminate habits that interfere with sleep	Promote habits that help sleep; eliminate habits that interfere with sleep
Cognitive Behavioral Therapy[a]	Combines sleep restriction, stimulus control, and sleep hygiene education with cognitive therapy	Combines sleep restriction, stimulus control, and sleep hygiene education with cognitive therapy

[a] Standard therapy (high clinical certainty).
   Data from Morgenthaler T, Kramer M, Alessi C, et al. Practice parameters for the psychological and behavioral treatment of insomnia: an update. An American Academy of Sleep Medicine report. Sleep 2006;29(11):1415–19.

efficacy across the night and minimum daytime residual effects. BzRA hypnotics should be used with caution in individuals with respiratory depression (eg, COPD and OSAS), in the elderly, in those with hepatic disease, in those with multiple medical conditions, and in those who are taking other medications that have CNS-depressant properties. Individuals who must awaken during the course of the drug's active period should not take these medications. All of the BzRAs are Drug Enforcement Administration (DEA) Schedule IV agents and carry a risk of abuse liability.

The most common adverse effects that are associated with ramelteon include somnolence, fatigue, and dizziness. It is not recommended for use with fluvoxamine because of a cytochrome P-450 1A2 interaction. A mild elevation in prolactin levels has been noted in a small number of women, and a mild decrease in testosterone values has been noted in elderly men; yet the clinical relevance of these changes remains unclear. Ramelteon does not demonstrate respiratory depression in mild-to-moderate OSAS or in mild-to-moderate COPD.

It is DEA nonscheduled and does not carry the risk of abuse liability.

Tolerance, a decrement in clinical efficacy following repeated use, and rebound insomnia, which is an escalation of insomnia beyond baseline severity levels following abrupt discontinuation, can occur even after a few weeks of administration and seems to be more pronounced after the administration of higher doses of hypnotics and after administration of the older benzodiazepine agents that have a short elimination half-life, such as triazolam, than after administration of the longer-elimination half-life benzodiazepines and some of the newer nonbenzodiazpine BzRAs.[57] Eszopiclone,[58] zolpidem ER,[59] and ramelteon[60] have been evaluated for up to 6 months in controlled studies and have demonstrated a low proclivity for the production of these effects. Nevertheless, clinical wisdom suggests that all hypnotics should be used for short periods of time as much as possible. Patients using these medications for longer periods of time should be evaluated periodically for tolerance and carefully monitored for withdrawal symptoms after abrupt discontinuation. The risk of rebound insomnia and withdrawal symptoms can be minimized by using the lowest effective dose and by gradually tapering the dose over the course of a few nights.

Hypnotics carry the potential for severe allergic reactions and complex sleep-related behaviors, which may include sleep driving. The latter may be associated with concomitant ingestion of alcohol and other sedating substances.[61] It may be useful, therefore, to advise patients to limit the use of such substances whenever possible.

Other prescription agents

These agents are used as hypnotics but are not indicated for this use by the FDA. Factors favoring their use include low abuse liability, availability of wide dose ranges, and, in some cases, low cost. These agents are used at doses that are subtherapeutic for the disorders for which they are intended, and there are limited data on their safety and efficacy in insomnia. They include the sedating antidepressants, most commonly trazodone, doxepin, and mirtazapine.[62] Trazodone, when used at low doses for insomnia, has been associated with rapid development of tolerance. Antidepressant use is also complicated by daytime sedation and cognitive impairment, anticholinergic effects, weight gain, and drug-drug interactions. The tricyclic antidepressants are also potentially fatal in an overdose.

Table 4
Hypnotic agents

Generic (Trade) Name	Dose Range[a] (mg)	Onset of Action	Half-Life (h)	Active Metabolites
Benzodiazpine receptor agonists				
Benzodiazpine agents				
Estazolam (ProSom)	1–2	Rapid	10–24	No
Flurazepam (Dalmane)	15–30	Rapid	47–100	Yes
Quazepam (Doral)	7.5–15	Rapid	39–73	Yes
Temazepam (Restoril)	7.5–30	Slow	3.5–18.4	No
Triazolam (Halcion)	0.125–0.25	Rapid	1.5–5.5	No
Nonbenzodiazpine agents				
Zolpidem (Ambien)	5–10	Rapid	2.5–2.6	No
Zolpidem ER (Ambien CR)	6.25–12.5	Rapid	2.8[b]	No
Zaleplon (Sonata)	5–20	Rapid	1	No
Eszopiclone (Lunesta)	1–3	Rapid	6	No
Melatonin receptor agonist				
Ramelteon (Rozerem)	8	Rapid	1–5	No

[a] Normal adult dose. Dose may require individualization.
[b] Modified formulation increases duration of action.

REFERENCES

1. Mahowald MW, Kader G, Schenck CH. Clinical categories of sleep disorders I. Continuum 1997; 3(4):35–65.
2. Mellinger GD, Balter MB, Uhlenhuth EH. Insomnia and its treatment. Prevalence and correlates. Arch Gen Psychiatry 1985;42(3):225–32.
3. International classification of sleep disorders. 2nd edition. Westchester (IL): American Academy of Sleep Medicine; 2005.
4. Diagnostic and statistical manual of mental disorders. Text Revision. 4th edition. Arlington (VA): American Psychiatric Association; 2000.
5. International statistical classification of diseases and related health problems. 10th revision edition. Geneva (Switzerland): World Health Organization; 1992.
6. Sutton DA, Moldofsky H, Badley EM. Insomnia and health problems in Canadians. Sleep 2001;24(6): 665–70.
7. Ohayon MM, Zulley J, Guilleminault C, et al. How age and daytime activities are related to insomnia in the general population: consequences for older people. J Am Geriatr Soc 2001;49(4):360–6.
8. Ohayon MM, Lemoine P, Arnaud-Briant V, et al. Prevalence and consequences of sleep disorders in a shift worker population. J Psychosom Res 2002; 53(1):577–83.
9. Li RH, Wing YK, Ho SC, et al. Gender differences in insomnia–a study in the Hong Kong Chinese population. J Psychosom Res 2002;53(1):601–9.
10. Kageyama T, Kabuto M, Nitta H, et al. A population study on risk factors for insomnia among adult Japanese women: a possible effect of road traffic volume. Sleep 1997;20(11):963–71.
11. Chevalier H, Los F, Boichut D, et al. Evaluation of severe insomnia in the general population: results of a European multinational survey. J Psychopharmacol 1999;13(4 Suppl 1):S21–4.
12. Leger D, Scheuermaier K, Philip P, et al. SF-36: evaluation of quality of life in severe and mild insomniacs compared with good sleepers. Psychosom Med 2001;63(1):49–55.
13. Weissman MM, Greenwald S, Nino-Murcia G, et al. The morbidity of insomnia uncomplicated by psychiatric disorders. Gen Hosp Psychiatry 1997;19(4): 245–50.
14. Ford DE, Kamerow DB. Epidemiologic study of sleep disturbances and psychiatric disorders. An opportunity for prevention? JAMA 1989;262(11): 1479–84.
15. Kripke DF, Garfinkel L, Wingard DL, et al. Mortality associated with sleep duration and insomnia. Arch Gen Psychiatry 2002;59(2):131–6.
16. Dew MA, Hoch CC, Buysse DJ, et al. Healthy older adults' sleep predicts all-cause mortality at 4 to 19 years of follow-up. Psychosom Med 2003;65(1): 63–73.
17. Espie CA, Inglis SJ, Harvey L, et al. Insomniacs' attributions. psychometric properties of the dysfunctional beliefs and attitudes about sleep scale and the sleep disturbance questionnaire. J Psychosom Res 2000;48(2):141–8.
18. Edinger JD, Means MK, Carney CE, et al. Psychomotor performance deficits and their relation to prior nights' sleep among individuals with primary insomnia. Sleep 2008;31(5):599–607.
19. Kales JD, Kales A, Bixler EO, et al. Biopsychobehavioral correlates of insomnia, V: clinical characteristics and behavioral correlates. Am J Psychiatry 1984;141(11):1371–6.
20. Merica H, Blois R, Gaillard JM. Spectral characteristics of sleep EEG in chronic insomnia. Eur J Neurosci 1998;10(5):1826–34.
21. Nofzinger EA, Buysse DJ, Germain A, et al. Functional neuroimaging evidence for hyperarousal in insomnia. Am J Psychiatry 2004;161(11):2126–8.
22. Vgontzas AN, Bixler EO, Lin HM, et al. Chronic insomnia is associated with nyctohemeral activation of the hypothalamic-pituitary-adrenal axis: clinical implications. J Clin Endocrinol Metab 2001;86(8): 3787–94.
23. Bonnet MH, Arand DL. Heart rate variability in insomniacs and matched normal sleepers. Psychosom Med 1998;60(5):610–5.
24. Bonnet MH, Arand DL. Physiological activation in patients with sleep state misperception. Psychosom Med 1997;59(5):533–40.
25. Watson NF, Goldberg J, Arguelles L, et al. Genetic and environmental influences on insomnia, daytime sleepiness, and obesity in twins. Sleep 2006;29(5): 645–9.
26. Hamet P, Tremblay J. Genetics of the sleep-wake cycle and its disorders. Metabolism 2006;55(10 Suppl 2):S7–12.
27. National Institutes of Health. National Institutes of Health State of the Science Conference Statement on Manifestations and Management of Chronic Insomnia in Adults, June 13–15, 2005. Sleep 2005; 28(9):1049–57.
28. Ohayon MM. Epidemiology of insomnia: what we know and what we still need to learn. Sleep Med Rev 2002;6(2):97–111.
29. Doghramji K, Choufani D. Taking a sleep history. In: Winkelman J, Plante D, editors. Foundations of psychiatric sleep medicine. Cambridge (MA): Cambridge University Press, in press.
30. Buysse DJ, Reynolds CF 3rd, Kupfer DJ, et al. Clinical diagnoses in 216 insomnia patients using the International Classification of Sleep Disorders (ICSD), DSM-IV and ICD-10 categories: a report from the APA/NIMH DSM-IV field trial. Sleep 1994; 17(7):630–7.

31. Ohayon MM, Caulet M, Lemoine P. Comorbidity of mental and insomnia disorders in the general population. Compr Psychiatry 1998;39(4):185–97.

32. Katz DA, McHorney CA. Clinical correlates of insomnia in patients with chronic illness. Arch Intern Med 1998;158(10):1099–107.

33. Reynolds CF 3rd, Kupfer DJ. Sleep research in affective illness: state of the art circa 1987. Sleep 1987;10(3):199–215.

34. Ohayon MM, Roth T. Place of chronic insomnia in the course of depressive and anxiety disorders. J Psychiatr Res 2003;37(1):9–15.

35. Benca RM. Mood disorders. In: Kryger MH, Roth T, Dement WC, editors. Principles and practice of sleep medicine. 4th edition. Elsevier Inc; 2009. p. 1311–26. Available at: www.sleepmedtext.com. Accessed March 1, 2010.

36. Nierenberg AA, Keefe BR, Leslie VC, et al. Residual symptoms in depressed patients who respond acutely to fluoxetine. J Clin Psychiatry 1999;60(4): 221–5.

37. Shapiro CM, Sloan EP. Nocturnal panic–an underrecognized entity. J Psychosom Res 1998;44(1): 21–3.

38. Belanger L, Morin CM, Langlois F, et al. Insomnia and generalized anxiety disorder: effects of cognitive behavior therapy for gad on insomnia symptoms. J Anxiety Disord 2004;18(4):561–71.

39. Krakow B, Hollifield M, Johnston L, et al. Imagery rehearsal therapy for chronic nightmares in sexual assault survivors with posttraumatic stress disorder: a randomized controlled trial. JAMA 2001;286(5): 537–45.

40. Kinsman RA, Yaroush RA, Fernandez E, et al. Symptoms and experiences in chronic bronchitis and emphysema. Chest 1983;83(5):755–61.

41. Klink M, Quan SF. Prevalence of reported sleep disturbances in a general adult population and their relationship to obstructive airways diseases. Chest 1987;91(4):540–6.

42. George CF, Bayliff CD. Management of insomnia in patients with chronic obstructive pulmonary disease. Drugs 2003;63(4):379–87.

43. Sateia MJ, Doghramji K, Hauri PJ, et al. Evaluation of chronic insomnia. An American Academy of Sleep Medicine review. Sleep 2000;23(2):243–308.

44. Schutte-Rodin S, Broch L, Buysse D, et al. Clinical guideline for the evaluation and management of chronic insomnia in adults. J Clin Sleep Med 2008; 4(5):487–504.

45. Bastien CH, Vallieres A, Morin CM. Validation of the insomnia severity index as an outcome measure for insomnia research. Sleep Med 2001; 2(4):297–307.

46. Krupp LB, LaRocca NG, Muir-Nash J, et al. The fatigue severity scale. Application to patients with multiple sclerosis and systemic lupus erythematosus. Arch Neurol 1989;46(10):1121–3.

47. Johns MW. A new method for measuring daytime sleepiness: the Epworth Sleepiness Scale. Sleep 1991;14(6):540–5.

48. Morin CM, Bootzin RR, Buysse DJ, et al. Psychological and behavioral treatment of insomnia: update of the recent evidence (1998–2004). Sleep 2006; 29(11):1398–414.

49. Morin CM, Hauri PJ, Espie CA, et al. Nonpharmacologic treatment of chronic insomnia. An American Academy of Sleep Medicine review. Sleep 1999; 22(8):1134–56.

50. Chesson AL Jr, Anderson WM, Littner M, et al. Practice parameters for the nonpharmacologic treatment of chronic insomnia. An American Academy of Sleep Medicine report. Standards of practice committee of the American Academy of Sleep Medicine. Sleep 1999;22(8):1128–33.

51. Morgenthaler T, Kramer M, Alessi C, et al. Practice parameters for the psychological and behavioral treatment of insomnia: an update. An American Academy of Sleep Medicine report. Sleep 2006; 29(11):1415–9.

52. Laurence LB. Goodman & Gilman's the pharmacological basis of therapeutics. 11th edition. New York: The McGraw-Hill Companies; 2006.

53. Sieghart W, Sperk G. Subunit composition, distribution and function of GABA(A) receptor subtypes. Curr Top Med Chem 2002;2(8):795–816.

54. Roth T, Stubbs C, Walsh JK. Ramelteon (TAK-375), a selective MT1/MT2-receptor agonist, reduces latency to persistent sleep in a model of transient insomnia related to a novel sleep environment. Sleep 2005;28(3):303–7.

55. Dubocovich ML, Rivera-Bermudez MA, Gerdin MJ, et al. Molecular pharmacology, regulation and function of mammalian melatonin receptors. Front Biosci 2003;8:d1093–108.

56. PDR.net. Available at: http://www.pdr.net/login/Login.aspx. Accessed February 26, 2010.

57. Soldatos CR, Dikeos DG, Whitehead A. Tolerance and rebound insomnia with rapidly eliminated hypnotics: a meta-analysis of sleep laboratory studies. Int Clin Psychopharmacol 1999;14(5): 287–303.

58. Krystal AD, Walsh JK, Laska E, et al. Sustained efficacy of eszopiclone over 6 months of nightly treatment: results of a randomized, double-blind, placebo-controlled study in adults with chronic insomnia. Sleep 2003;26(7):793–9.

59. Krystal AD, Erman M, ZOLONG Study Group, et al. Long-term efficacy and safety of zolpidem extended-release 12.5 mg, administered 3 to 7 nights per week for 24 weeks, in patients with chronic primary insomnia: a 6-month, randomized,

double-blind, placebo-controlled, parallel-group, multicenter study. Sleep 2008;31(1):79–90.

60. Mayer G, Wang-Weigand S, Roth-Schechter B, et al. Efficacy and safety of 6-month nightly ramelteon administration in adults with chronic primary insomnia. Sleep 2009;32(3):351–60.

61. Southworth MR, Kortepeter C, Hughes A. Nonbenzodiazepine hypnotic use and cases of "sleep driving". Ann Intern Med 2008;148(6):486–7.

62. James SP, Mendelson WB. The use of trazodone as a hypnotic: a critical review. J Clin Psychiatry 2004; 65(6):752–5.

Excessive Sleepiness

Sheila C. Tsai, MD

KEYWORDS

- Excessive sleepiness • Sleep deprivation
- Sleep management • Sleepiness assessment

Excessive sleepiness, or hypersomnia, is characterized by difficulty maintaining alertness during waking hours. Though brief periods of sleepiness can be normal, it is problematic when it interferes with daily activities and quality of life, manifests as inappropriate periods of drowsiness, or is chronic. Most people have experienced sleepiness at some point in their lives, and about two-thirds of Americans report experiencing sleep problems at least a few nights a week within the past month.[1] However, for millions of people, chronic sleepiness is a notable problem. Studies in developed countries have estimated the prevalence of daily or almost daily sleepiness at about 5% to 9% of the population.[2,3] When defined by at least 3 days of symptoms, about 20% of the population experiences chronic symptoms of sleepiness.[4] The prevalence of sleepiness is increasing and is likely exacerbated by an increase in work hours, work stress, family duties, and an increase in access to activities and entertainment that can extend waking periods and consequently decrease sleep time. The associated rise in sleepiness spans all age groups from children to elderly people. In the 2004 National Sleep Foundation (NSF) poll on Sleep in America, children who had a television or computer in their room slept less than those without such electronic devices.[5] Adolescents, as a group, also do not obtain enough sleep and notice the consequences as a result. In a 1998 study by Carskadon and colleagues,[6] earlier school start times led to less sleep rather than to a shift to an earlier bedtime. In another study, when adolescents were evaluated longitudinally, 54% to 74% of adolescents wished for more sleep while only 3% felt that they obtained enough sleep.[7] Likewise, adults do no obtain enough sleep each night; in the NSF's most recent poll on sleep,[1] 20% of American adults 18 year of age or older reported that they got an average of less than 6 hours of sleep. This percentage has increased significantly compared with 2001 when 13% reported getting less than 6 hours of sleep.[1]

PUBLIC HEALTH IMPLICATIONS

Not only does sleepiness limit the feeling of restfulness, there are other health consequences to the sleepy individual. When industrial workers were evaluated, daytime sleepiness was noted to have significant effects on worker's well-being with an increased rate of work accidents, decreased job satisfaction, increased amounts of drug usage, and more hospitalizations.[2] In evaluating sleep duration alone, shorter sleep time is associated with an increase in both systolic and diastolic blood pressure levels over a 5-year period, with an increased risk for developing hypertension.[8] Conversely, getting an adequate amount of sleep is associated with a lower incidence of coronary calcifications.[9] Sleepiness is also associated with metabolic effects, and decreased insulin sensitivity was noted when sleep was fragmented in healthy volunteers.[10] In addition, research suggests that chronic partial sleep loss may increase the risk of obesity and diabetes. Proposed mechanisms include effects on glucose regulation, insulin resistance, and alterations in appetite control via the neuroendocrine system.[11] More importantly, associations have been demonstrated between sleep length (too little and too much sleep) and mortality.[12] Finally, sleepiness is known to affect mood with an increase in sleepiness correlated with worsened mood. When sleep was restricted in healthy males from an average of 7.4 hours to 5 hours, sleepiness was noted along with increased complaints of anxiety, mood disturbances, and fatigue.[13]

Department of Internal Medicine, Division of Sleep Medicine, National Jewish Health, University of Colorado, Denver School of Medicine, 1400 Jackson Street, Denver, CO 80206, USA
E-mail address: tsais@njhealth.org

Clin Chest Med 31 (2010) 341–351
doi:10.1016/j.ccm.2010.02.007
0272-5231/10/$ – see front matter © 2010 Published by Elsevier Inc.

Sleepiness has major public health implications. Notable industrial accidents such as the Three-Mile Island nuclear meltdown and the Space Shuttle Challenger accident have been attributed to errors resulting from sleepiness or shift work.[14] Sleepiness in the transportation industry also poses a dangerous environment for the public. Sleepiness impairs reaction time and increases the propensity to fall asleep while driving. There is an increased risk of occupational accidents in men who both snore and report sleepiness.[15] In a study of bus drivers in a major city, 20% of drivers noted sleepiness, 8% reported falling asleep while driving at least once a month, 7% reported having an accident due to sleepiness during work, and 18% reported near-miss accidents at work due to sleepiness.[16] These results led the investigators to conclude that "professional drivers are at high risk of sleepiness due to a combination of factors including shift work and obstructive sleep apnea/hypopnea syndrome, and sleepiness in professional drivers is highly dangerous."[16]

Drowsy driving is not isolated to professional drivers. Approximately, 100,000 police-reported crashes, 71,000 injuries, and 1550 deaths occur yearly in the United States as a result of driver sleepiness.[17] In the 2009 NSF poll, a majority of adults (54%) surveyed reported drowsy driving at least once in the past year, and 28% reported driving while drowsy at least once a month.[1] The periods of greatest sleepiness during a 24-hour period correlate with the highest rates of motor vehicle accidents. Thus, there is an increase in single vehicle accidents between 1 and 4 AM and 1 and 4 PM.[14] More immeasurable are near-miss accidents due to sleepiness.

PATIENT SAFETY IMPLICATIONS

The implications of sleepiness on patient care and safety has been evaluated. In 1999, the Institute of Medicine published a document entitled "To Err is Human" estimating that about 98,000 in-hospital deaths yearly were related to medical errors and suggested that an important contributor to these errors was sleepiness among health care workers.[18] In a survey of medical residents, those who got 5 or fewer hours of sleep each night "were more likely to report serious accidents or injuries, conflict with other professional staff, use of alcohol, use of medications to stay awake, noticeable weight change, working in an 'impaired condition,' and having made significant medical errors."[19] As with other motorists, sleepiness affects the driving safety of medical trainees. In a survey of pediatric house staff, about half of

the respondents had fallen asleep at the wheel post-call.[20] As a result of increased concerns for patient and medical resident safety resulting from prolonged work hours and sleep restriction, the Accreditation Council on Graduate Medical Education (ACGME) recommended duty hour restrictions in 2003, which currently remain in place.[21] In addition the ACGME has mandated that programs educate their trainees on the importance of sleep and recognizing fatigue.

Despite the significant impact of sleepiness, only half of those individuals experiencing problems with sleepiness ever complain of these issues to their health care provider.[1] When they do discuss these complaints, about 40% are found to have a diagnosable sleep disorder.[2] Thus, the prevalence of sleep issues, including sleepiness, is likely significantly higher than estimated. Because of the implications of poor sleep and sleepiness, it is imperative for health care providers to recognize this common problem and evaluate their patients for sleep issues. It is also imperative that the public be educated on the serious effects of sleepiness and encouraged to address these issues. If chronic complaints exist, further investigation with a basic understanding of the various causes of sleepiness is necessary.

NORMAL SLEEP

Sleepiness is the most common complaint of patients presenting to sleep disorders centers. A general knowledge of what is defined as "normal sleep" is necessary to appropriately evaluate complaints of sleepiness. Sleep is recognized as an active process necessary for health and well-being. The specific role of sleep is debatable but it is generally felt to be restorative to the body, including the brain. Sleep is thought to be important in memory and learning, and rapid eye movement (REM) sleep may play an important role in learning and memory consolidation.[22,23]

Normal Circadian Rhythms

The body maintains circadian rhythms mainly through the suprachiasmatic nucleus of the hypothalamus. There is an increased propensity to sleep during normal sleep hours. In addition, normal peaks in sleepiness occur over a 24-hour period in a bimodal distribution. These peaks in sleepiness or dips in alertness occur in the early morning around 2 to 6 AM and less prominently in the midafternoon (around 2–6 PM).[24] These peaks have been correlated with unintentional sleep periods.[25] As mentioned above, these dips in alertness have been correlated with increased motor vehicle accidents.[14]

Sleep Duration

While significant individual and cultural variability exists, there are general norms for sleep duration. Newborns spend the majority of time sleeping. Sleep requirements gradually decrease until adulthood (**Fig. 1**). The average infant requires about 16 hours of sleep. This amount decreases to about 10 to 14 hours (or 13 hours on average) at 1 year of age, 12 hours at 2 years, 10 to 11 hours at 4 years, and 9 to 10 hours at 10 years of age. Adolescents require about 9 to 10 hours of sleep while adults average 7 to 8 hours.[26] Although normal in childhood, naps are not commonly needed by 5 to 6 years of age— though they continue to be a part of the culture in some societies.

CAUSES OF EXCESSIVE SLEEPINESS

Sleepiness is the most common complaint encountered in a sleep disorders center.[2] The differential diagnosis of sleepiness is quite broad. Sleepiness may occur because of disrupted sleep, circadian misalignment, or be attributed to a central cause.

Sleep Apnea Syndromes

Of the conditions causing sleepiness, the diagnosis of sleep apnea syndrome is the most frequently made and estimated to account for more than 40% of the diagnoses.[27] Repeated apneas and hypopneas cause sleep disruption and oxygen desaturations with daytime consequences.

Obstructive sleep apnea syndrome

Obstructive sleep apnea (OSA) is the most common sleep disordered breathing disorder. In OSA repeated apneas, hypopneas, or both disrupt

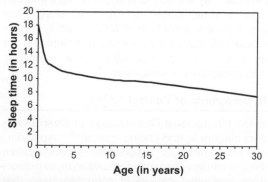

Fig. 1. Average sleep requirements decrease with age. The average adult needs 7 to 8 hours of sleep nightly. (*Data from* Aldrich MS. Ontogeny of Sleep. In: Aldrich MS, editor. Sleep medicine. New York: Oxford University; 1999. p. 70–81.)

sleep throughout the night. With an obstructive apnea, respiratory effort persists despite the cessation of airflow. In this syndrome, obstruction of the upper airway results in oxygen desaturation and arousal from sleep.[28] Witnessed pauses in breathing, or apneas, are common. Other presenting symptoms include loud snoring, awakening with a choking or gasping sensation, nonrestorative sleep, and excessive sleepiness. Risk factors for OSA include obesity, anatomic craniofacial abnormalities, and a positive family history. OSA contributes to other well-known complications including cardiovascular risk and is most closely correlated with systemic hypertension.[29] OSA is estimated to occur in about 2% of middle-aged women and 4% of middle-aged men based on previous estimates.[30] Prevalence is likely to increase due to the rising obesity rates across the country.

Central sleep apnea syndrome

In central sleep apnea syndromes, apneas are not associated with any respiratory effort. These apneas occur due to a high ventilatory response to carbon dioxide (CO_2) and are seen more commonly during wake-sleep transitions and non-REM sleep.[28] Frequent arousals may occur. Central sleep apnea is more commonly seen in patients with congestive heart failure due to a delay in circulation time and sensing of chemoreceptors, neurologic disorders, or ascent to high altitude. Cheyne-Stokes respiration, a form of central sleep apnea characterized by apneas or hypopneas alternating with hyperpneas in a crescendo-decrescendo pattern, has been shown to correlate with greater mortality in patients with systolic heart failure.[31] Central nervous system (CNS) depressants, such as narcotics, can also contribute to central sleep apnea as a result of depression of the hypercapnic ventilatory drive.

Sleep-related hypoventilation

Sleep-related nonobstructive hypoventilation is characterized by shallow breathing accompanied by an increase in CO_2 and a decrease in oxygenation. Hypoventilation may arise from an underlying medical condition, such as chronic lung disease or chest wall abnormalities, or may be idiopathic. CNS depressants can worsen hypoventilation. Frequent arousals and sleepiness are common complaints, as are headaches and nonrestorative sleep, which occur as a result of the elevated CO_2 levels and decreased oxygen levels during sleep.[28]

Circadian Rhythm Sleep Disorders

Sleepiness may result from a misalignment of an individual's intrinsic circadian rhythm with his or her environment. In circadian rhythm sleep disorders, patients may complain of insomnia or excessive sleepiness, both of which can affect various aspects of their lives.

Delayed sleep phase syndrome

In delayed sleep phase syndrome (DSPS) the sleep and wake times tend to be delayed at least 2 hours from normal societal bedtimes.[28] Patients with this disorder tend to have their peak in alertness in the evenings and are generally considered "night owls." People with this disorder may complain of insomnia and excessive sleepiness when asked to maintain conventional sleep-wake schedules. It may be influenced by social and environmental factors, and may have a familial component. This circadian rhythm disorder has an estimated prevalence of 0.15% in the general population; however, it is more prevalent in adolescents and may be seen in up to 7% to 16% of these individuals.[32]

Advanced sleep phase syndrome

In advanced sleep phase syndrome (ASPS), the circadian clock is advanced compared with conventional sleep-wake times. These individuals prefer to go to bed early and have early morning wakening. They tend to be most alert in the mornings. They may complain of the inability to stay awake for evening activities and difficulty staying asleep in the morning. This disorder is relatively uncommon. Unlike in DSPS, individuals with ASPS tend to be middle-aged or older, affecting about 1% of that population.[28]

Shift work sleep disorder

Shift workers, or those who work nonconventional hours, make up about 20% of the workforce.[32] Shift workers may experience circadian rhythm disorders resulting from their work schedules' affect on their sleep periods. Their work schedule occurs during typical sleep periods and consequently, they are expected to sleep during conventional awake periods during the day. Patients will complain of difficulty initiating sleep, difficulty maintaining sleep, or sleepiness. In addition to circadian misalignment with work hours, shift workers often have other personal obligations during their nonwork hours, which result in further sleep deprivation. When the American workforce was polled, shift workers got less sleep than non-shift workers. About one-third of shift workers reported sleeping less than 6 hours on a workday. Furthermore, shift workers were more likely to experience episodes of drowsy driving.[33] Shift workers also have an increased risk of traffic accidents when compared with workers with conventional work schedules.[34] The prevalence of shift work sleep disorder is estimated to be about 10% in night or rotating shift workers.[35]

Jet lag disorder

In jet lag disorder, a dyssynchrony exists between one's intrinsic circadian rhythm and the typical schedule of the new environment, which results from a rapid change in time zones. It is typically easier to travel in the westward direction, which allows the delay of sleep and wake times, than to travel in the eastward direction, which requires an advance in sleep and wake times.

Insomnia

Fatigue is generally a more common complaint than sleepiness in patients who have underlying insomnia. However, in a few patients, sleepiness results from the decrease in nocturnal sleep that is achieved due to the insomnia.

Sleep-related Movement Disorders

Sleep-related movement disorders may be associated with sleep-onset or sleep maintenance insomnia. They may cause sleep disruption and therefore sleepiness. The most commonly encountered sleep-related movement disorders are restless legs syndrome (RLS) and periodic limb movement disorder (PLMD). RLS is a clinical diagnosis based on a person's subjective complaints of an abnormal sensation in the legs. Patients may describe a "creepy-crawly" sensation and feel the need to move their legs. Occasionally it can involve the arms as well. Moving the legs tends to relieve the sensation. Although this discomfort may be noted at other times during sedentary periods, they are very prominent at night and can prevent sleep onset or return to sleep after a nocturnal arousal.[28] In PLMD, frequent, stereotypical limb movements are noted at night and are associated with a sleep disturbance, frequently with complaints of sleepiness.[28]

Hypersomnia of Central Origin

In the International Classification of Sleep Disorders diagnostic and coding manual,[28] "hypersomnias of central origin" are classified separately from sleep disordered breathing, circadian rhythm disorders, and other causes of disrupted sleep that contribute to hypersomnia. Diagnoses that fall into this category include behaviorally induced insufficient sleep syndrome, narcolepsy with and without cataplexy, recurrent hypersomnia, idiopathic hypersomnia, and medication-associated hypersomnia.

Insufficient sleep syndrome

Sleep deprivation resulting in insufficient sleep (behaviorally induced insufficient sleep syndrome) often results in sleepiness. This is the most common reason for sleepiness. As identified previously, the average amount of sleep that working Americans obtain on workdays is 6 hours 40 minutes, which is lower than the average 7 hours 18 minutes that Americans feel that they need to optimize alertness.[33] Patients do not intentionally deprive themselves of sleep and often do not recognize that their lack of sleep is contributing to symptoms.

Narcolepsy

Narcolepsy is estimated to occur in about 0.025% of the United States population, with slightly higher rates in Japan and lower rates in Israel.[36] Narcolepsy may present with or without cataplexy. About 20% to 50% of narcoleptics do not have cataplexy.[36] However, cataplexy is pathognomonic of narcolepsy. In cataplexy, periods of intense emotion or stress, such as anger or elation, will trigger a sudden loss of muscle tone or strength. Narcoleptics often complain of irresistible sleepiness that may be improved with a brief nap. Patients also frequently have disrupted sleep. Some may complain of sleep paralysis or hallucinations as they fall asleep or as they are awakening (hypnagogic or hypnopompic hallucinations, respectively).[37] Narcolepsy with cataplexy may be familial in some cases with a 1% to 2% risk for development of this disorder in first-degree relatives.[36] However, most cases are sporadic. The underlying pathology is felt to result from decreased hypocretin levels in the CNS.[36]

Recurrent hypersomnia

Recurrent hypersomnias are rare and are characterized by episodic hypersomnia. People may sleep up to 18 hours a day. Kleine-Levin syndrome is more common in males and is marked by abnormal behaviors during the episodes including hypersexuality, hyperphagia, aggressiveness and irritability, which are not present between episodes.[28] Menstrual-related hypersomnia also falls into this category. In general, the episodes in women with this disorder last about a week.[28]

Underlying medical condition

Patients may complain of sleepiness that results from a known underlying medical condition such as a stroke. However, some patients may have underlying medical conditions that are not yet diagnosed contributing to sleepiness, such as hypothyroidism. Mood disorders, such as depression contributing to early morning awakenings, can cause sleepiness, fatigue, or both. Other causes of hypersomnia include intracranial lesions, traumatic brain injury, and other neurologic diseases.[28]

Medication or substance use

Many commonly prescribed medications, such as certain antihypertensive medications, include sleepiness as a side effect (Table 1).[38] Nonprescription medications, such as antihistamines, and substances of abuse, such as cannabis, can also contribute to hypersomnia. Furthermore, when alerting medications or substances, such as methylphenidate or caffeine, are abruptly discontinued, sleepiness usually results.

Idiopathic hypersomnia

If no other primary sleep disorder and no other contributor to the sleepiness are determined, then the sleepiness may be classified as idiopathic. Idiopathic hypersomnia may be associated with or without long sleep episodes. In patients with long sleep, the sleep period typically is 12 to 14 hours in duration. Idiopathic hypersomnia is generally characterized by unrefreshing nap periods, undisrupted sleep periods, and postarousal confusion termed "sleep drunkenness."[28] This sleep disorder usually presents by young adulthood.

ASSESSMENT OF SLEEPINESS

It is important for clinicians to recognize complaints of sleepiness in their patients and to explore their sleep quality and quantity during an evaluation.

A Complete History and Thorough Physical Examination

The evaluation of sleepiness involves taking a thorough history and performing a good physical examination. As is true with the practice of medicine in general, much can be garnered from a thorough history. Questions regarding other medical problems, mood issues, duration of sleep issues, bedtime, wake time, sleep disruptors, snoring, apneas, work hours, and bedtime routine all assist in identifying problems (Fig 2). Specific questions may help pinpoint the cause: age of onset, witnessed apneas, restlessness during sleep, leg kicking, sleep paralysis, and cataplexy. In addition, consider the possibility that other medical conditions, prescription medications, or over-the-counter medications may be contributing to symptoms. Substance use should be explored as this

Table 1
Medications and substances commonly associated with sleepiness

Medications	Substances of Use/Abuse	Withdrawal of Substances
Alpha$_1$-adrenergic blockers	Alcohol	Amphetamine withdrawal
Alpha$_2$ agonists	Cannabis	Caffeine withdrawal
Anticholinergic medications	Narcotics	Cocaine withdrawal
Anti-epileptic medications		Abrupt discontinuation of modafinil
Anti-psychotics		Abrupt discontinuation of stimulants
Antihistamines		
Anxiolytics		
Beta-adrenergic blockers		
Benzodiazepines		
Dopaminergic agents		
Hypnotics		
Opiates or narcotics		
Selective serotonin reuptake inhibitors		
Tricyclic antidepressants		

Data from Schweitzer PK. Drugs that disturb sleep and wakefulness. In: Kryger MH, Roth T, Dement WD, editors. Principles and practice of sleep medicine. 4th edition. Philadelphia: Elsevier; 2005. p. 499–518.

can greatly influence symptoms. The effect of sleepiness on quality of life should be assessed (eg, traffic accidents, work, family). Family history can suggest diagnoses because many sleep disorders are considered to have at least some genetic propensity. The examination should include vitals signs, body mass index, measurement of neck circumference, an evaluation for oropharyngeal and nasopharyngeal abnormalities, a survey for facial abnormalities, a cardiac examination, pulmonary examination, an assessment for neurologic abnormalities, and psychiatric assessment.

Tools for Evaluating Sleepiness

Questionnaires
Questionnaires have been created in attempts to objectively quantify sleepiness. The Epworth Sleepiness Scale is a frequently used tool and assesses the propensity to fall asleep in various mundane activities that often occur during the week. The patient rates from zero to three their likelihood of falling asleep in eight situations; zero represents no possibility and three indicates a high probability of falling asleep. A score of 11 or greater out of a total of 24 is suggestive of sleepiness,[39] with a score of 16 or greater consistent with severe sleepiness. The Berlin Questionnaire screens for OSA with questions about the presence of snoring, obesity, and hypertension. A completed questionnaire that meets criteria for

the high-risk category has a positive predictive value of 0.89 for sleep OSA.[40]

Sleep logs or diaries
Sleep logs or diaries may assist in documenting sleep and provide a visual aid to the patient and physician. Patients record their bedtime, wake time, number of arousals, how long it took to return to sleep after any arousal, sleep aids used, and other subjective symptoms.

Actigraphy
Actigraphy may be helpful in providing more objective data regarding sleep episodes. Actigraphy is a device worn on the nondominant wrist that detects motion. Lack of motion is suggestive of sleep periods, whereas motion is consistent with wakefulness and movement. It can be particularly helpful in diagnosing circadian rhythm sleep disorders. Results may be less reliable in very sedentary patients or in those with limited physical activity.[41]

Pulse oximetry
Although nocturnal oximetry has been used as a screening tool for sleep-related breathing disorders, it has not been found to correlate well with the results of a polysomnography. Oximetry tends to over diagnose and under diagnose the presence of OSA.[42]

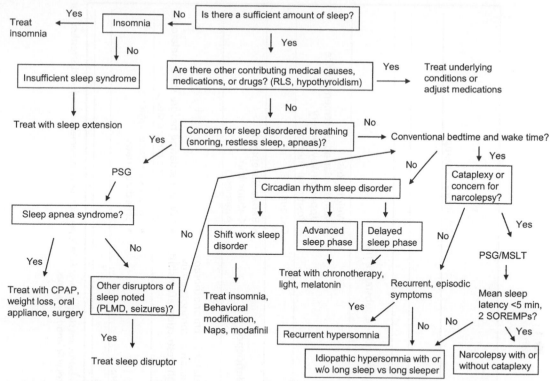

Fig. 2. An algorithm for the evaluation of excessive sleepiness. CPAP, continuous positive airway pressure; MSLT, multiple sleep latency test; PSG, polysomnography; SOREMP, sleep-onset REM period.

Polysomnography

After a general evaluation by a physician, a polysomnogram (PSG) is indicated for the evaluation of suspected sleep-related breathing disorders and PLMD.[43] It is not routinely needed to evaluate RLS or insomnia. An in-laboratory polysomnography provides data from various channels including electroencephalographic (EEG) monitoring to provide information on sleep staging, ECG, chin and leg electromyography (EMGs), respiratory effort monitoring, airflow channels, and pulse oximetry. OSA is diagnosed based on an apnea-hypopnea index of five or more events per hour in the presence of clinical symptoms or cardiovascular risks. In-laboratory polysomnography with a positive airway pressure titration study is indicated to determine effective treatment pressures and strategies for sleep apnea syndromes. Polysomnography is also routinely performed the night immediately preceding multiple sleep latency testing to confirm an adequate amount of sleep and to evaluate other causes of sleepiness.

Multiple sleep latency test

The multiple sleep latency test (MSLT) objectively assesses sleepiness by determining an individual's propensity to fall asleep. It is primarily indicated for the evaluation of narcolepsy and in suspected cases of idiopathic hypersomnia.[44] The MSLT consists of a series of four or five 20-minute nap periods, though generally five nap periods is more reliable. The test is performed following an overnight polysomnography with naps conducted 2 hours apart. The mean sleep latency is determined by averaging the time from lights out to sleep onset during each of the nap periods. Narcoleptic patients usually have a mean sleep latency of less than 8 minutes, which is consistent with pathologic sleepiness. A mean sleep latency of greater than 11 minutes over five nap periods is generally seen in normal controls.[44] In addition, each sleep-onset REM period (SOREMP), or the occurrence of REM sleep within 20 minutes of the start of the nap period, is also noted. The presence of two or more SOREMPs is highly suggestive of narcolepsy. The MSLT also assists in distinguishing idiopathic hypersomnia from narcolepsy without cataplexy. In idiopathic hypersomnia, mean sleep latency is less than 8 minutes but with less than two SOREMPs.[44] It is important to note the clinical context, however, because up to 30% of the general population may have a mean sleep latency of less than 8 minutes.[28]

Table 2
Common causes of sleepiness and their management

Cause of Sleepiness	Therapy	Additional Therapy
Insufficient sleep syndrome	• Sleep extension • Emphasize sleep hygiene	
Insomnia	Treat insomnia	
Hypersomnia due to a medical condition	Treat the underlying condition	
Hypersomnia due to medication or substance abuse	Change or discontinue medication; discontinue substance use	
OSA	Positive airway pressure therapy	• Weight loss • Mandibular advancement device • Upper airway surgery • Positional therapy
Central sleep apnea	• Positive airway pressure therapy • Treat underlying cause	Oxygen
RLS PLMD	• Dopamine agonists • Treat underlying cause (eg, iron deficiency)	• Benzodiazepines • Gabapentin • Analgesics
Circadian rhythm disorder • DSPS • ASPS • SWSD • Jet lag disorder	• DSPS: morning light, evening, melatonin, chronotherapy • ASPS: Evening light, morning melatonin, chronotherapy • SWSD: naps, light during shift, light restriction after shift • Melatonin	• SWSD: modafinil before shift; melatonin or hypnotic before sleep
Narcolepsy with and without cataplexy	• Cataplexy: TCAs, SSRIs • Sodium oxybate • Modafinil or stimulant medications	• Emphasize sleep hygiene • Scheduled naps
Idiopathic hypersomnia	Modafinil or stimulant medications	

Abbreviations: ASPS, advanced sleep phase syndrome; DSPS, delayed sleep phase syndrome; OSA, obstructive sleep apnea; PLMD, periodic limb movement disorder; RLS, restless legs syndrome; SSRIs, selective serotonin reuptake inhibitors; SWSD, shift work sleep disorder; TCAs, tricyclic antidepressants.

Maintenance of wakefulness test

Rather than assess the propensity to fall asleep, a maintenance of wakefulness test (MWT) provides information on an individual's ability to stay awake. The MWT is often performed on individuals in whom sleepiness would cause a significant public health risk, such as those in the transportation industry. It may also be used to assess response to therapy in patients with sleepiness.[44] The MWT protocol consist of four 40-minute trials conducted every 2 hours. A preceding night polysomnography is not required. The patient is seated in a dim, quiet room and asked to stay awake without doing any stimulating activity. A mean sleep latency of less than 8 minutes is considered abnormal. No recorded sleep in all four nap opportunities is the most reliable measure of an individual's ability to stay awake. A mean sleep latency value between 8 and 40 minutes is more difficult to assess and should be taken into clinical context.[44]

MANAGEMENT OF SLEEPINESS

Management of sleepiness is determined by the underlying contributing disorders (**Table 2**). A thorough evaluation for other underlying medical conditions such as thyroid abnormalities or medication use, such as antidepressants or pain medications, may suggest potential treatment options.

Positive airway pressure therapy is the mainstay of treatment for sleep apnea. However, other treatments may include positional therapy, weight management, mandibular advancement devices, or oral or upper airway surgery. Residual sleepiness despite adequate treatment of respiratory events and adequate sleep durations may require treatment with stimulants or wake-promoting agents. For hypoventilation syndromes or some forms of sleep apnea, oxygen or other modes of positive airway therapy (eg, bi-level positive airway pressure therapy or adaptive servo-ventilation) may be needed.

Extending sleep periods is recommended if sleepiness is related to sleep restriction or insufficient sleep. Sleep hygiene measures, referring to the practice of good sleep habits such as maintaining a set bedtime and wake time each day, may assist with sleep as well.

For circadian rhythm disorders, chronotherapy may be helpful in advanced and DSPS to realign the intrinsic clock with the external environment. Properly timed light therapy may also be considered. Morning light therapy helps advance the sleep-wake cycle in DSPS, whereas evening light helps in the management of advanced sleep phase syndrome. Properly timed administration

of exogenous melatonin also helps to advance or delay the sleep-wake schedule. For jet lag, appropriate use of melatonin and sleep aids may be beneficial. In shift-work sleep disorder, a well-lit work environment, and possibly scheduled napping may be helpful.

Therapy for narcolepsy is targeted at increasing alertness. Sodium oxybate is a sedative indicated in patients with narcolepsy; it seems to improve nocturnal sleep, which results in less daytime sleepiness.[45] Traditional stimulants and the non-amphetamine medication modafinil have also been used to manage sleepiness associated with narcolepsy. They appear to improve alertness as measured on the MWT and subjective sleepiness as determined by the Epworth Sleepiness Scale.[46] In those patients with cataplexy, tricyclic antidepressants and selective serotonin reuptake inhibitors can decrease the frequency of cataleptic episodes. Scheduled naps may be helpful in addition to medication therapy. For the idiopathic hypersomnias, amphetamine medications or modafinil are used to improve alertness.[46]

SUMMARY

Sleepiness presents a significant risk to the general population. It affects those who suffer from the disorder in terms of daily functioning, productivity, and mood. Sleepiness also contributes to systemic health effects and has been shown to contribute to mood disorders and cardiovascular risks. Conversely, optimizing sleep issues may improve secondary consequences such as improving blood pressure control or improving depression. Sleepiness not only affects the individual but it is also a danger to the public. As more information is obtained regarding the public health implications of sleepiness, such as major catastrophes, motor vehicle collisions, and patient safety, increasing efforts are being made to improve public safety. Safety regulations and work hour restrictions geared toward those in the transportation industry such as truck drivers and airline pilots have been instituted to decrease the dangers of sleepiness and improve public safety. Despite existing knowledge on the importance of good sleep and the hazards of sleepiness, more needs to be done. For instance, only 17 states currently require that issues related to drowsy driving be taught in driver's education.[17] Also, a survey of pediatric residents after the institution of ACGME work hour restrictions revealed that up to 56% continued to work shifts greater than 30 hours in duration and that average daily sleep duration, percentage of medication errors, and rates of motor vehicle crashes[47] were not significantly different than before the ACGME work hour restrictions. Thus, continued efforts at increasing awareness of the individual and public health implications of sleepiness are imperative to improving societal health and safety.

REFERENCES

1. National Sleep Foundation. Sleep in America poll: summary of findings. Available at: http://www. sleepfoundation.org/article/sleep-america-polls/2009-health-and-safety. 2009. Accessed August 18, 2009.
2. Lavie P. Sleep habits and sleep disturbances in industrial workers in Israel: main findings and some characteristics of workers complaining of excessive daytime sleepiness. Sleep 1981;4(2):147–58.
3. Ohayon MM. From wakefulness to excessive sleepiness: what we know and still need to know. Sleep Med Rev 2008;12(2):129–41.
4. Janson C, Gislason T, De Backer W, et al. Daytime sleepiness, snoring and gastro-oesophageal reflux amongst young adults in three European countries. J Intern Med 1995;237:277–85.
5. National Sleep Foundation. Final report. Sleep in America poll. Available at: http://www.sleepfoundation.org/article/sleep-america-polls/2004-children-and-sleep. 2004. Accessed August 18, 2009.
6. Carskadon MA, Wolfson AR, Acebo C, et al. Adolescent sleep patterns, circadian timing, and sleepiness at a transition to early school days. Sleep 1998;21(8):871–81.
7. Strauch I, Meier B. Sleep needs in adolescents: a longitudinal approach. Sleep 1988;11(4):378–86.
8. Knutson KL, Van Cauter E, Rathouz PJ, et al. Association between sleep and blood pressure in midlife: the CARDIA sleep study. Arch Intern Med 2009;169(11):1055–61.
9. King CR, Knutson KL, Rathouz PJ, et al. Short sleep duration and incident coronary artery calcification. JAMA 2008;300(24):2859–66.
10. Stamatakis K, Punjabi NM. Effects of sleep fragmentation on glucose metabolism in normal subjects. Chest 2010;137(1):95–101.
11. Knutson KL, Spiegel K, Penev P, et al. The metabolic consequences of sleep deprivation. Sleep Med Rev 2007;11(3):163–78.
12. Hublin C, Partinen M, Koskenvuo M, et al. Sleep and mortality: a population-based 22-year follow-up study. Sleep 2007;30:1245–53.
13. Dinges DF, Pack F, Williams K, et al. Cumulative sleepiness, mood disturbance, and psychomotor vigilance performance decrements during a week of sleep restricted to 4–5 hours per night. Sleep 1997;20(4):267–77.
14. Mitler MM, Carskadon MA, Czeisler CA, et al. Catastrophes, sleep and public policy: consensus report. Sleep 1988;11(1):100–9.
15. Lindberg E, Carter N, Gislason T, et al. Role of snoring and daytime sleepiness in occupational accidents. Am J Respir Crit Care Med 2001;164(1):2031–5.
16. Vennelle M, Engleman HM, Douglas NJ. Sleepiness and sleep-related accidents in commercial bus drivers. Sleep Breath 2010;14(1):39–42.
17. National Sleep Foundation. State of the states report on drowsy driving. Available at: http://drowsydriving.org/docs/2007%20State%20of%20the%20States%20Report.pdf. 2007. Accessed August 15, 2009.
18. Committee on Quality of Health Care in America, Institute of Medicine. Errors in healthcare: a leading cause of death and injury. In: Kohn L, Corrigan J, Donaldson M, editors. To err is human: building a safer health system. Washington, DC: National Academies Press; 2000. p. 26–48.
19. Baldwin DC Jr, Daugherty SR. Sleep deprivation and fatigue in residency training: results of a national survey of first- and second-year residents. Sleep 2004;27(2):217–23.
20. Marcus CL, Loughlin GM. Effect of sleep deprivation on driving safety in housestaff. Sleep 1996;19(10):763–6.
21. ACGME Common Program Requirements. Available at: http://www.acgme.org/acWebsite/dutyHours/dh_dutyhourscommonpr.pdf. Accessed September 2, 2009.
22. Siegel JM. The REM sleep-memory consolidation hypothesis. Science 2001;294:1058–63.
23. Stickgold R, Hobson JA, Fosse R, et al. Sleep, learning, and dreams: off-line memory reprocessing. Science 2001;294:1052–7.
24. Roehrs T, Carskadon MA, Dement WC, et al. Daytime sleepiness and alertness. In: Kryger MH, Roth T, Dement WD, editors. Principles and practice of sleep medicine. 4th edition. Philadelphia: Elsevier; 2005. p. 39–50.
25. Carskadon MA, Dement WC. Daytime sleepiness: quantification of a behavioral state. Neurosci Biobehav Rev 1987;111:307–17.
26. Aldrich MS. Ontogeny of sleep. In: Aldrich MS, editor. Sleep medicine. New York: Oxford University; 1999. p. 70–81.
27. Coleman RM, Roffwarg HP, Kennedy SJ, et al. Sleep-wake disorders based on a polysomnographic diagnosis. A national cooperative study. JAMA 1982;247(7):997–1003.
28. American Academy of Sleep Medicine. The international classification of sleep disorders. 2nd edition. Westchester (IL): American Academy of Sleep Medicine; 2005. Diagnostic and coding manual.
29. Peppard PE, Young T, Palta M, et al. Prospective study of the association between sleep-disordered

breathing and hypertension. N Engl J Med 2000; 342(19):1378–84.

30. Young T, Palta M, Dempsey J, et al. The occurrence of sleep-disordered breathing among middle-aged adults. N Engl J Med 1993;328(17):1230–5.

31. Javaheri S, Shukla R, Zeigler H, et al. Central sleep apnea, right ventricular dysfunction, and low diastolic blood pressure are predictors of mortality in systolic heart failure. J Am Coll Cardiol 2007; 49(20):2028–34.

32. Barion A, Zee PC. A clinical approach to circadian rhythm sleep disorders. Sleep Med 2007; 8(6):566–77.

33. National Sleep Foundation. Sleep in America poll: summary of findings. Available at: http://www.sleep foundation.org/article/sleep-america-polls/2008-sleep-performance-and-the-workplace. 2008. Accessed August 15, 2009.

34. Lyznicki JM, Doege TC, Davis RM, et al. Sleepiness, driving, and motor vehicle crashes. Council on Scientific Affairs, American Medical Association. JAMA 1998;279(23):1908–13.

35. Drake CL, Roehrs T, Richardson G, et al. Shift work sleep disorder: prevalence and consequences beyond that of symptomatic day workers. Sleep 2004;27(8):1453–62.

36. Mignot E. Narcolepsy: pharmacology, pathophysiology, and genetics. In: Kryger MH, Roth T, Dement WD, editors. Principles and practice of sleep medicine. 4th edition. Philadelphia: Elsevier; 2005. p. 761–79.

37. Guilleminault C, Fromherz S. Narcolepsy: diagnosis and management. In: Kryger MH, Roth T, Dement WD, editors. Principles and practice of sleep medicine. 4th edition. Philadelphia: Elsevier; 2005. p. 780–90.

38. Schweitzer PK. Drugs that disturb sleep and wakefulness. In: Kryger MH, Roth T,

Dement WD, editors. Principles and practice of sleep medicine. 4th edition. Philadelphia: Elsevier; 2005. p. 499–518.

39. Johns MW. A new method for measuring daytime sleepiness: the Epworth Sleepiness Scale. Sleep 1991;16:40–5.

40. Netzer NC, Stoohs RA, Netzer CM, et al. Using the Berlin Questionnaire to identify patients at risk for the sleep apnea syndrome. Ann Intern Med 1999; 131(7):485–91.

41. Morgenthaler T, Alessi C, Friedman L, et al. Practice parameters for the use of actigraphy in the assessment of sleep and sleep disorders: an update for 2007. Sleep 2007;30(4):519–29.

42. Golpe R, Jiménez A, Carpizo R, et al. Utility of home oximetry as a screening test for patients with moderate to severe symptoms of obstructive sleep apnea. Sleep 1999;22(7):932–7.

43. Kushida CA, Littner MR, Morgenthaler T, et al. Practice parameters for the indications for polysomnography and related procedures: an update for 2005. Sleep 2005;28(4):499–521.

44. Littner MR, Kushida C, Wise M, et al. Practice parameters for clinical use of the multiple sleep latency test and the maintenance of wakefulness test. Sleep 2005;28(1):113–21.

45. Mamelak M, Black J, Montplaisir J, et al. A pilot study on the effects of sodium oxybate on sleep architecture and daytime alertness in narcolepsy. Sleep 2004;27(7):1327–34.

46. Wise MS, Arand DL, Auger RR, et al. Treatment of narcolepsy and other hypersomnias of central origin. Sleep 2007;30(12):1712–27.

47. Landrigan CP, Fahrenkopf AM, Lewin D, et al. Effects of the accreditation council for graduate medical education duty hour limits on sleep, work hours, and safety. Pediatrics 2008;122(2): 250–8.

The Parasomnias: Epidemiology, Clinical Features, and Diagnostic Approach

Alon Y. Avidan, MD, MPH[a],*, Neeraj Kaplish, MD[b]

KEYWORDS

- Parasomnias • Confusional arousals • Sleepwalking
- Night terrors • Nightmares • RBD and sleep paralysis

Parasomnias are a group of disorders exclusive to sleep and wake-to-sleep transition that encompass arousals with abnormal motor, behavioral, or sensory experiences.[1–3] Sensory experiences often involve but are not limited to perceptions, dreamlike hallucinatory experiences, and autonomic symptoms. When accompanied with excessive motor activity and other complex motor behaviors, these parasomnias can be disruptive to the patient and bed partners. Motor behaviors may or may not be restricted to bed but can become dangerous when the subject ambulates or is agitated. In some parasomnias, it may be injury or concerns for physical injury to the patient or bed partner that brings them to the attention of physicians. The other presentations include disrupted nocturnal sleep of patients, bed partners, or family members sharing the sleeping quadrant. The behaviors are inappropriate for the time of occurrence but may seem purposeful or goal directed. In general, most parasomnias are more common in children and decrease in frequency as they get older.[4–6] Parasomnias have been reported in approximately 4% of the adult population.[7]

These complex motor behaviors occurring during sleep may have medicolegal implications, as violence could be a prominent component as documented in the case of Canadian Supreme Court case *Her Majesty the Queen v Kenneth Parks* and in the State Supreme Court case *State of Arizona v Scott Falater*. The incidence of violent behavior during sleep is generally presumed to be low, but recent reports indicate a prevalence of up to 2% in adults.[8] Sexual differences have also been noted in other parasomnias such as rapid eye movement (REM) sleep behavior disorder (RBD) and sleep-related eating disorder. Complex behaviors with sexual acts have been implicated in cases of sexual assault and rape.

PATHOPHYSIOLOGY

Sleep can be broadly divided in to non-REM (NREM) and REM sleep. NREM sleep is further divided into stage N1, stage N2, and stage N3 (slow wave sleep). Sleep stage shift is not a complete on-off switch phenomenon, but involves reorganization and transition of various neuronal centers for an equivocal stage to declare itself.[1,2] During this period of reorganization (a unique state of sleep dissociation) an admixture of 2 or 3 different states of being is observed. **Fig. 1** depicts the conceptualization of the overlapping states of being leading to parasomnias.[9] It is usually an arousal during these periods of

a Department of Neurology, UCLA Neurology Clinic, Sleep Disorders Center, University of California Los Angeles, 710 Westwood Boulevard, Room 1-169/RNRC, Los Angeles, CA 90095-1769, USA
b Department of Neurology, University of Michigan, 1500 East Medical Center Drive, SPC 5845, C 732, Med Inn Building, Ann Arbor, MI 48109-5845, USA
* Corresponding author.
E-mail address: avidan@mednet.ucla.edu

Clin Chest Med 31 (2010) 353–370
doi:10.1016/j.ccm.2010.02.015

Nocturnal Spells: overlapping states

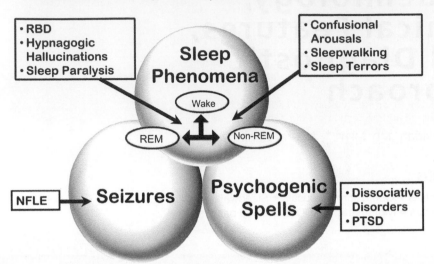

Fig. 1. Overlapping states of being. Parasomnias are explainable on the basic notion that sleep and wakefulness are not mutually exclusive states but may dissociate and oscillate rapidly. The abnormal admixture of the 3 states of being (NREM sleep, REM sleep, and wakefulness) may overlap, giving rise to parasomnias. REM parasomnias occur because of the abnormal intrusion of wakefulness into REM sleep and likewise NREM parasomnias such as sleepwalking occur because of abnormal intrusions of wakefulness into NREM sleep. Other nocturnal spells that may be confused with parasomnias include NFLE and psychogenic spells such as posttraumatic stress disorder (PTSD), dissociated disorders. (*Modified from* Mahowald MW, Schenck CH. Non-rapid eye movement sleep parasomnias. Neurol Clin 2005;23(4):1078, vii; with permission.)

reorganization that leads to complex motor behavior during sleep.[2,10]

Another hypothesis is the deafferentation of the locomotor centers from the generators of the different sleep states. Locomotor centers are present at spinal and supraspinal levels and this dissociation can explain motor activity or ambulation, especially in patients with disorders of arousals.[11]

Central pattern generators, which are located in the brain stem and spinal cord, are believed to be responsible for involuntary motor behaviors classified into:

(a) Oroalimentary automatisms, bruxism and biting;
(b) Ambulatory behaviors, ranging from the classic bimanual-bipedal activity of somnambulism to periodic leg movements; and
(c) Various sleep-related events associated with fear, such as sleep terrors, nightmares, and violent behaviors.[11]

CLASSIFICATION OF PARASOMNIAS
NREM Parasomnias

The International Classification of Sleep Disorders 2nd Edition (ICSD-II) categorizes NREM parasomnias (disorders of arousals) into 3 broad categories

(**Fig. 2**)[12]: confusional arousals, sleepwalking, and night terrors. These share several common features (such as having increased predilection in children, decreasing with age, and occurring in the first half of the night, typically within the first 2 hours of sleep) but have certain unique features: inconsolable crying and autonomic hyperactivity in night terrors and ambulation in sleep terrors, which helps differentiate them.

Confusional Arousals

Case history: A 56-year-old man with history of traumatic brain injury and noncompliance with positive airway pressure therapy for his sleep-disordered breathing, began experiencing nocturnal spells as frequently as multiple times per night, primarily during the first half of the night. These spells were characterized by sudden arousals associated with confusion and singing behavior.

During the diagnostic nocturnal polysomnogram (PSG) video recording (**Fig. 3**), multiple similar spells of arousals with confusion, along with side-to-side head movements, arm flapping, and talking occurred exclusively from NREM sleep, and in 1 event he was reported by the sleep technicians to be "quacking like a duck."

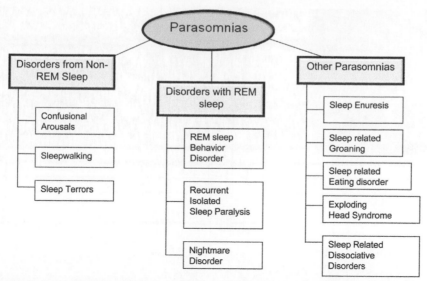

Fig. 2. ICSD-II classification of parasomnias showing all 11 of the 15 important parasomnias. Disorders from NREM sleep are also known as disorders of arousal. Parasomnias categorized as "other parasomnias" do not show a strong predilection for NREM or REM sleep. Other parasomnias also include: sleep-related hallucinations, parasomnias due to drug or substance, parasomnias due to medical conditions, parasomnias unspecified.

Approximately 20 of these nocturnal episodes were recorded with and without preceding respiratory effort related arousal. No epileptiform activity was recorded on the limited electroencephalogram (EEG) recording during these episodes. The events were clinically suspected of being consistent with the diagnosis of confusional arousals and were resolved with the application of continuous positive airway pressure during the titration phase of the study. This suggested that sleep-disordered breathing was probably a precipitating factor for the patient's nocturnal events.

Confusional arousals (also known as sleep drunkenness or excessive sleep inertia) consist of arousals originating from NREM sleep (usually slow wave sleep) associated with an arousal linked to confusion and disorientation. The associated behaviors may be inappropriate and patients have slow mentation in responding to questioning from the observer. Usually these behaviors are noted in the first half of the night but forced and anticipatory awakenings during slow wave sleep may result in confusional arousal induction. Aggression or violent behavior is atypical, but may follow forced awakening from sleep. Confusional arousals are associated with amnesia of the event, and recollection in the morning is absent or sketchy Associated motor behavior may be simple and nongoal oriented and, less commonly, complex and associated with aggression, violence, or inappropriate sexual activity.[12] When sexual behavior is encountered along the spectrum of

confusional arousals, the parasomnia is further defined as a sexsomnia.[13]

There is no sexual predilection in confusional arousals. High prevalence is observed at a prevalence of 17.3% in children 3 to 13 years of age, after which the prevalence decreases.[12] Prevalence among adults 15 years and older is estimated at 2.9% to 4.2%.[7] Genetic factors play a significant predisposing role, as there may be a familial history of similar childhood nocturnal behaviors.[14] In adults, a variety of factors that lead to arousals from sleep have the potential to precipitate confusional arousals. These factors include sleep deprivation, fever, infections, centrally active medications (hypnotics, antidepressants, and tranquilizers), sleep-disordered breathing, and periodic limb movements of sleep.[15]

Confusional arousal variants

ICSD-II describes 2 variants of confusional arousals in adults and adolescents: sleep-related sexual behaviors and severe morning sleep inertia.[12]

- Abnormal sexual behavior has been reported to occur during sleep and this is now classified in ICSD-II as a variant of confusional arousals in adults and adolescents. In 2002 Guilleminault and colleagues[17] described 11 subjects (7 men and 4 women) with atypical sexual behaviors during sleep. The range of abnormal

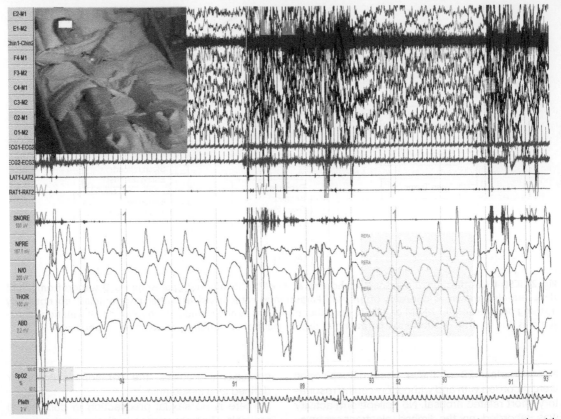

Fig. 3. A 120-second epoch of a diagnostic PSG from a 54-year-old man conducted to evaluate for arousals with confusion and singing behavior. The figure illustrates 1 of the patient's representative events: an arousal from slow wave sleep with the patient's arms abducted (flapping his arms and described by the technicians to be "quacking like a duck"). Channels are as follows: electro-oculogram (*left*: E1-M2, *right*: E2-M1), chin electromyogram (EMG) (Chin1-Chin2), EEG (*left*: frontal-F3, central-C3, occipital-O1, left mastoid-M1 and *right*: frontal-F4,central-C4, occipital-O2, right mastoid-M2), 2 electrocardiogram (ECG) channels, 2 limb EMG (LAT, RAT), snore channel, nasal-oral airflow (N/O), nasal pressure signal (NPRE), respiratory effort (thoracic, abdominal) and oxygen saturation (SaO2).

sexual behaviors is wide and includes violent masturbations, sexual assaults and loud sexual vocalizations, fondling the bed partner, sexual intercourse with or without orgasm, and agitated sexual behaviors, which may have considerable medicolegal implications. In addition to occurring in confusional arousals, sexsomnias have been reported with other NREM parasomnias such as somnambulism.[13] Treatment with medications such as clonazepam with simultaneous psychotherapy is an effective treatment combination in these patients.[16]

- Another variant in adults of confusional arousals is severe morning sleep inertia.[17] This variant remains clinically similar to typical confusional arousal and arises from light NREM sleep, but does not occur out of slow wave sleep.

Sleepwalking

Case history: A 67-year-old woman presented with a history of "difficulties with her sleep since she was a toddler." She complained of multiple arousals in the night with associated "uncomfortable feeling in her legs." She reported that the symptoms have been there for many years but gradually this has been getting worse. The patient's niece, who accompanied her to the clinic, said that the patient wakes up in multiple spots in the house, calling these her "little nests." She does not remember moving around the house at night and does not have any idea why she wakes up in different locations. In the morning, she also reports finding bed sheets, pillows, and covers at different spots in her house.

The sleep disorders clinic managed her for restless leg syndrome, a possible factor contributing to her sleepwalking behaviors, and the therapy completely resolved her spells, which were clinically believed to represent somnambulism. Her sleep and daytime functioning improved. She reported that her sleep was more consolidated and she slept in her bed throughout the night.

Sleepwalking (also known as somnambulism) arises out of slow wave sleep and is noticed usually in the first third of the nocturnal sleep, as there is more abundance of slow wave sleep, which serves as a substrate for these spells.[18,19] The episodes are characterized as an ambulatory phenomenon during sleep. Patients with sleepwalking behaviors are typically calm; however, more complex behaviors such as eating, cooking, cleaning the house, unlocking doors, sexual activities, and even driving have been reported.[20,21] If awakened, patients are observed to be confused and can become violent or agitated.[22] The ambulation usually terminates spontaneously but may occur in unusual places such as the bathroom or kitchen. Most often, patients return to their bed and have no recollection of the episodes the following morning.

Sleepwalking is common in children, with prevalence as high as 17%, decreasing to about 3% in adults.[23,24] Sleepwalking in men can be associated with injury and violence.[25] Children between 4 and 6 years of age form the major group exhibiting sleepwalking behavior. With advancing age, especially after puberty, sleepwalking decreases significantly.[4,5] Patients are at risk of injury from falls while going downstairs, running into closed doors or windows, or jumping out of windows.[26]

Genetic factors play a significant risk for sleepwalking, especially if a first-degree relative is affected with this parasomnia, as the risk increases 10-fold when compared with the general population.[27] In a twin study, monozygotic twins exhibited 6 times greater concordance for sleepwalking compared with dizygotic twins.[28] Precipitating factors for sleepwalking include sleep deprivation, fever, centrally active substances, hypnotic medications (such as zolpidem), stress, and sleep-disordered breathing, sharing a similar predisposing factor as in patients with confusional arousals.[29] Genetic susceptibility to develop sleepwalking has been linked to *DQB1* genes, with 35% of White sleepwalkers testing positively compared with only 13.3% of controls.[30]

Delta power density during spectral analysis is reduced in children who sleepwalk and adults with persistent sleepwalk.[31–33] Patients who experience sleepwalking had increased power of low delta just before the confusional arousal in the first sleep cycle, suggesting a chronic inability to sustain slow wave sleep.[32,34] Increased blood flow in the thalamus and cingulated cortex has been seen on a single photon emission-computed tomography (SPECT) scan during sleepwalking in a 16-year-old boy.[35]

Sleep Terrors

Case history: A 4-year-old boy experienced episodes of nighttime arousals with severe agitation and a piercing scream occurring within the first 2 to 3 hours of sleep onset, which lasted approximately 5 to 10 minutes. The frequency of these spells was once to twice per night. The episodes were first noted when he went on an overseas trip and his sleep-wake cycle was altered. Following an arousal with loud scream, his crying was inconsolable but had a waxing and waning pattern. At the time, he was also suffering from symptoms of upper respiratory infection (URI). On consultation with the pediatrician, his parents were given reassurance, and symptomatic treatment of his URI was initiated. In addition, better sleep hygiene, including attaining a regular sleep-wake schedule, turning off the lights, and limiting physical activity close to bedtime were discussed, including measures on how to best readjust the child's altered circadian rhythm. Gradually as the child recovered from URI and his circadian rhythm became more synchronized, his nocturnal episodes resolved completely.

Sleep terrors, also known as night terrors or pavor nocturnes, are parasomnias arising out of slow wave sleep. Affected children are usually 4 to 12 years old and the estimated prevalence is between 1% and 6.5% of children.[12] Although sleep terrors tend to resolve spontaneously during adolescence, they may persist and can be seen in 4% of adults as well.[36] Psychopathology is rare in the affected children but may have a more significant factor in adults with sleep terrors [7]

Sleep terrors are characterized by a sudden arousal associated with a piercing scream or cry in the first few hours of sleep onset (**Fig. 4**).[19] During a sleep terror, the patient may act in an afraid, agitated, anxious, and panicky manner.[37] Inconsolability is a striking feature. Typically, the child does not want to be touched or comforted during the event, to the surprise of the parents. Verbalization during the episode is incoherent and perception of the environment seems altered. The child may run into walls or in circles and even run outside, possibly as a result of altered perception and panic. These events can be potentially dangerous, when ambulation is present, and may result in physical harm to self or their bed partners.[25,38]

Sleep terrors typically last from 30 seconds up to 5 minutes. Most patients with sleep terrors are amnesic to the event in the morning but some

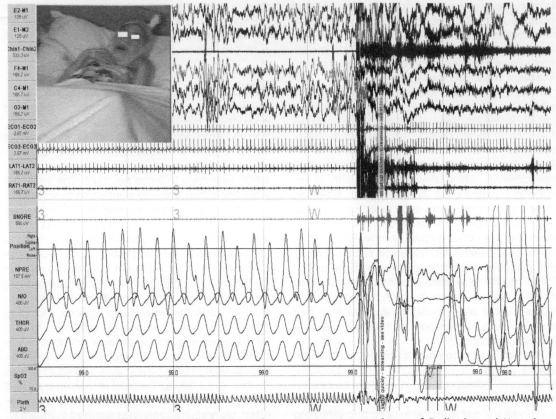

Fig. 4. PSG slide provided courtesy of Timothy Hoban, MD, Associate Professor of Pediatrics and Neurology, University of Michigan, Ann Arbor, MI, USA. Two-minute epoch of a diagnostic PSG from a 9-year-old boy performed to evaluate for arousals associated with screaming and inconsolable crying. The figure illustrates 1 of the patient's representative spells: an arousal with screaming arising out of slow wave sleep with the patient's arms flexed and held close to chest (as if afraid and protecting himself). Channels are as follows: electro-oculogram (*left*: E1-M2, *right*: E2-M1), chin EMG (Chin1-Chin2), EEG (*right*: frontal-F4,central-C4, occipital-O2, right mastoid-M2), 2 ECG channels, 2 limb EMG (LAT, RAT), snore channel, nasal-oral airflow (N/O), nasal pressure signal (NPRE), respiratory effort (thoracic, abdominal) and oxygen saturation (SaO2).

maintain dream imagery or fragments of dream.[39] A strong component of sympathetic activation characterized by tachycardia, tachypnea, sweating, flushed skin, or mydriasis is present in almost all patients, and is typically a key distinguishing factor. In adults, associated behaviors may be violent and may result in injury to the patient or the bed partner.[25] Injury to self may appear as an apparent suicide (pseudosuicide) in some cases.[38]

Somniloquy

Somniloquy, also known as sleep talking, is not listed under the category of traditional parasomnias in ICSD-II. In this manual it is classified under "sleep disorders associated with conditions classified elsewhere".[12] However, it is a common sleep-related behavior involving vocalization of sounds, speech, or at times conversations without any awareness of the event, and hence it is

reminiscent of a parasomnia in its semiology. Events of somniloquy have the potential to lead to legal ramification if any confidential material is uttered. Diagnostic polysomnography reveals that the events most commonly occur during stage N1, N2, and REM sleep.[40] The prevalence of this condition is not certain; however, it is estimated to be 4.9% in Chinese children between 2 and 12 years of age.[41] In older adults, somniloquy is also associated with obstructive sleep apnea, other disorders of arousals, or RBD. No specific treatment exists but if there is suspicion for coexistent sleep disorder, diagnostic work-up and management of the underlying comorbid conditions is warranted.

Nocturnal Frontal Lobe Epilepsy

Nocturnal frontal lobe epilepsy (NFLE), including supplementary motor area seizures, are episodes which may closely mimic the NREM parasomnias and pose a tough diagnostic challenge.[42–44] The episodes are sudden, brief, spanning less than a minute in duration with little or no ictal confusion and occur exclusively or predominantly during sleep.[45] The main distinguishing features between parasomnias and nocturnal seizures are shown in **Table 1**.[44] The semiology suggests a frontal lobe origin involving the orbitofrontal or mesial frontal regions.[45] There is often vocalization of variable complexity, frequent warning, usually nonspecific, the attacks seem to be bizarre and hysterical, the unique feature is a stereotypical pattern, and the interictal and ictal surface EEG are often normal.[46,47] These episodes can be misdiagnosed during wakefulness as pseudoseizures and during sleep as movement disorders.

NFLE is 1 clinical example of localization-related epilepsy, which shares a strong interface with sleep. Three major clinic semiologies have been described in patients with NFLE: paroxysmal arousals, characterized by brief and sudden recurrent motor paroxysmal behavior; nocturnal paroxysmal dystonia (NPD) (discussed in further detail in the next section) and motor attacks with complex dystonic-dyskinetic features; and episodic nocturnal wanderings (stereotyped, agitated somnambulism).[48]

An NFLE with strong genetic predisposition, autosomal-dominant NFLE (ADNLE) is a channelopathy with a defect in the neuronal nicotinic acetylcholine receptor. Video electroencephalography monitoring and video PSG with full EEG are useful in distinguishing NFLE and ADNFLE from other conditions such as parasomnias.[44] Treatment with carbamazepine is effective in many patients with frontal lobe seizures.[49]

NPD

NPD was listed as a motor disorder of sleep in the earlier version of the ICSD,[50] and the most recent edition classifies it as a form of frontal lobe epilepsy: sleep-related epilepsy.[12] NPD consists of a sudden arousal, occurring during NREM sleep, associated with a complex sequence of movements, repeated dystonia or dyskinetic (ballistic or chorioathetotic).[51] Patients may also move their legs and arms with cycling or kicking movements, rock their trunks, and show tonic asymmetric or dystonic posture of the limbs. A few cases are characterized by a violent ballistic pattern with flaying of the limbs.[51] Differential diagnosis includes REM sleep behavior disorder and sleep terrors. Treatment with carbamazepine is often effective.[52]

REM PARASOMNIAS

The ICSD-II distinguishes among 3 separate REM parasomnias: nightmares, recurrent isolated sleep paralysis, and RBD.[12]

Nightmares

Nightmares are common, affecting between 10% and 50% of children and up to two-thirds of the general population can recall at least 1 or a few nightmares in the course of their childhood. Half of all adults recall an occasional nightmare, whereas 1% report more than an occasional nightmare a week.[53] Nightmares present as a vivid and prolonged dream sequence that tends to become progressively more intense, complex, and anxiety provoking, eventually terminating in an arousal and vivid recall. Episodes may increase during times of

Table 1
Differences between sleep terrors and nightmares

Characteristic	Sleep Terror	Nightmare
Timing during the night	First third (deep slow wave sleep)	Last third (REM sleep)
Movements	Common	Rare
Severity	Severe	Mild
Vocalizations	Common	Rare
Autonomic discharge	Severe and intense	Mild
Amnesia	Absent	Present
State on waking	Confused/disoriented	Function well
Injuries	Common	Rare
Violence	Common	Rare
Displacement from bed	Common	Very rare

stress, particularly following traumatic events.[53,54] Some medications such as levodopa, β-adrenergic blockers, and abrupt withdrawal of REM-suppressant medications may precipitate nightmares. The PSG shows an abrupt awakening from REM sleep associated with an increased REM sleep density and variability in heart and respiratory rates.[55] Reassurance is often the main management necessary, but when episodes are severe and refractory, the use of REM-suppressing agents such as tricyclic antidepressants (TCAs) or selective serotonin reuptake inhibitors (SSRIs) may be needed.[56–58] Differentiation between sleep terrors and nightmares is shown in **Table 1.**

Recurrent Isolated Sleep Paralysis

Sleep paralysis is defined as an inability to perform voluntary motor function at sleep onset or on awakening. The disorder occurs at least once in a lifetime in 40% to 50% of normal subjects. Patients report frightening episodes in which movements of the skeletal muscles are not possible, although ocular and respiratory movements and cognition usually remain intact. Episodes last a few minutes and may be aborted spontaneously or on external stimulation (vigorous eye movements). Episodes may occur in isolation, in healthy patients, as a genetically transmitted familial form, and as 1 of the narcolepsy symptoms. Depending on the meaning given to and cause of the sleep paralysis experience, which is largely culturally determined, patients may react to the event in specific ways. Predisposing factors include acute sleep deprivation and sleep-wake cycle disturbances (jet lag, shift work). In 1 study of first-year medical students, sleep paralysis episodes (predormital, postdormital, or both types of sleep paralysis) occurred in up to 16.25% of individuals.[59] The underlying cause for sleep paralysis may be attributed to abnormalities in the mechanism controlling REM sleep muscle atonia and it is probably a result of abnormal activation of limbic system structures.[60] Pharmacotherapy for sleep paralysis is often unnecessary when episodes are infrequent and in most cases reassurance is all that is needed. Management is most successful when patients avoid irregular sleep schedules but when sleep paralysis is severe, the use of anxiolytic medications and fluoxetine may be indicated.[61,62]

RBD

RBD is characterized by abnormal elevation of limb or chin electromyography tone during REM sleep and by complex and elaborate motor activity associated with agitated and violent dream mentation. Patients with RBD report a wide spectrum of abnormal dream experiences, ranging from simple and relatively benign verbalizations, singing, yelling, shouting, and screaming to more complex motor phenomena such as walking, running, kicking, punching, jumping, and violent agitated behaviors that correlate with the reported aggressive dream imagery experience.[63–65] The injury associated with the spells is often what brings the patient to the care and attention of the physician.

The prevalence of RBD is estimated to be 0.5%.[8] The disorder has an increased gender predilection in that it affects men more than women (9:1 ratio), and has a higher prevalence in older age, usually in men more than 60 years old.[63,65] The specific reason for the gender predilection in men is a mystery.[66–68] Subjective reports indicate that about 25% of patients with Parkinsonism have dream enactment behaviors suggestive of RBD, and sleep evaluation in patients with Parkinson disease who experience sleep disturbances found RBD to be present in up to 47%.[69,70]

Case history: A 68-year-old man presented with violent dreams reported by his wife. His dreams became extremely aggressive and "dramatic" in the last few months before presentation for sleep medicine evaluation. His wife reported that there is not 1 night that her husband wakes up without "kicking and cursing as if in an intense argument." One episode led to his punching a lamp and sustaining severe cuts in his wrist, necessitating surgical repair. He had purchased 2 sleeping bags which he tied to the mattress o prevent himself from moving and hurting himself and his wife.

Patients with RBD may experience their spells as early as 90 minutes after falling asleep and more frequently during the second half of night, as REM sleep is denser in the later part of the night. The frequency of episodes varies from once a month to nightly episodes, as in this case history, which result in more significant sleep disruption and are more likely to be brought to medical attention. RBD may be further classified into an acute and a chronic form. The acute form of RBD may be seen in the setting of substance- or medication-related cases, injury of the central nervous system (CNS) (stroke, demyelination), or metabolic derangements. The most common drug-related forms include rapid withdrawal from alcohol, abrupt discontinuation of sedative-hypnotics agents (which result in REM rebound), and cases related to TCAs, biperiden, monoamine oxidase inhibitors (MAOIs), cholinergic agents, and SSRIs (resulting in loss of REM atonia).[71–81]

Exposure to caffeine (sometimes in the form of chocolate) has also been implicated in RBD.[82,83] A prodromal history of other, and sometimes milder, forms of nocturnal spells such as sleep talking, yelling, or limb jerking may be present. With time, the dream content and enactment often become increasingly more aggressive, complex, action-filled, violent, or unpleasant, coinciding with the onset of RBD. Hypersomnolence may emerge if sleep becomes disrupted with dream enactment spells, leading to frequent arousals and nonrestorative sleep. The potential for bodily injury, skin lacerations, face ecchymoses, and skull fractures to patients and bed partners are a major safety concern and may necessitate preemptive pharmacologic interventions. Safety measures such as protective barricades around the bed, heavy curtains over the windows, removing sharp objects from the bedroom area, and sleeping on the ground floor in a sleeping bag (as in this case history) should be recommended until the disorder is fully managed.

Older age is a predisposing factor for the chronic or idiopathic form of RBD, which is generally more frequent, occurs later in life, becomes progressively more severe with time, and eventually stabilizes. Approximately 60% of patients who present with RBD are classified as idiopathic; the remaining cases are associated with underlying neurologic diseases and injury such as neurodegenerative disorders, cerebrovascular accidents, and multiple sclerosis. Dementias implicated in RBD include the synucleinopathies such as olivopontocerebellar atrophy and Lewy body disease with a characteristic α-synuclein inclusion in the nerve cell bodies. The condition has also been reported in Machado-Joseph disease (spinocerebellar ataxia type 3) and the Guillain-Barré syndrome.[68,84] Acute neurologic insult such as brainstem lesions caused by demyelination in multiple sclerosis, subarachnoid hemorrhage, pontine stroke, and brainstem neoplasm have been all implicated in the acute form of RBD.[68,85–87] Recent findings have also identified patients with tauopathies such as progressive supranuclear palsy[88] and probable Alzheimer disease.[89]

RBD typically begins in the sixth or seventh decade of life and may precede clinical manifestation of the underlying neuropathologic lesion process by several years to more than a decade.[90–94] Patients with narcolepsy experience a higher incidence of RBD, and RBD may be the first sign of disease onset in children.[95] Medications that act on the CNS and psychiatric medications such as TCAs, SSRIs, and MAOIs, which can be used to treat cataplexy, can sometimes exacerbate or trigger RBD in these patients.[96]

The underlying pathophysiology of RBD may be related to abnormal brainstem control of medullary inhibitory regions (Fig. 5). An identical syndrome was reported by Jouvet 4 decades ago.[97] The studies involved an animal preparation, in cats, in which experimentally induced bilateral lesions of pontine regions adjacent to the locus coeruleus

Events Typically Last 3-5 minutes

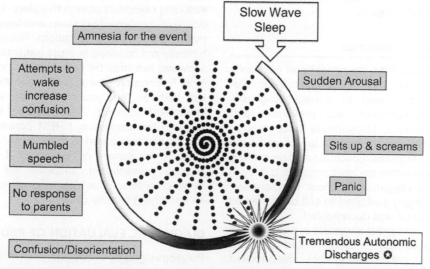

Fig. 5. Characteristic pattern of sleep terror. Sleep terrors are characterized by a sudden arousal associated with a scream, agitation, panic, and heightened autonomic activity. Inconsolability is almost universal. The child is incoherent and has altered perception of the environment, appearing confused. This behavior may potentially be dangerous and could result in injury.

produced absence of REM-related muscle atonia associated and abnormal motor behaviors during REM sleep.[97] In this experimental preparation, the cat slept until its first REM period, when it was noted to jump, with eyes still closed, and run around the cage, making attack motions. Two decades later, in 1986, the condition was eventually characterized as a new parasomnia by Schenck and colleagues,[98] reporting a series of patients, mainly older men, with aggressive nocturnal behaviors. RBD is currently viewed as a complex sleep phenomenon with a possible mechanism related to either a reduction of REM atonia or an abnormal augmentation of locomotor intermittent excitatory influences during REM sleep, or both.[99,100]

Recent brain imaging data, based on SPECT studies, show a possible mechanism relating to dopaminergic abnormalities and decreased striatal dopaminergic innervation as well as reduced striatal dopamine transporters.[101–103] Positron emission tomography and SPECT studies further confirm reduced nigrostriatal dopaminergic projections in patients with multiple system atrophy and RBD.[104] RBD is believed to be mediated neither by direct abnormal α-synuclein inclusions nor alone, by striatonigral dopaminergic deficiency as it probably reflects a more complex multiple neurotransmitter dysfunction involving GABAergic (γ-aminobutyric acid-mediated), glutamatergic, and monoaminergic systems.[105] In patients with idiopathic RBD, impaired cortical activation as determined by EEG spectral analysis supports the relationship between RBD and neurodegenerative disorders.[106] The potential pathophysiology of RBD is depicted in **Fig. 6**.

Evaluation of Parasomnias

A detailed history from the patient and especially from the witness of these events can provide valuable insight and lead to correct diagnosis, rewarding management, and preventive and safety interventions. Home-made video recordings if available can be used to lend support the presumptive diagnosis. Education and counseling the patient and family are key components in evaluation and management of most parasomnias. Any physical injury sustained to self or to the bed partner should be well documented.

The major differential diagnosis in patients with NREM parasomnias is sleep-related epilepsy. Differentiating parasomnias from sleep-related epilepsy can be challenging, especially when the patient lives alone or these nocturnal behaviors are unwitnessed. However, even when these behaviors are recorded during long-term video EEG monitoring, diagnosis can still remain uncertain. Up to 44% of patients with a diagnosis of NFLE can have a normal ictal EEG during video EEG recording.[48] Similarly, a substantial number of patients with NFLE can have a personal and a family history of parasomnias.[48]

A detailed personal history (sleep and nonsleep related) is critical to the diagnosis of NREM parasomnias. Family history, if available, can be helpful to support the clinical diagnosis. Recently a Frontal Lobe Epilepsy and Parasomnias (FLEP) scale has been reported to have higher accuracy in differentiating NFLE from parasomnias.[44] The scale consists of several key questions based on the semiologic features of NFLE and parasomnias. The FLEP scale is designed to discriminate between features that are universally problematic based on clinical experience and the medical literature.[44] Responses favoring nocturnal epilepsy (spells that are of brief duration, occurring several times per night, with a high degree of stereotypy) are scored positively, whereas those favoring parasomnias (amnesia, recall) are scored negatively. A score of 3 or higher is highly suggestive of epilepsy, whereas a positive score is more likely to represent a parasomnia.[44] The FLEP scale may have some limitations in differentiating sleepwalking from episodic nocturnal wanderings (a form of NFLE) and RBD from seizures.[107] For nocturnal frontal lobe seizures, the FLEP scale has a sensitivity of 71.4%, a specificity of 100%, a positive predictive value of 100%, and a negative predictive value of 91.1%.[44]

Factors that may precipitate NREM parasomnias as mentioned earlier should be explored, including comorbid obstructive sleep apnea, periodic limb movements of sleep, and temporal association with certain medications. Neuroimaging is typically not required in most patients with parasomnias, but may be necessary in patients with focal findings on neurologic examination or atypical features (eg, younger women with dream enactment behavior). The nocturnal PSG is not required for diagnosing NREM parasomnias but should be considered if there is concern about injury to the patient or spouse, or if there is an unusual presentation, suspicion for coexistent sleep disorders, or a high level of suspicion for an underlying seizure disorder.

DIAGNOSTIC EVALUATION OF RBD

Polysomnography is obligatory for RBD, revealing abnormal muscle augmentation during REM sleep; exceeding the normal REM sleep-related phasic electromyography twitches (**Fig. 7**). These motor phenomena may be simple (talking, laughing) or

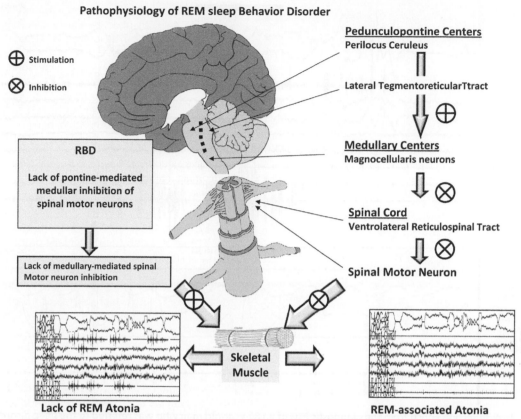

Fig. 6. The normally generalized muscle atonia during REM sleep results from pontine-mediated perilocusceru-leus inhibition of motor activity. This pontine activity exerts an excitatory influence on medullary centers (mag-nocellularis neurons) via the lateral tegmentoreticular tract. These neuronal groups, in turn, hyperpolarize and the spinal motor neuron postsynaptic membranes via the ventrolateralreticulospinal tract. In RBD, the brainstem mechanisms generating the muscle atonia normally seen in REM sleep may be disrupted. The pathophysiology of RBD in humans is based on the cat model. In the cat model, bilateral pontine lesions result in a persistent absence of REM atonia associated with prominent motor activity during REM sleep, similar to that observed in RBD in humans. The pathophysiology of the idiopathic form of RBD in humans is still not well understood but may be. (*Adapted from* Avidan AY. Sleep disorders in the older patient. Prim Care 2005;32:536–87; with permission.)

complex (limb and trunk movements, repeated punching, kicking, or yelling) and are sometimes associated with emotionally charged utter-ances.[100,108–110] When the patient wakes up from the episode they may have vivid recall and report dream mentation, which sometimes correlates with the observed behavior (trying to kick or protect themselves from an aggressive intruder). As in the NREM parasomnias the results of the neurologic history and examination may further indicate the need for other neurologic testing, including computed tomography or magnetic resonance imaging of the brain to identify struc-tural lesion of underlying neurodegenerative processes. This procedure is especially important if the episodes are acute, are temporally related, follow neurologic injury, or occur in younger patients and women.[87,111,112]

The differential diagnosis of RBD includes nocturnal frontal lobe seizures, somnambulism, sleep terrors, confusional arousals, posttraumatic stress disorders, and nightmares. RBD is often distinguished based on the complex nature of the spells, occurrence later in the night when REM density is highest, and the characteristic patient profile (ie, older men).[65,86] Differentiation among the key parasomnias and nocturnal seizures is shown in **Table 2**. **Table 3** summarizes the differentiation between NREM parasomnias, REM parasomnias, and nocturnal seizures.

Treatment of Parasomnias

Successful management of disturbing paras-omnias depends on establishing an accurate diag-nosis. Reassurance, nonpharmacologic therapy,

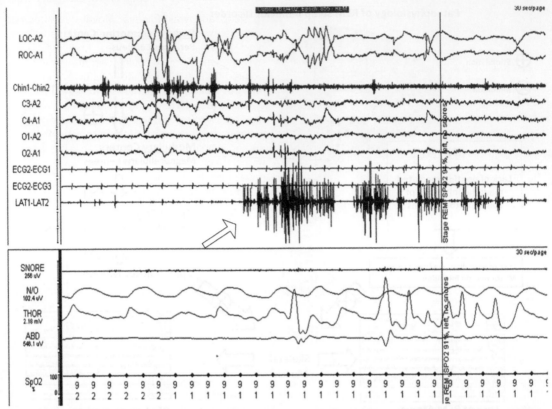

Fig. 7. A 30-second epoch from the diagnostic PSG of an 80-year-old man who was referred to the sleep disorders clinic for evaluation of recurrent violent nighttime awakenings. Illustrated in this figure is a typical spell that this patient was experiencing. He was noted to yell, jump from bed, and have complex body movements. The open arrow shows the point during REM sleep at which the patient had abnormal dream enactment behavior associated with REM-associated muscle atonia in the left anterior tibialis muscle. Channels are as follows: electro-oculogram (*left:* LOC-A2, *right:* ROC-A1), chin EMG, EEG (left central, right central, left occipital, right occipital), 2 ECG channels, limb EMG (LAT), snore channel, nasal-oral airflow, respiratory effort (thoracic, abdominal) and oxygen saturation (SaO2). (*Adapted from* Avidan AY. Sleep disorders in the older patient. Prim Care 2005;32:536–87; with permission.)

and intervention measured to address safety issues are important for the less dramatic parasomnias. When the patient's parasomnias are associated with displacement from the bedroom, the patient and the family need to maintain a safe bedroom environment, relocating the bedroom to the ground floor of the house and if possible, blocking all windows with heavy drapes. The patient should be warned to avoid precipitating events of parasomnias, including unusual stress, sleep deprivation, and ingestion of substances believed to promote arousal disorders such as alcohol (which is known to increase slow wave sleep and may promote parasomnias such as sleepwalking) and caffeine-containing substances (which have been implicated in parasomnias such as RBD).

Treatment of NREM Parasomnias

Counseling and support are the key elements for the treatment of NREM parasomnias. Improving

sleep hygiene (keeping a regular sleep-wake cycle and limiting exercise, caffeine, alcohol, and exposure to bright light before bedtime) should be stressed to the patient and bed partners. Educating the patient and family members about taking necessary safety precautions when these episodes occur is helpful in most cases. Removing dangerous objects from the immediate vicinity, locking mediation cabinets, locking doors and windows, hiding car keys, and placing the mattress on the ground floor are a few examples that limit the risk of injury. Forced awakenings, which risk precipitating some parasomnias during slow wave sleep, should be discouraged.

Pharmacotherapy is typically not needed for patients who present with mild or infrequent episodes. However, when there is a concern for physical injury or if the episodes involve potentially dangerous complex activities, pharmacotherapy is a necessity. Low-dose clonazepam and other benzodiazepines such as temazepam or

Table 2
Key similarities and differentiating features between NREM and REM parasomnias as well as nocturnal seizures

	Confusional Arousals	Sleep Terrors	Sleepwalking	Nightmares	RBD	Nocturnal Seizures
Time	Early	Early	Early-Mid	Late	Late	Any
Sleep stage	SWA	SWA	SWA	REM	REM	Any
EEG discharges	–	–	–	–	+	+
Scream	–	++++	–	++	+	+
Autonomic activation	+	++++	+	+	+	+
Motor activity	–	+	+++	+	++++	++++
Awakens	–	–	–	+	+	+
Duration (minutes)	0.5–10	1–10	2–30	3–20	1–10	5–15
Postevent confusion	+	+	+	–	–	+
Age	Child	Child	Child	Child-Young Adult	Older Adult	Young Adult
Genetics	+	+	+	–	–	±
Organic CNS lesion	–	–	–	–	++	++++

Abbreviations: REM, rapid eye movement; SWA, slow wave arousal

Table 3
Differentiating patterns between NFLE and parasomnias: discriminatory components on history

	NFLE	Parasomnia
Duration	Duration <2 min	Duration >10 min
Timing at night	Events in first 30 minutes	Events later in the night
Number of events	Multiple events per night	One or 2 events per night only
Complexity	Complex behavior uncommon	Often wandering and complex behavior
Semiology	Highly stereotyped	Variable semiology
Recall	Often full recall of event and speech	Event and speech during event not recalled

Data from Derry CP, Davey M, Johns M, et al. Distinguishing sleep disorders from seizures: diagnosing bumps in the night. Arch Neurol 2006;63(5):708.

diazepam have been used to limit nocturnal arousals.[113] Trazodone and certain SSRIs such as paroxetine are effective as well.[114,115] Other co-morbid sleep disorders such as obstructive sleep apnea and periodic limb movements of sleep may be viewed as possible precipitating factors. Management of comorbid sleep disturbances in these patients results in a significant decline in frequency or disappearance of the NREM parasomnias.[116] Cognitive behavioral therapy, biofeedback, relaxation therapy, and hypnosis are helpful in children and adults.[117,118] Interventions such as anticipatory arousal therapy are beneficial, especially in children. Anticipatory awakening is believed to work by either preventing or interrupting the altered underlying electrophysiology of partial arousal, interrupting the disturbing behavioral features of the parasomnia.[119]

Management of RBD

Patients with RBD should be carefully assessed for risks for injury, particularly given the aggressive nature of the events and the potential for displacement and violent behaviors. Active and passive safety measures are a necessity in every patient with possible RBD who experiences aggressive spells and affliction of harm to the bed partner. Practice guidelines are currently being written, and are not yet available in publishable form; the most extensive studies to date include pharmacotherapy with clonazepam (0.25–1 mg by mouth every bedtime), which achieved improvement in most (90%) patients with little evidence of tolerance or abuse.[2,63,120]

Although clonazepam does not normalize abnormal muscle augmentation during REM sleep, it probably exerts its function in preventing the arousals associated with the REM sleep disassociation at the level of the pons.[63,121] Treatment of RBD with melatonin may help normalize or perhaps even restore REM sleep electromyography atonia and may be effective in 87% of patients taking doses of between 3 and 12 mg at bedtime.[122,123] Over-the-counter melatonin is not regulated or approved by the US Food and Drug Administration (FDA), is considered a dietary supplement, may have poor regulations in terms of pharmacologic preparation, and side effects have not been widely studied. Research into treatment with melatonin receptor agonists in patients with RBD is under way, but results are not yet available in publishable form. Other agents that may be helpful for RBD include imipramine (25 mg by mouth every bedtime), carbamazepine (100 mg by mouth 3 times a day) as well as dopamine agonists and precursors (ie, pramipexole and levodopa, respectively).[124–126] One recent study described successful amelioration of RBD with sodium oxybate when other treatments are ineffective or poorly tolerated.[127] This finding also suggests that RBD and cataplexy may in part share a common underlying mechanism.[127]

SUMMARY

Much has been learned in the last few decades about pathogenesis of parasomnias, especially RBD. However, the role of central pattern generators as progenitors for disorders of arousal remains unclear. Although there are pharmacologic and nonpharmacologic management strategies, well-researched standard of practice guidelines, including strategies for evaluation and management, are not yet available in this domain of sleep medicine. Violent behaviors associated with parasomnia probably remain underreported and the forensic implications will undoubtedly continue to challenge the sleep physician as an expert witness.

REFERENCES

1. Mahowald MW, Bornemann MC, Schenck CH. Parasomnias. Semin Neurol 2004;24(3):283–92.
2. Mahowald MW, Ettinger MG. Things that go bump in the night: the parasomnias revisited. J Clin Neurophysiol 1990;7(1):119–43.
3. Brooks S, Kushida CA. Behavioral parasomnias. Curr Psychiatry Rep 2002;4(5):363–8.
4. Fisher C, Kahn E, Edwards A, et al. A psychophysiological study of nightmares and night terrors. I. Physiological aspects of the stage 4 night terror. J Nerv Ment Dis 1973;157(2):75–98.
5. Fisher C, Kahn E, Edwards A, et al. A psychophysiological study of nightmares and night terrors. 3. Mental content and recall of stage 4 night terrors. J Nerv Ment Dis 1974;158(3):174–88.
6. Klackenberg G. Somnambulism in childhood–prevalence, course and behavioral correlations: a prospective longitudinal study (6–16 years). Acta Paediatr Scand 1982;71(3):495–9.
7. Ohayon MM, Guilleminault C, Priest RG. Night terrors, sleepwalking, and confusional arousals in the general population: their frequency and relationship to other sleep and mental disorders. J Clin Psychiatry 1999;60(4):268–76 [quiz 277].
8. Ohayon MM, Caulet M, Priest RG. Violent behavior during sleep. J Clin Psychiatry 1997;58(8):369–76 [quiz: 377].
9. Mahowald MW, Schenck CH. Non-rapid eye movement sleep parasomnias. Neurol Clin 2005;23(4):1077–106, vii.
10. Mahowald MW. Overview of parasomnias. American Academy of Sleep Medicine. 1999 (National Sleep Medicine Course, Westchester (IL)).
11. Tassinari CA, Cantalupo G, Hogl B, et al. Neuroethological approach to frontolimbic epileptic seizures and parasomnias: the same central pattern generators for the same behaviours Rev Neurol (Paris) 2009;165(1):762–8.
12. American Academy of Sleep Medicine. The international classification of sleep disorders: diagnostic and coding manual. 2nd edition. Westchester (IL): American Academy of Sleep Medicine; 2005 . p. 139–47.
13. Shapiro CM, Trajanovic NN, Fedoroff JP. Sexsomnia–a new parasomnia? Can J Psychiatry 2003; 48(5):311–7.
14. Kotagal S. Parasomnias in childhood. Sleep Med Rev 2009;13(2):157–68.
15. Ohayon MM, Priest RG, Zulley J, et al. The place of confusional arousals in sleep and mental disorders: findings in a general population sample of 13,057 subjects. J Nerv Ment Dis 2000;188(6):340–8.
16. Guilleminault C, Moscovitch A, Yuen K, et al. Atypical sexual behavior during sleep. Psychosom Med 2002;64(2):328–36.
17. Roth B, Rechtsch A, Nevsimal S. Hypersomnia with sleep drunkenness. Arch Gen Psychiatry 1972; 26(5):456.
18. Mehlenbeck R, Spirito A, Owens J, et al. The clinical presentation of childhood partial arousal parasomnias. Sleep Med 2000;1(4):307–12.
19. Sheldon SH. Parasomnias in childhood. Pediatr Clin North Am 2004;51(1):69–88, vi.
20. Ebrahim IO. Somnambulistic sexual behaviour (sexsomnia). J Clin Forensic Med 2006;13(4): 219–24.
21. Pillmann F. Complex dream-enacting behavior in sleepwalking. Psychosom Med 2009;71(2):231–4.
22. Schenck CH, Pareja JA, Patterson AL, et al. Analysis of polysomnographic events surrounding 252 slow-wave sleep arousals in thirty-eight adults with injurious sleepwalking and sleep terrors. J Clin Neurophysiol 1998;15(2):159–66.
23. Mahowald MW, Cramer-Bornemann M. NREM sleep-arousal parasomnias. In: Principles and practice of sleep medicine, 4th edition. 2005. p. 889–96
24. Hublin C, Kaprio J, Partinen M, et al. Prevalence and genetics of sleepwalking: a population-based twin study. Neurology 1997;48(1):177–81.
25. Mahowald MW, Bundlie SR, Hurwitz TD, et al. Sleep violence forensic-science implications–polygraphic and video documentation. J Forensic Sci 1990;35(2):413–32.
26. Kotagal S. Parasomnias of childhood. Curr Opin Pediatr 2008;20(6):659–65.
27. Kales A, Soldatos CR, Bixler EO, et al. Hereditary factors in sleepwalking and night terrors. Br J Psychiatry 1980;137:111–8.
28. Bakwin H. Sleep-walking in twins. Lancet 1970; 2(7670):446–7.
29. Broughton RJ. Parasomnias. In: Chokroverty S, editor. Sleep disorders medicine 1994. p. 381–99.
30. Lecendreux M, Bassetti C, Dauvilliers Y, et al. HLA and genetic susceptibility to sleepwalking. Mol Psychiatry 2003;8(1):114–7.
31. Espa F, Ondze B, Deglise P, et al. Sleep architecture, slow wave activity, and sleep spindles in adult patients with sleepwalking and sleep terrors. Clin Neurophysiol 2000;111(5):929–39.
32. Guilleminault C, Poyares D, Abat F, et al. Sleep and wakefulness in somnambulism: a spectral analysis study. J Psychosom Res 2001;51(2):411–6.
33. Gaudreau H, Joncas S, Zadra A, et al. Dynamics of slow-wave activity during the NREM sleep of sleepwalkers and control subjects. Sleep 2000;23(6): 755–60.
34. Szelenberger W, Niemcewicz S, Dabrowska AJ. Sleepwalking and night terrors: psychopathological and psychophysiological correlates. Int Rev Psychiatry 2005;17(4):263–70.
35. Bassetti C, Vella S, Donati F, et al. SPECT during sleepwalking. Lancet 2000;356(9228):484–5.

36. Crisp AH. The sleepwalking/night terrors syndrome in adults. Postgrad Med J 1996; 72(852):599–604.

37. Pressman MR. Disorders of arousal from sleep and violent behavior: the role of physical contact and proximity. Sleep 2007;30(8):1039–47.

38. Mahowald MW, Schenck CH, Goldner M, et al. Parasomnia pseudo-suicide. J Forensic Sci 2003; 48(5):1158–62.

39. Rosen G, Mahowald MW, Ferber R. Sleepwalking, confusional arousals, and sleep terrors in the child. In: Principles and practice of sleep medicine in the child.1995. p. 99–106.

40. Arkin AM. Sleep-talking: a review. J Nerv Ment Dis 1966;143(2):101–22.

41. Liu X, Ma Y, Wang Y, et al. Brief report: an epidemiologic survey of the prevalence of sleep disorders among children 2 to 12 years old in Beijing, China. Pediatrics 2005;115(1 Suppl):266–8.

42. Bae CJ, Lee JK, Foldvary-Schaefer N. The use of sleep studies in neurologic practice. Semin Neurol 2009;29(4):305–19.

43. Derry CP, Duncan JS, Berkovic SF. Paroxysmal motor disorders of sleep: the clinical spectrum and differentiation from epilepsy. Epilepsia 2006; 47(11):1775–91.

44. Derry CP, Davey M, Johns M, et al. Distinguishing sleep disorders from seizures: diagnosing bumps in the night. Arch Neurol 2006;63(5):705–9.

45. Ryvlin P, Rheims S, Risse G. Nocturnal frontal lobe epilepsy. Epilepsia 2006;47(Suppl 2):83–6.

46. Malow BA. Sleep and epilepsy. Neurol Clin 2005; 23(4):1127–47.

47. Bazil CW. Nocturnal seizures. Semin Neurol 2004; 24(3):293–300.

48. Provini F, Plazzi G, Tinuper P, et al. Nocturnal frontal lobe epilepsy: a clinical and polygraphic overview of 100 consecutive cases. Brain 1999;122(6): 1017–31.

49. Herman ST. Epilepsy and sleep. Curr Treat Options Neurol 2006;8(4):271–9.

50. American Sleep Disorders Association. International classification of sleep disorders: diagnostic and coding manual. Rochester (MN): American Sleep Disorders Association; 1997.

51. Sellal F, Hirsch E. Nocturnal paroxysmal dystonia. Mov Disord 1993;8(2):252–3.

52. Bhatia KP. The paroxysmal dyskinesias. J Neurol 1999;246(3):149–55.

53. Levin R, Fireman G. Nightmare prevalence, nightmare distress, and self-reported psychological disturbance. Sleep 2002;25(2):205–12.

54. Nguyen TT, Madrid S, Marquez H, et al. Nightmare frequency, nightmare distress, and anxiety. Percept Mot Skills 2002;95(1):219–25.

55. Woodward SH, Arsenault NJ, Murray C, et al. Laboratory sleep correlates of nightmare complaint in PTSD inpatients. Biol Psychiatry 2000;48(11): 1081–7.

56. Mahowald MW, Schenck CH. NREM sleep parasomnias 1996;14(4):675–96.

57. Aldrich MS. Sleep medicine, vol. 53. Oxford New York USA: Oxford University Press, Inc; 1999.

58. Wise MS. Parasomnias in children. Pediatr Ann 1997;26(7):427–33.

59. Penn NE, Kripke DF, Scharff J. Sleep paralysis among medical students. J Psychol 1981;107(Pt 2):247–52.

60. Buzzi G, Cirignotta F. Isolated sleep paralysis: a web survey. Sleep Res Online 2000;3(2):61–6.

61. Snyder S, Hams G. Serotoninergic agents in the treatment of isolated sleep paralysis. Am J Psychiatry 1982;139(9):1202–3.

62. Koran LM, Raghavan S. Fluoxetine for isolated sleep paralysis. Psychosomatics 1993;34(2): 184–7.

63. Schenck CH, Mahowald MW. Polysomnographic, neurologic, psychiatric, and clinical outcome report on 70 consecutive cases with REM sleep behavior disorder (RBD): sustained clonazepam efficacy in 89.5% of 57 treated patients. Cleve Clin J Med 1990;57(Suppl):s9–23.

64. Mahowald MW, Schenck CH. REM sleep behavior disorder. In: Thorpy MJ, editor. Handbook of sleep disorders. New York: Marcel Dekker; 1990. p. 567–93.

65. Schenck CH, Hurwitz TD, Mahowald MW. REM sleep behavior disorder. Am J Psychiatry 1988; 145(5):652.

66. Abad VC, Guilleminault C. Review of rapid eye movement behavior sleep disorders. Curr Neurol Neurosci Rep 2004;4(2):157–63.

67. Ozekmekci S, Apaydin H, Kilic E. Clinical features of 35 patients with Parkinson's disease displaying REM behavior disorder. Clin Neurol Neurosurg 2005;107(4):306–9.

68. Schenck CH, Bundlie SR, Patterson AL, et al. Rapid eye movement sleep behavior disorder. A treatable parasomnia affecting older adults. JAMA 1987;257(13):1786–9.

69. Comella CL, Nardine TM, Diederich NJ, et al. Sleep-related violence, injury, and REM sleep behavior disorder in Parkinson's disease. Neurology 1998;51:526–9.

70. Eisehsehr I, Parrino L, Noachtar S, et al. Sleep in Lennox-Gastaut syndrome: the role of the cyclic alternating pattern (CAP) in the gate control of clinical seizures and generalized polyspikes. Epilepsy Res 2001;46:241–50.

71. Tachibana M, Tanaka K, Hishikawa Y, et al. A sleep study of acute psychotic states due to alcohol and meprobamate addiction. Adv Sleep Res 1975;2: 177–205.

72. Passouant P, Cadilhac J, Ribstein M. Les priva-
tions de sommeil avec mouvements oculaires
par les anti-depresseurs [Sleep privation with
eye movements using antidepressive agents].
Rev Neurol 1972;127:173–92 [in French].

73. Guilleminault C, Raynal D, Takahashi S, et al. Evaluation of short-term and long-term treatment of the
narcolepsy syndrome with clomipramine hydrochloride. Acta Neurol Scand 1976;54:71–87.

74. Besset A. Effect of antidepressants on human
sleep. Adv Biosci 1978;21:141–8.

75. Shimizu T, Ookawa M, Iijuma S, et al. Effect of clomipramine on nocturnal sleep of normal human
subjects. Annu Rev Pharmacopsychiat Res Found
1985;16:138.

76. Bental E, Lavie P, Sharf B. Severe hypermotility
during sleep in treatment of cataplexy with clomipramine. Isr J Med Sci 1979;15:607–9.

77. Akindele MO, Evans JI, Oswald I. Mono-amine
oxidase inhibitors, sleep and mood. Electroencephalogr Clin Neurophysiol 1970;29:47–56.

78. Carlander B, Touchon J, Ondze B, et al. REM sleep
behavior disorder induced by cholinergic treatment in Alzheimer's disease. J Sleep Res 1996;
5(Suppl 1):28.

79. Ross JS, Shua-Haim JR. Aricept-induced nightmares in Alzheimer's disease: 2 case reports.
J Am Geriatr Soc 1998;46:119–20.

80. Schenck CH, Mahowald MW, Kim SW, et al. Prominent eye movements during NREM sleep and REM
sleep behavior disorder associated with fluoxetine
treatment of depression and obsessive-compulsive
disorder. Sleep 1992;15:226–35.

81. Schutte S, Doghramji K. REM behavior disorder
seen with venlafaxine (Effexor). Sleep Res 1996;
25:364.

82. Stolz SE, Aldrich MS. REM sleep behavior disorder
associated with caffeine abuse. Sleep Res 1991;
20:341.

83. Vorona RD, Ware JC. Exacerbation of REM sleep
behavior disorder by chocolate ingestion: a case
report. Sleep Med 2002;3:365–7.

84. Friedman JH. Presumed rapid eye movement
behavior disorder in Machado-Joseph disease
(spinocerebellar ataxia type 3). Mov Disord 2002;
17(6):1350–3.

85. Xi Z, Luning W. REM sleep behavior disorder in
a patient with pontine stroke. Sleep Med 2009;
10(1):143–6.

86. Schenck CH, Mahowald MW. Rapid eye movement
sleep parasomnias. Neurol Clin 2005;23(4):1107–
26.

87. Plazzi G, Montagna P. Remitting REM sleep
behavior disorder as the initial sign of multiple sclerosis. Sleep Med 2002;3(5):437–9.

88. Arnulf I, Merino-Andreu M, Bloch F, et al. REM
sleep behavior disorder and REM sleep without
atonia in patients with progressive supranuclear
palsy. Sleep 2005;28(3):349–54.

89. Gagnon JF, Petit D, Fantini ML, et al. REM sleep
behavior disorder and REM sleep without atonia
in probable Alzheimer disease. Sleep 2006;
29(10):1321–5.

90. Pareja JA, Caminero AB, Masa JF, et al. A first case
of progressive supranuclear palsy and pre-clinical
REM sleep behavior disorder presenting as inhibition of speech during wakefulness and somniloquy
with phasic muscle twitching during REM sleep.
Neurologia 1996;11:304–6.

91. Boeve BF, Silber MH, Ferman JT, et al. Association
of REM sleep behavior disorder and neurodegenerative disease may reflect an underlying synu-
cleinopathy. Mov Disord 2001;16:622–30.

92. Boeve BF, Silber MH, Parisi JE, et al. Synucleinop-
athy pathology often underlies REM sleep behavior
disorder and dementia or parkinsonism. Neurology
2003;61:40–5.

93. Schenck CH, Bundlie SR, Mahowald MW. Delayed
emergence of a parkinsonian disorder in 38% of 29
older men initially diagnosed with idiopathic rapid
eye movement sleep behavior disorder. Neurology
1996;46:388–93.

94. Montplaisir J, Petit D, Decary A, et al. Sleep
and quantitative EEG in patients with progressive supranuclear palsy. Neurology 1997;49:
999–1003.

95. Nevsimalova S, Prihodova I, Kemlink D, et al. REM
behavior disorder (RBD) can be one of the first
symptoms of childhood narcolepsy. Sleep Med
2007;8(7–8):784–6.

96. Schenck CH, Mahowald MW. Motor dyscontrol in
narcolepsy: rapid-eye-movement (REM) sleep
without atonia and REM sleep behavior disorder.
Ann Neurol 1992;32:3–10.

97. Jouvet M, Delorme F. Locus coeruleus et sommeil
paradoxal. C R Soc Biol 1965;159:895–9.

98. Schenck CH, Bundlie SR, Ettinger MG, et al. Chronic
behavioral disorders of human REM sleep: a new
category of parasomnia. Sleep 1986;9:293–308.

99. Paparrigopoulos TJ. REM sleep behaviour
disorder: clinical profiles and pathophysiology. Int
Rev Psychiatry 2005;17(4):293–300.

100. Mahowald M, Schenck C. REM sleep parasomnias.
In: Kryger MH, Roth T, Dement WC, editors. Princi-
ples and practice of sleep medicine. 3rd edition.
Philadelphia: W.B. Saunders; 2000. p. 724–37.

101. Eisensehr I, Linke R, Noachtar S, et al. Reduced
striatal dopamine transporters in idiopathic rapid
eye movement sleep behavior disorder. Comparison with Parkinson's disease and controls. Brain
2000;123:1155–60.

102. Eisehsehr I, Linke R, Tatsch K, et al. Increased
muscle activity during rapid eye movement sleep
correlates with decrease of striatal presynaptic

dopamine transporters. IPT and IBZM SPECT imaging in subclinical and clinically manifest idiopathic REM sleep behavior disorder, Parkinson's disease, and controls. Sleep 2003;26:507–12.

103. Albin RL, Koeppe RA, Chervin RD, et al. Decreased striatal dopaminergic innervation in REM sleep behavior disorder. Neurology 2000;55:1410–2.

104. Gilman S, Koeppe RA, Chervin R, et al. REM sleep behavior disorder is related to striatal monoaminergic deficit in MSA. Neurology 2003;61:29–34.

105. Iranzo A, Santamaria J, Tolosa E. The clinical and pathophysiological relevance of REM sleep behavior disorder in neurodegenerative diseases. Sleep Med Rev 2009;13(6):385–401.

106. Fantini ML, Gagnon JF, Petit D, et al. Slowing of electroencephalogram in rapid eye movement sleep behavior disorder. Ann Neurol 2003;53(6):774–80.

107. Raffaele M, Michele T, Alessandra R. The FLEP scale in diagnosing nocturnal frontal lobe epilepsy, NREM and REM parasomnias: data from a tertiary sleep and epilepsy unit. Epilepsia 2008;49(9):1581–5.

108. Schenck CH, Mahowald MW. REM parasomnias. Neurol Clin 1996;14:697–720.

109. Schenck CH, Mahowald MW. REM sleep behavior disorder: clinical, developmental, and neuroscience perspectives 16 years after its formal identification in SLEEP. Sleep 2002;25(2):120–38.

110. Mahowald MW. Parasomnias. Med Clin North Am 2004;88(3):669–78, ix.

111. Bonakis A, Howard RS, Ebrahim IO, et al. REM sleep behaviour disorder (RBD) and its associations in young patients. Sleep Med 2009;10(6):641–5.

112. Stores G. Rapid eye movement sleep behaviour disorder in children and adolescents. Dev Med Child Neurol 2008;50(10):728–32.

113. Schenck CH, Mahowald MW. Long-term, nightly benzodiazepine treatment of injurious parasomnias and other disorders of disrupted nocturnal sleep in 170 adults. Am J Med 1996;100(3):333–7.

114. Balon R. Sleep terror disorder and insomnia treated with trazodone: a case report. Ann Clin Psychiatry 1994;6(3):161–3.

115. Lillywhite AR, Wilson SJ, Nutt DJ. Successful treatment of night terrors and somnambulism with paroxetine. Br J Psychiatry 1994;164(4):551–4.

116. Guilleminault C, Kirisoglu C, Bao G, et al. Adult chronic sleepwalking and its treatment based on polysomnography. Brain 2005;128(5):1062–9.

117. Sadeh A. Cognitive-behavioral treatment for childhood sleep disorders. Clin Psychol Rev 2005;25(5):612–28.

118. Hurwitz TD, Mahowald MW, Schenck CH, et al. A retrospective outcome study and review of hypnosis as treatment of adults with sleepwalking and sleep terror. J Nerv Ment Dis 1991;179(4):228–33.

119. Tobin JD Jr. Treatment of somnambulism with anticipatory awakening. J Pediatr 1993;122(3):426–7.

120. Mahowald MW, Schenck CH. REM sleep behavior disorder. Philadelphia: WB Saunders; 1994.

121. Lapierre O, Montplaisir J. Polysomnographic features of REM sleep behavior disorder: Development of a scoring method. Neurology 1992;42:1371–4.

122. Takeuchi N, Uchimura N, Hashizume Y, et al. Melatonin therapy for REM sleep behavior disorder. Psychiatry Clin Neurosci 2001;55(3):267–9.

123. Boeve B. Melatonin for treatment of REM sleep behavior disorder: response in 8 patients. Sleep 2001;24(Suppl):A35.

124. Schmidt MH, Koshal VB, Schmidt HS. Use of pramipexole in REM sleep behavior disorder: results from a case series. Sleep Med 2006;7(5):418–23.

125. Fantini ML, Gagnon J-F, Filipini D, et al. The effects of pramipexole in REM sleep behavior disorder. Neurology 2003;61:1418–20.

126. Tan A, Salgado M, Fahn S. Rapid eye movement sleep behavior disorder preceding Parkinson's disease with therapeutic response to levodopa. Mov Disord 1996;11(2):214–6.

127. Shneerson JM. Successful treatment of REM sleep behavior disorder with sodium oxybate. Clin Neuropharmacol 2009;32(3):158–9.

Clinical Features, Diagnosis and Treatment of Narcolepsy

Imran Ahmed, MD[a,b,*], Michael Thorpy, MD[a,b]

KEYWORDS

- Narcolepsy • Symptoms • Genetics
- Epidemiology • Pathophysiology
- Differential diagnosis • Pediatric • Treatment

HISTORY

Narcolepsy, from the Greek words "narco," meaning numbness, stupor, or stiffness, and "lepsy," meaning fit or seizure, literally translates to mean a fit of stupor or stiffness. The attacks of stupor were identified as sleep episodes. Narcolepsy was originally described by Gelineau in 1880 as a disorder involving excessive sleepiness and sleep attacks associated with a variety of emotional states. He also described episodes of falls or astasia, which were later termed cataplexy. Westphal, in 1877, further detailed these episodes of muscle weakness emphasizing preservation of consciousness during the attacks. Before these accounts, in the early nineteenth century, there were reports describing automatic behavior, sleep paralysis, and hypnagogic hallucinations; however, these phenomena were not depicted in Gelineau's or Westphal's description of narcolepsy. More than half a century later, Daniels, in 1930, reported the relationship between the daytime sleepiness, cataplexy, hypnagogic/hypnapompic hallucinations, and sleep paralysis in narcolepsy. About 3 decades later (1960), Vogel demonstrated the connection between narcolepsy and sleep onset rapid eye movement (REM) sleep. The International Symposium on Narcolepsy, in 1975, characterized narcolepsy by excessive sleepiness and sleep (particularly REM sleep)-wake cycle instability. Excessive sleepiness and the pathologic manifestations of REM sleep, including cataplexy, sleep paralysis, and hypnagogic hallucinations were identified as its major symptoms. In the 1980s, research in narcolepsy found an association with HLA-DR2 (later renamed DR15 and then with DRB1*1501/DRB1*1503). Further studies identified an association with HLA DQB1*0602. Although these leukocyte antigens are found in many non-narcoleptic individuals, their discovery in patients with narcolepsy suggested a possible genetic susceptibility for some event, such as autoimmune activation. Decades later, non–sleep-related research led to the accidental discovery of a neuropeptide, hypocretin/orexin, by 2 independent groups in 2005, which is now believed to be responsible for many of the symptoms of narcolepsy. Also in this year, the International Classification of Sleep Disorders, second edition, divided narcolepsy into 2 subtypes: narcolepsy with cataplexy and narcolepsy without cataplexy. Currently, further research is underway to better understand the pathophysiology and other aspects of the disorder.

CLINICAL FEATURES

Narcolepsy is a disorder of the central nervous system for which there is no known cure. The

a Montefiore Medical Center, Albert Einstein College of Medicine, Bronx, NY, USA
b Neurology Department, Sleep-Wake Disorders Center, 111 East 210th Street, Bronx, NY 10467, USA
* Corresponding author. Neurology Department, Sleep-Wake Disorders Center, 111 East 210th Street, Bronx, NY 10467.
E-mail address: iahmed00@yahoo.com

Clin Chest Med 31 (2010) 371–381
doi:10.1016/j.ccm.2010.02.014
0272-5231/10/$ – see front matter © 2010 Published by Elsevier Inc.

effects of narcolepsy are largely manifested during periods of wakefulness. Narcolepsy is described as a syndrome consisting of excessive daytime sleepiness (EDS) (including periods of irresistible sleep), cataplexy, sleep paralysis, and hypnagogic hallucinations; additional features include automatic behaviors and fragmented or disrupted nighttime sleep.

Narcolepsy typically begins with the symptom of excessive sleepiness and other symptoms of variable severity may develop slowly, suddenly, or not at all. Excessive sleepiness is common to other illnesses and can occur under certain circumstances in normal individuals. Patients with narcolepsy often have an irresistible urge to sleep at inopportune times whether it is during monotonous sedentary tasks or while performing mentally or physically demanding activities. For instance, they may fall asleep while eating, while listening to a lecture, during conversations, during sexual intercourse, while driving a car, or while operating heavy machinery. These sleep episodes occur about 3 to 5 times per day in most patients and usually vary from a few minutes to several hours in duration.[1] It is typically reported that after these sleep episodes or after taking scheduled naps, patients wake up refreshed and may not feel sleepy again for up to a few hours later; however, there are many patients who indicate persistent sleepiness despite taking these naps (albeit their sleepiness becomes less severe). Patients may also experience microsleep events, which are split seconds of sleep that intrude into the waking state. On awaking from these episodes, the patients may not be aware that they were asleep and continue the activity they were performing before the sleep event. It is likely that such episodes are at least partially associated with patients' complaints of difficulty concentrating, inattention, or memory impairment.

Cataplexy is the most specific symptom of narcolepsy consisting of an abrupt, bilateral (occasionally unilateral) loss of skeletal muscle tone. When severe, an episode of cataplexy may cause a patient to collapse to the ground, sometimes suffering injury. During a cataplexy attack, which may last up to several minutes, the patient is unable to move; however, the diaphragm and ocular muscles are unaffected. During this time, the patient remains awake, aware of their surroundings and able to remember the details of the event. If the attack is prolonged, however, sleep may follow. More commonly, attacks of cataplexy are partial, affecting only certain muscle groups, such as the arms, neck, or face. During partial cataplexy attacks, the jaw may sag, the head may droop, and speech becomes garbled.[2]

An unusual aspect of cataplexy is that it is triggered by the occurrence of sudden emotion. Most commonly, cataplexy is caused by laughter or humorous experiences although sometimes even the memory of a humorous event can precipitate an attack. Other triggers for cataplexy include anger, embarrassment, surprise, stress, or even sexual arousal.[3] Physicians who treat these patients often encounter distressing stories about the effect of cataplexy on patient's lives. For example, the excitement of feeling the tug of a fish on a line, or bowling a strike, may limit their ability to participate in these activities because of the likelihood of suffering attacks of cataplexy.

Similar to cataplexy, patients with sleep paralysis experience a brief loss of voluntary muscle control with an inability to move or speak and retention of awareness during the event. Unlike, cataplexy, these episodes are not provoked by intense emotion or stress. The phenomena usually occur during sleep-wake transitions and are often associated with fearful hypnapompic or hypnagogic hallucinations. The events typically remit on their own within 1 to 10 minutes, but can also be terminated when someone touches the patient.

Narcolepsy patients also experience hallucinations or intense dreamlike states when falling asleep (hypnagogic), or more commonly when awaking from sleep (hypnopompic).[4] These dreams may occasionally be pleasant; however, usually they are frightening or disturbing to the patient. They are usually visual or auditory and occasionally involve other senses, for example, tactile or vestibular. The visual hallucinations may be in color or appear as dark shadows and typically consist of simple forms, for example, circles or multisided geometric figures, but can be more intricate, for instance, animals or people. Similarly, the auditory hallucinations may manifest as simple sounds, such as knocking on a door or a phone ring, or more complex tunes, such as a musical composition. The auditory hallucinations may be threatening or derogatory statements or words that can leave patients upset or even terrified. Occasionally, patients report hallucinations such as smelling smoke (or other scent/odor) or having a sense of falling or feeling that someone or something is touching them.

Automatic behavior is the performance of simple or complex routine tasks by individuals who remain unaware of the activity. These behaviors range from activities such as talking on the phone or writing to walking, cooking, driving, or operating heavy machinery. Some patients report that they have ordered items by phone and did not remember doing so; or being unable to read the notes they took in class because it was in chicken scratch; or driving home from work and not realizing how they got there. The personal and public hazards of such behaviors are self- evident.

It is generally understood that narcolepsy is a disorder of excessive sleepiness; accordingly, many people are often surprised to learn that patients with narcolepsy often report difficulty in maintaining sleep at night. The dysfunction of central sleep regulation causes frequent inappropriate transitions between sleep and wakefulness. Narcolepsy results in sleep and wake episodes that occur throughout the 24-hour cycle; thus, most patients with narcolepsy have difficultly maintaining sleep or full alertness for consolidated periods. They report frequent nocturnal awakenings and occasionally indicate that they do not sleep for long periods during the night.

EPIDEMIOLOGY

Narcolepsy can begin in infancy (rarely) or as late as old age, but most commonly before age 25 years, and usually in the first 2 decades of life.[5] It affects men and women equally; however, some studies indicate a slightly greater prevalence in men.[6] Although the exact number of patients with narcolepsy is not known with certainty, it is by definition a rare disorder, affecting approximately 1 in 2000 people in the United States. Although there is a greater incidence of narcolepsy among first-degree relatives, it occurs less frequently than would be predicted based on normal patterns of inheritance.[7] Therefore, it has been suggested that there may be a genetically controlled susceptibility to an environmentally controlled event, such as an autoimmune process. There is reportedly a predisposition for narcolepsy based on race and ethnicity as a review of the literature indicates that the prevalence of narcolepsy/cataplexy ranges from a low of 0.002% among Israeli Jews to a high of 0.15% among the Japanese general population. More recently, a general population study with a representative sample of more than 18,000 individuals in 5 European countries estimated a prevalence of 0.047%.[8]

The true prevalence of narcolepsy is difficulty to assess as some of its clinical and polysomnographic/multiple sleep latency test (MSLT) features overlap with other disorders, such as depression, epilepsy, psychiatric illness, or other sleep disorders, and even with normal individuals. Accordingly, an accurate diagnosis can often require 10 years after the onset of symptoms. It is estimated that less than 50% of patients with narcolepsy have been diagnosed.[9,10]

The prevalence of cataplexy among patients with narcolepsy varies widely with estimates ranging from 60% to 90%[11,12] of narcoleptics. Once present, patients generally report that cataplexy remains persistent with only minor fluctuations in severity; however, the severity and frequency of attacks may vary widely and range from occasional to many attacks daily. A few patients have reported spontaneous remission of cataplexy attacks. It has been suggested that a decline in cataplexy over time represents the ability of patients to adapt to their illness and learning to avoid those situations where cataplexy is most likely to occur.

The prevalence of sleep paralysis in patients with narcolepsy ranges from 28% to 46%[1,13]; however, it may be seen in 3% to 6% of the normal population.[14] Hypnopompic/hypnagogic hallucinations have a prevalence in narcolepsy of about 25%.[13] Automatic behaviors prevalence rate in narcolepsy varies from 20% to 40%.[12]

GENETICS

Many studies suggest a genetic influence to narcolepsy. An early study by Kessler and colleagues[15] identified 9 patients with narcolepsy and 17 patients with EDS among first-degree relatives of 50 narcoleptic probands. Guilleminault and colleagues[16] showed that 40% of probands (out of a clinic population of 334 unrelated patients with narcolepsy) had at least 1 family member with an isolated daytime sleepiness complaint and 6% had a positive family history of narcolepsy. Mignot[17] reported that 1% to 2% of first-degree relatives have narcolepsy with cataplexy and 4% to 6% of first-degree relatives may have isolated symptoms of narcolepsy.

Narcolepsy with cataplexy is closely associated with the human leukocyte antigen (HLA) subtypes DR2 (DRB1*1501) and DQ (DQB1*0602). Both these subtypes are present in most patients with narcolepsy; however, DQB1*0602 is more specifically associated with narcolepsy in African American patients. The most common HLA marker associated with narcolepsy with cataplexy is DQB1*0602 with a prevalence ranging from 85% to 95%. In patients with narcolepsy without cataplexy, the HLA DQB1*0602 prevalence is also increased (about 40%), but clearly less so than in patients with cataplexy. Unfortunately, it is a poor screening or diagnostic test because it also has a high prevalence of approximately 26% in the general population. Some studies have suggested that individuals with this HLA subtype are predisposed to developing narcolepsy.[18]

Genetic factors other than HLA-DQ and DR probably play a role in the development of narcolepsy. Nakayama and colleagues[19] and others have reported an association between narcolepsy and chromosome 4p13-q21. Polymorphisms in the tumor necrosis factor (TNF) alpha and TNF receptor 2 genes have also been implicated.[20,21] A case report by Peyron and colleagues[22] described a patient with early onset narcolepsy with a mutation of the hypocretin gene.

PATHOPHYSIOLOGY

The pathophysiology of narcolepsy with cataplexy has recently been better understood with the discovery of the neuropeptide hypocretin.[23,24] Hypocretin-containing neurons are located in the perifornical and lateral hypothalamus where they project widely to communicate with numerous brain nuclei including those responsible for the regulation of sleep and alertness. Current evidence suggests that most cases of narcolepsy with cataplexy are associated with loss of hypocretin-containing hypothalamic neurons. These patients display unusually low or undetectable concentrations (≤ 110 pg/mL) of hypocretin in cerebrospinal fluid (CSF) and postmortem binding studies have demonstrated an 85% to 95% decrease in hypocretin-containing neurons in narcolepsy patients.[25,26] Another study also found a loss of about a third of the hypothalamic hypocretin-containing cells in 1 patient with narcolepsy without cataplexy.[27] This suggests that narcolepsy without cataplexy may be caused by a partial loss of hypocretin cells. An autoimmune process may be responsible for the loss of the hypocretin neurons; however, antibodies to hypocretin and hypocretin receptors have not been found.[28–31] Recently, increased antistreptococcal antibodies were reported in patients with recent onset of narcolepsy, suggesting streptococcal infections may be an inciting event that is initiating an autoimmune process.[32]

Cataplexy can be viewed as REM sleep atonia that intrudes into wakefulness during episodes of, among other emotions, laughter. Hypocretin release is usually maximal during periods of normal wakefulness and is believed to increase muscle tone through activation of a motor facilitatory system in the locus coeruleus and the raphe nuclei.[33] These neurons increase the activity of motor neurons through the release norepinephrine and serotonin. These same neurons are inhibited during REM sleep by γ-aminobutyric acid (GABA)-containing neurons that are activated by the pontine REM sleep generator. In the absence of sufficient levels of hypocretin, the balance of motor excitation and inhibition elicited by emotional stimuli is altered, causing inactivation of the facilitatory system and activation of the

inhibitory system. The net result is a decrease in muscle tone resulting in cataplexy in narcoleptic patients. For a detailed discussion on the mechanism of REM sleep atonia, see Houghton and colleagues.[33]

As mentioned earlier, there is a higher occurrence of HLA DQB1*0602 in narcolepsy patients than in the general population, and a somewhat higher prevalence of among first-degree relatives, although less than would be expected from normal inheritance patterns.[30] Therefore, it is suspected that patients with this HLA marker (and likely other currently unknown genetic link) may possess a genetic susceptibility for some event that leads to the development of narcolepsy. Environmental insults such as infections,[32,34] head trauma,[35,36] or even a change in sleeping habits[34] have been associated with the onset of narcolepsy.

DIAGNOSIS

There are 3 main types of narcolepsy: narcolepsy with cataplexy, narcolepsy without cataplexy, and secondary narcolepsy (**Box 1**). Narcolepsy with cataplexy is defined as excessive sleepiness that occurs for at least 3 months and is associated with definite cataplexy. The diagnosis may be confirmed by polysomnography followed by a MSLT.[37] Alternatively, a low CSF hypocretin level (≤ 110 pg/mL or one-third of mean normal control values) is diagnostic.[26] The polysomnography should confirm at least 6 hours of sleep and exclude other sleep disorders that could account for the symptoms, such as obstructive sleep apnea syndrome. The polysomnograph usually shows a short sleep latency and may show early REM sleep onset. Further analysis of the sleep architecture can also reveal increased stage 1 sleep and frequent arousals. The MSLT should exhibit 2 or more sleep onset REM periods with a mean sleep latency of 8 minutes or less.[8]

Patients who do not have cataplexy or have atypical cataplexy-like events, and in whom other sleep disorders have been excluded, require confirmatory sleep studies (nocturnal polysomnography followed by an MSLT) or CSF hypocretin levels for the diagnosis. Similarly, such studies are required to establish the diagnosis of secondary narcolepsy that temporally occurs with an underlying neurologic disorder.

As mentioned earlier, HLA testing is not a useful screening or diagnostic tool; however, it might be useful in atypical narcolepsy with cataplexy presentations. A negative test should encourage the physician to make certain other sleep disorders are excluded before assigning a diagnosis of narcolepsy.

Box 1
Diagnostic criteria for narcolepsy

Narcolepsy with cataplexy

1. Excessive daytime sleepiness of at least 3 months duration
2. A definite history of cataplexy is present

May be confirmed by

3. Polysomnogram ruling out other causes of disrupted nocturnal sleep and demonstrating at least 6 hours of sleep followed by an MSLT showing a sleep latency of less than or equal to 8 minutes and 2 or more sleep onset REM periods or
4. A CSF hypocretin-1 level less than or equal to 110 pg/mL

Narcolepsy without cataplexy

1. Excessive daytime sleepiness of at least 3 months duration
2. No cataplexy or questionable or atypical cataplexy-like episodes

Must be confirmed by

3. Polysomnogram ruling out other causes of disrupted nocturnal sleep and demonstrating at least 6 hours of sleep followed by an MSLT showing a sleep latency of less than or equal to 8 minutes and 2 or more sleep onset REM periods

Narcolepsy caused by a medical condition

1. Excessive daytime sleepiness of at least 3 months duration
2. A significant underlying medical or neurologic condition accounts for the daytime sleepiness
3. A definite history of cataplexy is present or
4. When there is no cataplexy or questionable/atypical cataplexy-like episodes are present, a polysomnogram ruling out other causes of disrupted nocturnal sleep and demonstrating at least 6 hours of sleep followed by an MSLT showing a sleep latency of less than or equal to 8 minutes and 2 or more sleep onset REM periods must be present
5. If either condition 3 or 4 is not met, CSF hypocretin-1 levels must be less than 110 pg/mL (or 30% of normal control values) in a noncomatose patient

Adapted from American Academy of Sleep Medicine. International classification of sleep disorders. 2nd edition. Westchester (IL): American Academy of Sleep Medicine; 2005; with permission.

PEDIATRIC CONSIDERATIONS

Generally speaking, narcolepsy is rare in children less than 5 years of age. In a meta-analysis of 235 patients, Challamel and colleagues[38] reported that 4.6% of the patients were younger than 5 years of age at the time of the diagnosis. Furthermore, it is difficult to identify narcolepsy symptoms in preschool children as they are not able to provide an accurate history of cataplexy, hypnagogic hallucinations, or sleep paralysis, and many normal children in this age group take habitual naps (making it difficult to identify excessive sleepiness). School-aged children may present with the reappearance of daytime naps after they had previously discontinued regular napping. Often the sleepiness presents as behavioral problems, decreased performance, inattentiveness, lack of energy, or bizarre hallucinations. It is not uncommon for physicians to misinterpret some of these symptoms as primarily psychological or psychiatric and this may lead to inappropriate management including initial referral to psychiatric or educational rather than neurologic or sleep disorder services.

A diagnosis of narcolepsy can be made based on the presence of cataplexy (if clearly identified by history or documented on video polysomnogram), a positive MSLT study (a negative MSLT does not necessarily exclude a diagnosis of narcolepsy in children) or by demonstrating a low CSF hypocretin-1 level. An assessment of the child's Tanner stage of sexual development is necessary to compare sleep study results with normal values of nocturnal total sleep time, daytime sleep latency, and daytime REM sleep latency as these are closely linked to the Tanner stages.[39] Nevertheless, normal values on sleep studies, namely the MSLT, have not been standardized in subjects younger than 8 years of age and results should be interpreted with care.

DIFFERENTIAL DIAGNOSIS

The individual symptoms of narcolepsy are also seen in other disorders and can be a normal phenomenon in certain circumstances (eg, sleep deprivation). **Table 1** lists some other disorders associated with narcolepsy symptoms.

TREATMENT

There is no known cure for narcolepsy and therefore treatment is targeted at symptom management. Even with optimum management, EDS and cataplexy are seldom completely controlled.

Nonpharmacologic management should be initiated in all patients. Patient education is an important component of any treatment plan for narcolepsy. Good sleep habits with avoidance of sleep deprivation and/or irregular sleep patterns should be emphasized. The scheduling of short

Table 1
Differential diagnosis of narcolepsy

	Some Differentiating Features
EDS	
Other sleep disorders	
Idiopathic hypersomnia	Naps are unrefreshing, less than 2 SOREMs, may be associated with autonomic system dysfunction
Sleep-related breathing disorder	Respiratory events present during PSG, RDI>5
Recurrent hypersomnia	Normal sleep between periods of hypersomnia
Environmental sleep disorder	History of disruptive environmental feature during sleep
Behaviorally induced, insufficient sleep syndrome	History and/or sleep logs or actigraphy reveal decreased sleep
Circadian rhythm disorders	Sleep cycle is advanced, delayed, irregular or disrupted by shift work
Other	
Recreational drugs or medications	History of drug or substance use that may cause sleepiness, serum or urine drug screen may be revealing
Thalamic stroke	Other neurologic deficits are usually present
Tumor	Imaging studies may be revealing
Metabolic encephalopathy	Metabolic derangements present
Encephalitis	CSF studies often revealing
Depression (or other psychiatric disorder)	Identify by history
Malingering	Identify by history
Cataplexy	
Transient ischemic attack	Usually other vascular risk factors and/or stroke symptoms present; not typically provoked by emotion
Syncope	Consciousness typically not preserved
Seizures (atonic, gelastic)	Positive EEG, consciousness may not be preserved
Sleep paralysis	Not associated with emotion
Diencephalic/brainstem tumors	Imaging may be revealing; other neurologic symptoms may be present
Psychiatric disorders	Identify by history
Hypnagogic/Hypnapompic Hallucinations	
Sleep onset rumination	Hallucination-like events not visual or auditory
Behaviorally induced insufficient sleep syndrome	Can occur normally in sleep-deprived individuals; demonstrated by sleep logs and/or actigraphy and history
Sleep terrors	Individuals typically do not recall event
Nightmares	Associated with intense fear
Peduncular hallucinosis	Imaging may be revealing
Seizures	Positive EEG
Recreational drugs or medications	History of drug or substance use that may cause sleepiness, serum or urine drug screen revealing
Metabolic encephalopathy	Metabolic derangements present
Psychiatric disorders (eg, schizophrenia)	Identify by (psychiatric) history

(continued on next page)

Table 1
(continued)

	Some Differentiating Features
Sleep Paralysis	
Fatigue	Not frightening
Sleep drunkenness	Weakness, not paralysis, present
Recurrent isolated sleep paralysis	Not typically associated with EDS
Automatic Behaviors	
Complex partial seizures	Positive EEG
Extreme absent-mindedness	Complex activities unusual
Psychiatric disorders	Identify by history
Metabolic encephalopathy	Metabolic derangements present

Abbreviations: CSF, cerebrospinal fluid; EDS, excessive daytime sleepiness; EEG, electroencephalography; PSG, polysomnogram; RDI, Respiratory Disturbance Index; SOREM, sleep onset REM periods.

naps (15–20 minutes) 2 to 3 times per day can help control EDS and improve alertness, but this is impractical in many settings. Patients and family members should also be warned about the potential dangers of sleepiness relative to driving or in other hazardous settings. Unfortunately, lifestyle changes are rarely sufficient to adequately control the symptoms of narcolepsy and most patients require life-long medication to cope with the debilitating effects of the disorder.

Currently, sodium oxybate, amphetamines, methylphenidate, modafinil, and armodafinil are the only medications approved by the US Food and Drug Administration (FDA) for the treatment of narcolepsy. Other medications have been used for years with beneficial results.[40]

EDS

EDS has traditionally been treated with stimulants, such as methylphenidate or dextroamphetamine, but more recently, modafinil or armodafinil have become the first-line treatment of most patients.[41,42] Amphetamines and methylphenidate are indirect sympathomimetics that increase the level of monoamines within the synaptic cleft by enhancing the release of norepinephrine, dopamine, and serotonin, while also blocking their reuptake. The main action responsible for the psychomotor stimulatory effects of these agents is on central dopamine systems. Most clinical studies of stimulant medications report objective improvements in somnolence in 65% to 85% of patients.

Common adverse effects associated with stimulants include nervousness, headaches, irritability, tremor, insomnia, anorexia, gastrointestinal upset, and cardiovascular stimulation.[43] The development of drug tolerance can also occur. Serious problems with long-term stimulant use are uncommon in most patients with narcolepsy. The risk of addiction with stimulant drugs is relatively low (<1% to 3% of cases), and is not higher than that in other patient groups; however, the risk is greater in patients taking high dosages of stimulants, in patients who have received long-term treatment with stimulants, and in those with an underlying psychiatric disorder. Methylphenidate has similar efficacy to dextroamphetamine but has a better therapeutic index because of a lower propensity to produce adverse effects. There is little evidence to support an increased risk of increased blood pressure in normotensive individuals with commonly used dosages of stimulants.

Selegiline, a monoamine oxidase B inhibitor, has produced statistically and clinically significant improvement in narcoleptic symptoms and polysomnographic measures in patients with narcolepsy, but is rarely used in the United States. The main advantage of this agent is its anticataplectic anticataleptic activity in addition to its relatively good alerting effect; however, the main disadvantage is having to maintain a diet low in tyramine.

Modafinil is chemically unrelated to central nervous system (CNS) stimulants, and is the first-line medication in the treatment of daytime sleepiness. It has a low abuse potential and is not associated with rebound hypersomnolence, as are other stimulants. The exact mechanism of action of modafinil is unknown. Modafinil may indirectly increase wakefulness partly through inhibition of GABA release via serotonergic mechanisms, or indirectly on dopaminergic stimulation. It also stimulates norepinephrine inhibition of the sleep-promoting nucleus, the ventrolateral prepotic nucleus.

Modafinil has an elimination half-life of 9 to 14 hours, permitting once-daily administration, although some patients prefer to have a second dose at midday.[44] Usual doses of modafinil are

200 mg/d or 400 mg/d, but higher doses may be required in some patients.[45] The drug is well tolerated, with headache and nausea being the most common side effects. A long-acting isomeric form of modafinil, called armodafinil, has recently become available.[46]

Armodafinil is the dextro-enantiomer component of modafinil. It has a similar therapeutic and side effect profile to modafinil but with the advantage of having a longer elimination half-life. Armodafinil has a T_{max} of about 2 hours and a half-life of about 10 to 14 hours compared with 3 to 4 hours with S-modafinil. This modification of modafinil has a more prolonged effect during the day and may improve daytime sleepiness in the late afternoon and early evening in some patients with narcolepsy. It has been shown to be effective and produces longer wakefulness than modafinil in patients with sleepiness caused by acute sleep loss.[47]

Sodium oxybate, the sodium salt of γ-hydroxy-butyrate (GHB), an endogenous substance in the brain, is an effective medication in the treatment of daytime sleepiness in narcolepsy.[41,48] GHB inhibits the release of several neurotransmitters, including GABA, glutamate, and dopamine. Supraphysiologic concentrations seem necessary in order for GHB to bind to GABA(B) receptors, which are responsible for sleep induction and an increase in slow-wave sleep. The nocturnal sleep effects have been correlated with the improvement in daytime sleepiness in patients with narcolepsy. Sodium oxybate was first described 50 years ago when used as a general anesthetic agent.[49] Consequently, it was administered therapeutically at bedtime to patients suffering from disorders of nocturnal sleep, including narcolepsy; it was found to reduce nocturnal awakenings, increase stage non-REM 3 (delta or slow-wave) sleep, and consolidate REM sleep periods. In addition, the improvements in nocturnal sleep were associated with improvements in the daytime symptoms including cataplexy and EDS. Sodium oxybate's adverse events include dizziness (23% incidence), headache (20%), nausea (16 %), pain (12%), somnolence (9%), sleep disorder (9%), confusion (7%), infection (7%), vomiting (6%), and enuresis (5%) with most described as mild or moderate in severity. Dizziness, nausea, vomiting, and enuresis may be dose-related.[50]

Cataplexy

Although treatment of sleepiness can have a mild beneficial effect on cataplexy, most wake-promoting agents/stimulants do not provide sufficient relief from cataplexy. Most medications used for the treatment of cataplexy have REM sleep suppressant properties and/or increase aminergic (especially by blocking the norepinephrine transporter) transmission.[51] Tricyclic antidepressant agents and serotonin reuptake inhibitors (SSRIs) have been successfully used for decades for the treatment of cataplexy. More recently, sodium oxybate, as mentioned earlier, has been found to be highly efficacious for the treatment of cataplexy in narcolepsy, and is also effective for the treatment of excessive sleepiness as well as improving sleep quality in these patients.

The tricyclic antidepressants (TCAs) were the first drugs discovered to have anticataplectic activity. The anticataplectic effects of TCAs are generally attributed to their ability to block the presynaptic reuptake of catecholamines, thereby enhancing their postsynaptic activity. Several small open-label studies and several decades of use have demonstrated that desmethylimipramine, protriptyline, imipramine, and desipramine have beneficial anticataplectic effects[33]; however, clomipramine remains the most efficacious and widely used. Clomipramine at doses of 10 to 75 mg daily has the most REM-suppressing activity, which may be related to its greater ability to block serotonin reuptake.[51–53] Adverse events commonly associated with TCA therapy include nausea, anorexia, dry mouth, urinary retention, and tachycardia. Men may encounter decreased libido, impotency, or delayed ejaculation. An unusual property of TCAs is the rebound cataplexy phenomenon that occurs on abrupt discontinuation of TCA therapy. When severe, this is known as status cataplecticus and can be disabling for several days.[54]

Like the TCAs, SSRIs also block the presynaptic reuptake of catecholamines, thereby increasing their activity; however, they are much more selective for serotonin than TCAs. Like the TCAs, the SSRIs also inhibit nocturnal REM sleep. Fluvoxamine, zimeldine, femoxetine, paroxetine, and fluoxetine have all been shown to have anticataplectic activity; however, fluoxetine seems to be the most commonly used of the SSRIs for the treatment of cataplexy.[55] As a class, the SSRIs are generally less efficacious than TCAs; however, they are safer and better tolerated than the older antidepressants. Reported adverse events include headache, nausea, weight gain, dry mouth, and delayed ejaculation.[55,56] Other antidepressant medications have also been found to have some anticataplectic activity; these include monoamine oxidase inhibitors such as phenelzine and selegiline, atypical antidepressants such as venlafaxine and atomoxetine, as well as other sympathomimetics such as mazindol (not available in the United States).

Sodium oxybate is the only medication approved by the FDA in the United States for the treatment of cataplexy. Several double-blind placebo-controlled studies have demonstrated its efficacy at nightly doses of 4.5, 6, and 9 g.[57–59]

Fragmented Nocturnal Sleep

As mentioned earlier, sodium oxybate taken at bedtime and again during the night increases slow-wave sleep, decreases light sleep (stage N1 sleep), and decreases the number of arousals. REM sleep is initially increased, but after increasing the dose and duration of therapy, it is decreased.[57]

Other medications have also been tried in the management of the fragmented sleep of patients with narcolepsy. A study evaluating 0.25 mg of triazolam taken at bedtime showed improved sleep efficiency and overall sleep quality.[60] Other medications such as zolpidem, eszopiclone, or clonazepam have been used with varying success in some patients (personal experience and conversations with other sleep medicine physicians).

Sleep Paralysis and Hypnagogic Hallucinations

As described earlier, the use of TCAs or other REM suppressant medications may also result in a decrease in other REM-related narcolepsy symptoms, including sleep paralysis and hypnagogic hallucinations.[61,62] Imipramine and viloxazine have been shown to be effective for hallucinations.[51] Venlafaxine has also been shown to be helpful.

SPECIAL CONSIDERATION
Narcolepsy and Obstructive Sleep Apnea

EDS is a common symptom in narcolepsy and obstructive sleep apnea. When both disorders are present in the same patient, it poses a diagnostic and treatment challenge. The frequency of this co-occurrence and its clinical significance is not known. From the prevalence of obstructive sleep apnea's alone (about 4% of the general population[8]), it is likely that this co-occurrence is not uncommon. Sleep apnea may be seen more frequently with narcolepsy.[63] The pathogenesis for obstructive sleep apnea in patients with narcolepsy seems similar to that of the typical obstructive sleep apnea syndrome.[64] Accordingly, 1 possible reason for this increased prevalence is the increased occurrence of obesity in patients with narcolepsy, especially in children.[65–67] It has been suggested from mice models that hypocretin deficiency may contribute to irregular respirations and apneas.[68] There are also reports that sodium oxybate used to treat narcolepsy symptoms may result in or exacerbate obstructive sleep apnea[69,70]; however, other studies contradict this finding.[71]

It is usually not possible to differentiate the excessive sleepiness caused by obstructive sleep apnea from that caused by narcolepsy. The MSLT criteria used to diagnose narcolepsy (specifically, the presence of 2 or more sleep onset REM periods) can also be present in about 5% of patients with untreated obstructive sleep apnea.[72] Therefore, it is prudent to diagnose and treat a patient's obstructive sleep apnea before confirming a diagnosis of narcolepsy with an MSLT. Residual sleepiness if present can then be pursued with, among other things, a repeat polysomnogram followed by an MSLT. Unfortunately, when obstructive sleep apnea is present in an undiagnosed narcoleptic, it may delay the narcolepsy diagnosis by several years and interfere with its proper management.[73] Accordingly, a physician should always entertain the possibility of narcolepsy in a patient with sleep apnea with residual sleepiness and be vigilant in inquiring about cataplexy.

SUMMARY

Narcolepsy is characterized by EDS, cataplexy, sleep paralysis, and hypnagogic/hypnapompic hallucinations. It is currently believed to be caused by a deficiency in hypocretin-producing neurons in the lateral hypothalamus. Diagnosis is by the presence of appropriate clinical symptoms and confirmation by a polysomnogram followed by an MSLT. The MSLT shows a short sleep latency ($\leq$8 minutes) and 2 or more sleep onset REM periods. In patients with cataplexy, CSF hypocretin levels are typically less than 110 pg/mL. There are nonpharmacologic (eg, scheduled naps, following proper sleep hygiene) and symptom-directed pharmacologic (eg, CNS stimulants, modafinil, sodium oxybate, certain antidepressants) treatments that are usually used together for optimal management of narcolepsy.

REFERENCES

1. Roth B. Narcolepsy and hypersomnia. Basel (Switzerland): S Karger; 1980;66:77.
2. Overeem S, Mignot E, van Dijk JG, et al. Narcolepsy: clinical features, new pathological insights, and future perspectives. J Clin Neurophysiol 2001;18:78–105.
3. Krahn LE, Lymp JF, Moore WR, et al. Characterizing the emotions that trigger cataplexy. J Neuropsychiatry Clin Neurosci 2005;17:45–50.

4. Guilleminault C, Fromherz S. Narcolepsy: diagnosis and management. In: Kryger MH, Roth TA, Dement WC, editors. Principles and practice of sleep medicine. Philadelphia: WB Saunders; 2005. p. 780.

5. Ohayon MM, Ferini-Strambi L, Plazzi G, et al. Frequency of narcolepsy symptoms and other sleep disorders in narcoleptic patients and their first-degree relatives. J Sleep Res 2005;14(4):437–45.

6. Honda Y, Asaka A, Tanimura M, et al. A genetic study of narcolepsy and excessive daytime sleepiness in 308 families with a narcolepsy or hypersomnia proband. In: Guilleminault C, Lugaresi E, editors. Sleep/wake disorders: natural history, epidemiology, and longterm evolution. New York: Raven Press; 1983. p. 187–99.

7. Ohayon MM, Ferini-Strambi L, Plazzi G, et al. How age influences the expression of narcolepsy. J Psychosom Res 2005;59(6):399–405.

8. American Academy of Sleep Medicine. International classification of sleep disorders. 2nd edition. Westchester (IL): American Academy of Sleep Medicine; 2005.

9. Mayer G, Kesper K, Peter H, et al. [Comorbidity in narcoleptic patients]. Dtsch Med Wochenschr 2002;127(38):1942–6 [in German].

10. Kryger MH, Walid R, Manfreda J. Diagnoses received by narcolepsy patients in the year prior to diagnosis by a sleep specialist. Sleep 2002;25(1):36–41.

11. Silber MH, Krahn LE, Olson EJ, et al. The epidemiology of narcolepsy in Olmsted County, Minnesota: a population-based study. Sleep 2002;25(2):197–202.

12. Parkes D. Sleep, its disorders. Philadelphia: WB Saunders; 1985.

13. Yoss RE, Daly DD. Narcolepsy. Arch Intern Med 1960;106:168–71.

14. Goode GB. Sleep paralysis. Arch Neurol 1962;6: 228–34.

15. Kessler S, Guilleminault C, Dement W. A family study of 50 REM narcoleptics. Acta Neurol Scand 1974; 50(4):503–12.

16. Guilleminault C, Mignot E, Grumet FC. Familial patterns of narcolepsy. Lancet 1989;2(8676):1376–9.

17. Mignot E. Genetic and familial aspects of narcolepsy. Neurology 1998;50(2 Suppl 1):S16–22.

18. Mignot E, Lin L, Rogers W, et al. Complex HLA-DR and –DQ interactions confer risk of narcolepsy-cataplexy in three ethnic groups. Am J Hum Genet 2001; 68:686–99.

19. Nakayama J, Miura M, Honda M, et al. Linkage of human narcolepsy with HLA association to chromosome 4p13-q21. Genomics 2000;65:84–6.

20. Wieczorek S, Gencik M, Rujescu D, et al. TNF alpha promoter polymorphisms and narcolepsy. Tissue Antigens 2003;61:437–42.

21. Kato T, Honda M, Kuwata S, et al. Novel polymorphism in the promoter region of the tumor necrosis factor alpha gene: no association with narcolepsy. Am J Med Genet 1999;88(4):301–4.

22. Peyron C, Faraco J, Rogers W, et al. A mutation in a case of early onset narcolepsy and a generalized absence of hypocretin peptides in human narcoleptic brains. Nat Med 2000;6:991–7.

23. Nishino S, Ripley B, Overeem S, et al. Hypocretin (orexin) deficiency in human narcolepsy. Lancet 2000;355:39–40.

24. Zeitzer JM, Nishino S, Mignot E. The neurobiology of hypocretins (orexins), narcolepsy and related therapeutic interventions. Trends Pharmacol Sci 2006; 27(7):368–74.

25. Thannickal TC, Moore RY, Niehus R, et al. Reduced number of hypocretin neurons in human narcolepsy. Neuron 2000;27:469–74.

26. Mignot E, Lammers GJ, Ripley B, et al. The role of cerebrospinal fluid hypocretin measurement in the diagnosis of narcolepsy and other hypersomnias. Arch Neurol 2002;59:1553–62.

27. Thannickal TC, Nienhuis R, Siegel JM. Localized loss of hypocretin (orexin) cells in narcolepsy without cataplexy. Sleep 2009;32(8):993–8.

28. Scammell TE. The frustrating and mostly fruitless search for an autoimmune cause of narcolepsy. Sleep 2006;29(5):601–2.

29. Black JL 3rd. Narcolepsy: a review of evidence for autoimmune diathesis. Int Rev Psychiatry 2005; 17(6):461–9.

30. Dauvilliers Y, Tafti M. Molecular genetics and treatment of narcolepsy. Ann Med 2006;38(4):252–62.

31. Tanaka S, Honda Y, Inoue Y, et al. Detection of autoantibodies against hypocretin, hcrtrl, and hcrtr2 in narcolepsy: anti-Hcrt system antibody in narcolepsy. Sleep 2006;29(5):633–8.

32. Aran A, Lin L, Nevsimalova S, et al. Elevated anti-streptococcal antibodies in patients with recent narcolepsy onset. Sleep 2009;32(8):979–83.

33. Houghton WC, Scammell TE, Thorpy M. Pharmacotherapy for cataplexy. Sleep Med Rev 2004;8:355–66.

34. Picchioni D, Hope CR, Harsh JR. A case-control study of the environmental risk factors for narcolepsy. Neuroepidemiology 2007;29(3–4):185–92.

35. Castriotta RJ, Wilde MC, Lai JM, et al. Prevalence and consequences of sleep disorders in traumatic brain injury. J Clin Sleep Med 2007;3(4):349–56.

36. Gill AW. Idiopathic and traumatic narcolepsy. Lancet 1941;1:474.

37. Rack M, Davis J, Roffwarg HP, et al. The multiple sleep latency test in the diagnosis of narcolepsy. Am J Psychiatry 2005;162(11):2198–9.

38. Challamel MJ, Mazzola ME, Nevsimalova S, et al. Narcolepsy in children. Sleep 1994;17S:17–20.

39. Carskadon MA. The second decade. In: Guilleminault C, editor. Sleeping and waking disorders: indications and techniques. Menlo Park (CA): Addison-Wesley; 1982. p. 99–125.

40. Morgenthaler TI, Kapur VK, Brown T, et al. Practice parameters for the treatment of narcolepsy and

other hypersomnias of central origin. Sleep 2007; 30(12):1705–11.

41. Black J, Guilleminault C. Medications for the treatment of narcolepsy. Expert Opin Emerg Drugs 2001;6(2):239–47.

42. Didato G, Nobili L. Treatment of narcolepsy. Expert Rev Neurother 2009;9(6):897–910.

43. Mitler MM, Hayduk R. Benefits and risks of pharmacotherapy for narcolepsy. Drug Saf 2002;25:791–809.

44. U.S. Modafinil in Narcolepsy Multicenter Study Group. Randomized trial of modafinil as a treatment for excessive daytime somnolence of narcolepsy. Neurology 2000;54:1166–75.

45. Schwartz JR, Feldman NT, Bogan RK. Dose effects of modafinil in sustaining wakefulness in narcolepsy patients with residual evening sleepiness. J Neuropsychiatry Clin Neurosci 2005;17(3):405–12 [Erratum in: J Neuropsychiatry Clin Neurosci 2005; 17(4):561].

46. Harsh JR, Hayduk R, Rosenberg R, et al. The efficacy and safety of armodafinil as treatment for adults with excessive sleepiness associated with narcolepsy. Curr Med Res Opin 2006;22(4):761–74.

47. Dinges DF, Arora S, Darwish M, et al. Pharmacodynamic effects on alertness of single doses of armodafinil in healthy subjects during a nocturnal period of acute sleep loss. Curr Med Res Opin 2006;22(1):159–67.

48. U.S. Xyrem International Study Group. A double blind placebo controlled study demonstrates sodium oxybate is effective for the treatment of excessive sleepiness in narcolepsy. J Clin Sleep Med 2005;1(4):391–7.

49. Wedin GP, Hornfeldt CS, Ylitalo LM. The clinical development of γ-hydroxybutyrate (GHB). Curr Drug Saf 2006;1:99–106.

50. Xyrem Prescribing Information, Jazz Pharmaceuticals, Palo Alto, California.

51. Guilleminault C, Raynal D, Takahashi S, et al. Evaluation of short-term and long-term treatment of the narcolepsy syndrome with clomipramine hydrochloride. Acta Neurol Scand 1976;54:71–87.

52. Shapiro WR. Treatment of cataplexy with clomipramine. Arch Neurol 1975;32:653–6.

53. Chen SY, Clift SJ, Dahlitz MJ, et al. Treatment in the narcoleptic syndrome: self assessment of the action of dexamphetamine and clomipramine. J Sleep Res 1995;4:113–8.

54. Martinez-Rodriguez J, Iranzo A, Santamaria J, et al. Status cataplecticus induced by abrupt withdrawal of clomipramine. Neurologia 2002;17:113–6.

55. Frey J, Darbonne C. Fluoxetine suppresses human cataplexy: a pilot study. Neurology 1994;44:707–9.

56. Langdon N, Shindler J, Parkes JD, et al. Fluoxetine in the treatment of cataplexy. Sleep 1986;9:371–3.

57. U.S. Xyrem Multicenter Study Group. Sodium oxybate demonstrates long-term efficacy for the

treatment of cataplexy in patients with narcolepsy. Sleep Med 2004;5:119–23.

58. Xyrem International Study Group. Further evidence supporting the use of sodium oxybate for the treatment of cataplexy: a double-blind, placebo-controlled study in 2228 patients. Sleep Med 2005; 6:415–21.

59. U.S. Xyrem Multicenter Study Group. A randomized, double blind, placebo-controlled multicenter trial comparing the effects of three doses of orally administered sodium oxybate with placebo for the treatment of narcolepsy. Sleep 2002;25(1):42–9.

60. Thorpy MJ, Snyder M, Aloe FS, et al. Short-term triazolam use improves nocturnal sleep of narcoleptics. Sleep 1992;15(3):212–6.

61. Hishikawa Y, Ida H, Nakai K, et al. Treatment of narcolepsy with imipramine (Tofranil) and desmethylimipramine (Pertofran). J Neurol Sci 1966;3:453–61.

62. Guilleminault C, Wilson RA, Dement WC. A study on cataplexy. Arch Neurol 1974;31:255–61.

63. Chakravorty SS, Rye DB. Narcolepsy in the older adult: epidemiology, diagnosis and management. Drugs Aging 2003;20(5):361–76.

64. Inoue Y, Nanba K, Higami S, et al. Clinical significance of sleep-related breathing disorder in narcolepsy. Psychiatry Clin Neurosci 2002;56(3):269–70.

65. Dahmen N, Bierbrauer J, Kasten M. Increased prevalence of obesity in narcoleptic patients and relatives. Eur Arch Psychiatry Clin Neurosci 2001;251(2):85–9.

66. Kotagal S, Krahn LE, Slocumb N. A putative link between childhood narcolepsy and obesity. Sleep Med 2004;5(2):147–50.

67. Kok SW, Overeem S, Visscher TL, et al. Hypocretin deficiency in narcoleptic humans is associated with abdominal obesity. Obes Res 2003;11(9):1147–54.

68. Williams RH, Burdakov D. Hypothalamic orexins/hypocretins as regulators of breathing. Expert Rev Mol Med 2008;10:e28.

69. Seeck-Hirschner M, Baier PC, von Freier A, et al. Increase in sleep-related breathing disturbances after treatment with sodium oxybate in patients with narcolepsy and mild obstructive sleep apnea syndrome: two case reports. Sleep Med 2009;10(1):154–5.

70. Feldman NT. Clinical perspective: monitoring sodium oxybate-treated narcolepsy patients for the development of sleep-disordered breathing. Sleep Breath 2010;14(1):77–9.

71. Sériès F, Sériès I, Cormier Y. Effects of enhancing slow-wave sleep by gamma-hydroxybutyrate on obstructive sleep apnea. Am Rev Respir Dis 1992; 145(6):1378–83.

72. Chervin RD, Aldrich MS. Sleep onset REM periods during multiple sleep latency tests in patients evaluated for sleep apnea. Am J Respir Crit Care Med 2000;161(2 Pt 1):426–31.

73. Sansa G, Iranzo A, Santamaria J. Obstructive sleep apnea in narcolepsy. Sleep Med 2010;11(1):93–5.

All the Wrong Moves: A Clinical Review of Restless Legs Syndrome, Periodic Limb Movements of Sleep and Wake, and Periodic Limb Movement Disorder

Rachel E. Salas, MD[a],*, Russell Rasquinha, MSE[b],
Charlene E. Gamaldo, MD[a]

KEYWORDS

- Restless legs syndrome (RLS)
- Periodic limb movements of sleep (PLMS)
- Periodic limb movements in wake (PLMW)
- Periodic limb movement disorder (PLMD)
- Dopaminergic agents

Sleep disorders affect millions of American annually, which makes encountering a patient in a medical practice with a comorbid sleep condition inevitable. Common sleep disorders such as restless legs syndrome (RLS) can often manifest with the disease progression or treatment of several other medical conditions. Another clinical sleep condition, periodic limb movement disorder (PLMD), can also be associated with sleep-disruptive limb movements, and these limb movements referred to in the literature as periodic limb movements (PLM) can be seen in sleep and wake (PLMS and PLMW, respectively). PLMS and PLMW can be associated with clinical conditions such as RLS or PLMD, various medical conditions, several medications, and in some cases, as an incidental finding on a sleep study without any specific clinical correlate. Deciphering between the different terms related to abnormal limb movements and their related clinical conditions can often be daunting for the novice health care provider. Therefore, the first step in becoming proficient in diagnosing, treating, and managing the abnormal limb movements of sleep is a proper grasp of the definitions of these commonly confused acronyms relating to limb movements.

RLS

RLS is a clinically diagnosed condition that is defined by the International Classification of Sleep Disorder 2nd Edition (ICSD-2)[1] as a sensorimotor

[a] Department of Neurology, Division of Pulmonary and Critical Care, Johns Hopkins Sleep Disorders Center at Johns Hopkins Hospital, 600 North Wolfe Street, Suite 1261, Baltimore, MD 21287, USA
[b] Department of Biomedical Engineering, Johns Hopkins University, 3400 North Charles Street, Baltimore, MD 21218, USA
* Corresponding author.
E-mail address: rsalas3@jhmi.edu

Clin Chest Med 31 (2010) 383–395
doi:10.1016/j.ccm.2010.02.006

condition whereby patients often complain of uncomfortable sensations associated with an urge to move (**Box 1**). These sensations are most prominent in the evenings and are brought on with rest and relieved with movements. The sensations can take on a variety of characterizations, ranging from paresthesias to frank pain. As long as the patient moves, the discomfort is usually completely and immediately relieved but returns when the patient is resting, thus resulting in the significant sleep disturbance that often accompanies those with frequent and severe symptoms. Often the subjective complaints related to these sensations manifest with physical signs of involuntary limb twitching and jerking most commonly seen in the legs during sleep (PLMS) and during wakefulness (PLMW).

PLMS

PLMS are a series of stereotypical limb movements identified on a polysomnogram (PSG). PSG recording for PLMS is based on uncalibrated anterior tibialis surface electromyography (EMG) recordings. The American Academy of Sleep Medicine (AASM) scoring manual[2] defines an eligible leg movement to be 0.5 to 10 seconds in duration, with a minimum amplitude of 8 μV increase above the resting baseline EMG. To be considered as part of a periodic chain of PLMS, there must be a minimum of 4 repetitive eligible limb movements reoccurring every 5 to 90 seconds (**Fig. 1**). Both legs should be monitored for the presence of the leg movements. Separate channels for each leg are strongly preferred because combining electrodes from the 2 legs may reduce the number of detected overall LMs. Moreover, movements of the upper limbs may be sampled if clinically indicated.

There are special circumstances to be aware of when scoring LMs as recommended by the AASM scoring manual. First, LMs should not be scored if they occur 0.5 seconds before or after an apnea or hypopnea. LMs occurring within 0.5 seconds before or after a respiratory event such as an apnea or

hypopnea are considered to be associated with the respiratory event and are not counted. LMs associated with respiratory events tend to improve once the sleep-disordered breathing events are treated with continuous positive airway pressure (CPAP). In addition, an arousal and a PLM should be considered associated with each other when there is less than 0.5 seconds between the end of 1 event and the onset of the other event, regardless of which is first.

PLMW

PLMW are a series of limb movements observed in a periodic series based on the same AASM scoring criteria as PLMS. However, these limb movements are observed during the wake portion of a PSG or during a suggested immobilization test (SIT).[3] The SIT was originally developed as an objective research diagnostic tool for RLS based on measuring PLMW. The general protocol for conducting the SIT involves placing the patient in a soporific setting while they are sitting up with legs outstretched. The individual is instructed to stay awake and refrain from moving their legs for 1 hour. Leg movements are measured by EMG on the anterior tibialis and in some cases the patient records their level of discomfort every 5 minutes.[4] To ensure that alertness is maintained, EEG along with EMG are monitored and recorded during the procedure by a technician.[5]

PLMW are considered more specific for RLS than PLMS and therefore can be useful when seeking supportive diagnostic information. According to the ICSD-2, PLMW of 5 per hour or greater on a PSG and 40 per hour or greater on the SIT are considered suggestive of RLS.[1]

PLMD

PLMD is a sleep disorder characterized by periodic episodes of repetitive, highly stereotyped PLMS. It is often associated with insomnia, nonrestful sleep, or daytime dysfunction that cannot be accounted for by another primary sleep disorder. To that end, PLMD is essentially a diagnosis of exclusion.

BEYOND DEFINITIONS: STRATEGIES FOR MANAGING SLEEP-RELATED MOVEMENTS AND THEIR ASSOCIATED CLINICAL DISORDERS (RLS, PLMS, AND PLMD)
RLS

Diagnosing RLS: supportive features and diagnostic tools

RLS, which often occurs in otherwise healthy people, can have a significant effect on sleep

---

Box 1
RLS essential diagnostic criteria

(1) Uncomfortable sensations with an urge to move legs
(2) Sensations worsen during periods of rest or inactivity
(3) Sensations are relieved by movement, such as walking or getting up
(4) Sensations are worse in the evening or at night

Inter-Leg Movement Duration (I-LMD)
Leg Movement Duration (LMD)
Duration Between Offset and Onset

5 s < I-LMD< 90 s

0.5 s < LMD < 10 s

0.5 s < LMD < 10 s

> 0.5 s

< 0.5s

onset threshold: baseline + 8 µV
offset threshold: baseline + 2 µV
baseline: <5 µV
0 µV

10 µV
1 s

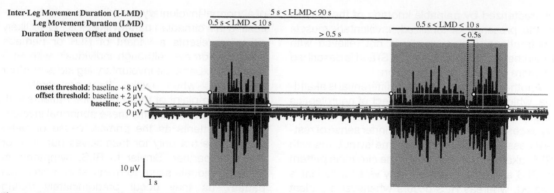

Fig. 1. Demonstration of periodic limb movements by criteria.

quality, daytime functioning, and overall quality of life. Although RLS affects mostly the legs (as the name suggests), it can also affect the arms, trunk, or multiple body parts simultaneously. Patients with RLS may experience their symptoms in many different ways, but all generally describe unpleasant, in some cases creepy-crawly, sensations that occur in the legs when they are sitting or lying still (at rest), especially at bedtime. Although, the sensations may be described as painful in some instances, the painful sensations associated with RLS should be distinct in quality from the pain experienced from other painful conditions such as leg cramps, radiculopathy, or arthritis. RLS sensations are also different from the pins and needles or the burning feeling a patient with diabetic neuropathy may experience. The uncomfortable feelings of RLS appear most often in the calves of the legs and are relieved, or at least improved slightly, as long as the individual continues to move. In severe instances, RLS sensations with the associated circadian component result in significant sleep disturbance and insomnia.

A PSG can be helpful in the diagnosis of RLS, as approximately 80% of patients with RLS have accompanied limb movements documented on PSG. Symptom severity has also been measured objectively by an overnight in-home PSG in a community population.[6] In this study, sleep architecture on the PSG and RLS questionnaires was compared, and results revealed that the single-night PSG was able to detect a significant difference in sleep latency in RLS (40 minutes) compared with controls (26 minutes), and that delayed sleep latency was associated with severity of subjective RLS symptoms. However, no association was found between RLS symptom severity and other measures of sleep disruption (wake after sleep onset) after the patient initiated sleep.[7]

As mentioned earlier, the SIT has been used as an objective measure and tool for diagnosing RLS

and has been shown to have high RLS sensitivity and specificity.[3,5]

Differential diagnosis

Various conditions that can mimic the sensorimotor disturbances of RLS must be considered and excluded before a conclusive diagnosis of RLS can be made. Several rheumatologic, neurologic, and psychiatric conditions can share 1 or more of the complaints related to the 4 RLS clinical criteria (see **Box 1**). Some of these conditions include but are not limited to the following: positional discomfort, sleep-related leg cramps, painful legs and moving toes, PLMS, akathisia, Vesper's curse, vascular diseases, peripheral neuropathies (especially small-fiber), hypnic (sleep) jerks, generalized anxiety disorder, depression, and leg pain from osteoarthritic conditions, sciatica, or pruritus.

Excluding common conditions in the differential diagnosis usually involves more in-depth clinical queries to determine whether all 4 RLS criteria are present. For instance, positional discomfort may be experienced at night while lying down; however, it occurs when pressure is applied, resulting in a compressed nerve. Improvement is usually noted when the individual changes position. Unlike RLS the improvement of symptoms continues to be experienced as long as this new position is maintained. Painful legs and moving toes are a syndrome of involuntary and irregular movements of the toes, and sometimes the foot, with severe diffuse pain felt deeply in the foot and sometimes proximally in the leg. The disorder may affect 1 leg alone, or can spread to involve both. The involuntary movements usually occur after the onset of pain. The cause of this condition is unknown and there are no treatments for permanent pain relief. Moreover, painful legs and moving toes do not exhibit a circadian pattern and are not associated with an urge to move. Sleep-related leg cramps are also a common sleep-related problem characterized by palpable knotting of the muscle in the presence of localized, involuntary muscle contractions, which usually is not relieved with movement or walking (unlike RLS) and is described as more of a cramping sensation.

Another consideration in the differential is akathisia, which is a possible side effect of neuroleptics and dopaminergic blockers that is characterized by excessive movement and an inner sense of restlessness. Although sharing some symptoms with RLS, akathisias do not exhibit the circadian pattern of RLS and usually present only when a patient is seated, whereas RLS occurs whenever a patient is at rest. Moreover, in comparison with RLS, usually akathisia does not cause sleep disturbance.

Vesper's curse is a transient lumbar stenosis, caused by an increase in right atrial filling pressure, which results in leg pain, lumbosacral discomfort, and/or paresthesias that may cause sleep disturbance. Vesper's curse involves sensory symptoms that are painful rather than uncomfortable. These painful sensations occur in the recumbent position, which may be confused with the circadian feature of RLS even although it does not have a circadian pattern. Vascular diseases such as deep venous thrombosis, intermittent claudication, and varicose veins may cause sensations that mimic RLS symptoms, but usually do not take on a clear circadian pattern, with worsening in the evening and relative improvement early in the day like RLS.

Peripheral neuropathy also often results in sensory complaints of numbness, tingling, or pain, which can be associated with worsening symptoms at night. Neuropathy can pose a particular challenge for the diagnostician because it can be the underlying cause of secondary RLS. However, primary neuropathy with the overlapping sensory symptoms independent of RLS is usually not relieved by movement.

As described earlier, PLMS are periodic, highly repetitive limb movements occurring during sleep that can be found on a PSG, in relation to other medical conditions, medications, or as part of an RLS presentation. PLMS can be present in approximately 80% of patients with RLS and therefore represent a sensitive but nonspecific marker of RLS. PLMS are also linked to other sleep disorders, such as sleep apnea and narcolepsy. Therefore, it is crucial that the treating health care provider consider these other disorders or the diagnosis of idiopathic PLMS in the absence of the essential diagnostic criteria of RLS.

Recently, a clinical presentation known as, quiescegenic nocturnal dyskinesia (QND) was described and should be considered in the RLS differential as well. QND refers to the presentation of abnormal involuntary periodic movements manifesting in a circadian pattern like RLS.[7] QND likely either represents a variant of RLS or perhaps a new syndrome. Although individuals with RLS may also experience involuntary leg kicks or other dyskinesias when awake, they are rarely the primary complaint of these patients. Patients with QND consistently identify these abnormal involuntary movements as the primary cause of sleep disturbance not only for themselves but also for their bed-partner. Similar to RLS, symptoms in these individuals seem to manifest in a circadian pattern, as they occur predominately during relaxed wakefulness in the evening or night, including, but not limited to, the time before sleep onset. The distinguishing feature between the two is that patients with QND do not report the uncomfortable sensations or the urge to move that patients with RLS endure.

How common is RLS?

Seven to 10 of every 100 individuals experience the discomfort of RLS at some time in their lives. Approximately 2 to 5 of every 100 individuals experience symptoms severe enough to require medical attention. RLS is more common in women and older individuals, but can occur at any age in men and women. RLS can also present initially during pregnancy, and can be severe, especially during the last 6 months of the pregnancy. The course of RLS can range from episodic (especially in pregnancy), to intermittent (with waxing and waning severity), or chronically progressive.

Approximately 30% of RLS cases are hereditary. In hereditary RLS cases, RLS symptoms are more likely to begin earlier in life (usually before the age of 45 years) and are more likely to be associated with iron deficiency. Childhood conditions and risk factors that may be associated with RLS include growing pains and history of restless sleep, although these findings have been mixed.[8,9]

RLS and associated comorbid sleep and medical conditions

In recent years RLS has been linked with the manifestation and progression of several medical conditions (**Box 2** for full list). These associated conditions often negatively affect the individual's morbidity and mortality, thus further underscoring the importance of properly diagnosing and treating RLS. This section discusses the current findings regarding some of the conditions whose links with RLS are particularly compelling.

Circadian rhythm and RLS Disturbances in circadian rhythms may affect the prevalence and

Box 2
Conditions associated with or exacerbating RLS

Alcoholism

Anemia

Apnea

Attention deficit hyperactivity disorder (ADHD)

Bruxism

Circadian rhythm disorders

Celiac disease

Diabetes

Fatigue

Iron deficiency anemia

Kidney disease

Lyme disease

Magnesium deficiency

Medications

Muscle disorders

Neuropathy

Opiate withdrawal

Parkinson's disease (PD)

Peripheral neuropathy

Pregnancy

Renal disease

Rheumatoid arthritis

Sleep deprivation

Smoking

Vitamin or mineral deficiencies

intensity of RLS symptoms. One study found that those individuals who work rotational shifts appeared to be disproportionately affected by RLS, especially those who primarily work a night shift compared with individuals with conventional work hours.[10] Investigators in this study concluded that rotational shift work acts as a risk for RLS, and suggest it may be linked via disruption of circadian rhythms. Therefore, screening shift workers may help with management of RLS in these populations.

Apnea and RLS Sleep apnea often accompanies leg movement disorders such as RLS and is a strong predictor of RLS (3.5 odds ratio [OR]) and PLMD (1.5).[11] Although the causation has not been linked, it has been suggested that the brainstem may be involved in both pathologies.[12] This study found that CPAP therapy reduced RLS severity in those individuals concurrently suffering

with sleep apnea and RLS, before introducing RLS-specific treatment.[13] Although no reason for this improvement has been suggested, it could be speculated that the improvement in sleep quality with CPAP may inadvertently improve perception or tolerance of RLS symptoms.

Bruxism and RLS A recent study estimating the prevalence of RLS with bruxism[14] surveyed factory workers with regular and irregular work shift schedules and reported that RLS was significantly associated with the presence of bruxism and perceived dissatisfaction with work shift schedule, implying some comorbidity between RLS and bruxism. The investigators propose that perceived bruxism may indicate increased stress, often associated with alternative work schedules, and that RLS, an independent entity, might negatively affect sleep quality, further aggravating stress.[14]

RLS and cardiovascular disease Several studies have investigated associations between cardiovascular disorders and RLS, but causality has not been established. In a cross-sectional study, Winkelman and colleagues[15] observed an increased likelihood (OR ≈ 2) of cardiovascular disease (CVD) and coronary artery disease (CAD) in patients with RLS (RLS prevalence of 6.8% in women and 3.3% in men), even after controlling for sex, diabetes, total/high-density lipoprotein cholesterol ratio, sleep onset latency, smoking, use of antihypertensive medication, and apnea hypopnea index. The association was stronger in those older than 65 years (OR ≈ 2.4), in those with RLS symptoms that occurred more than 15 times per month (OR ≈ 2.3–4), and in those who reported that their RLS symptoms were severely bothersome (OR ≈ 2.4). The causality between the 2 is not known, but these associations are believed to be mediated through increased autonomic arousals during sleep observed in patients with RLS and associated PLMS. Alternatively, CVD could produce vascular changes in the nervous system, causing RLS, or a third factor might influence RLS and CVD.

RLS and gastrointestinal disease In a community study led by Weinstock and colleagues[16] patients with celiac disease were evaluated for RLS. There was a markedly increased incidence of RLS in these patients, which occurred mainly after the onset of gastrointestinal symptoms. The proposed link between the RLS and celiac disease is that both conditions have concomitant iron deficiency, although this is not universal. The study did, however, find a 50% improvement of RLS symptoms after gluten withdrawal, perhaps because of improved iron absorption as well as other factors. Investigators recommend that screening for celiac disease in patients with RLS may help with uncovering this silent disease. Furthermore, recognition that RLS occurs in patients with celiac disease could yield potential diagnostic and therapeutic benefits for both groups of patients.

RLS and mood disorders Patients with RLS and PLMS have been shown to present with increased depressive symptoms. Moreover, antidepressants may precipitate or exacerbate PLMS. The effect of RLS on the quality of life and daily functioning has also been investigated in several studies. Abetz and colleagues[17] and Allen and colleagues[18] assessed the quality of life using the short-form 36-item health survey (SF-36) and reported significant diminished physical functioning, role-physical, bodily pain, general health, vitality, social functioning, and role-emotional scores. These variables are presumed to be a result of RLS through disrupted sleep and insufficient hours of sleep. RLS sufferers also reported daytime sleepiness and difficulty in paying attention the following day. Thus, this study definitively showed the negative effect that RLS can have on the quality of life and attentiveness of sufferers.

RLS and cognitive disturbance

Individuals with moderate to severe RLS symptoms may reportedly obtain as little as 3 to 5 hours of sleep daily, representing a degree of chronic sleep loss arguably more profound than any other sleep disorder.[19] Significant cognitive disturbances have been demonstrated when individuals in the general population are subjected to this degree of sleep loss even in the short-term.[20,21] On the other hand, investigations regarding the effect of chronic sleep loss from RLS have revealed mixed results, with increased daytime sleepiness documented in patients with RLS relative to normal controls in some studies and no differences in other studies.[17,18,22–25] One study comparing the sleep latency of patients with RLS, off medications, relative to sleep-restricted controls using the SIT revealed longer sleep latencies and greater objective alertness in patients with RLS relative to their matched sleep-deprived controls. The heightened degree of alertness amongst patients with RLS was especially compelling considering that the patients with RLS often endured a greater degree of sleep deprivation than their matched controls.[26] Thus it has been proposed that patients with RLS may display a compensatory mechanism that enhances alertness despite significant sleep

loss.[26] Another study comparing the cognitive function between patients with RLS and sleep-restricted controls specifically measured the performance on prefrontal lobe-specific tasks because the prefrontal lobe has been shown to be exquisitely sensitive to sleep loss. Similar to their enhanced alertness compared with controls on the SIT test, the patients with RLS performed better on 2 of the prefrontal lobe function tasks compared with matched sleep-restricted controls.[27] These findings again suggest a compensatory mechanism in individuals with RLS regarding cognitive function in the face of chronic sleep loss. Edinger[28] reported that patients with RLS/PLMD display many of the cognitive and behavioral anomalies believed to perpetuate primary insomnia. Patients with primary insomnia have also shown hyperarousal characteristics as shown by autonomic and metabolic patterns, which may suggest a common neurobiological link between the 2 conditions.[28]

RLS is also common in children with ADHD,[29] and ADHD is common in adults with RLS. Zak and colleagues[30] recently published a preliminary study that suggested an inverse relationship may also exist (RLS is common in adults with ADHD). They found a significantly larger prevalence of RLS in a group of 30 patients with ADHD and that ADHD was more severe in those with both disorders. ADHD is more prevalent in young people and in men, whereas RLS is more prevalent in women and increases with age. Although a larger study is required, these results suggest that RLS may exacerbate the symptoms of ADHD.

RLS treatment and management considerations

Patients with any degree of RLS should be able to obtain substantial symptom relief, as there are many suitable therapies. Successful management is often attained when the treatment is tailored to the patient's specific symptoms. Specific factors to consider when devising an individualized treatment strategy include iron status, disease severity, the frequency and duration of symptoms, symptoms onset, presence of pain, and medication side effect profile.[31] All patients with RLS should be screened and treated for iron deficiency with new onset or a noted change in RLS symptoms. Ferritin levels less than 50 μg/L have been correlated with increased symptom severity, decreased sleep efficiency, and increased PLMS associated with arousals. Therefore, iron status should always be included in the RLS evaluation[32] and iron supplementation should be recommended in patients with RLS with a low ferritin. Furthermore, an appropriate evaluation for iron deficiency anemia should also be performed in those individuals meeting the criteria for iron deficiency. Currently, there are no data linking absolute iron levels with RLS severity. Treatment plans usually include a combination of aggravator reduction (**Table 1**) along with nonpharmacologic and pharmacologic therapy. The current available treatments for RLS are discussed later.

Nonpharmacologic therapy Nonpharmacologic therapies may be effective for some patients with RLS; however, this is more anecdotal. Some of these therapies include hot or cold baths, leg massages, applied heat, ice packs, aspirin or other over-the-counter pain relievers, regular exercise, stimulating activities, and the elimination of caffeine.

Iron supplementation Iron deficiency is widespread among patients with RLS. Oral iron supplementation is generally recommended for patients with RLS with morning fasting serum ferritin level less than 18 µg/L and a percent iron saturation less than 16%. Ferrous sulfate at a dose of 325 mg twice or thrice daily with a vitamin C tablet or a glass of orange juice is recommended to increase iron absorption. The goal for ferritin levels should be more than 50 µg/L. A fasting morning iron panel including ferritin and percentage of transferrin saturation should be checked every 3 months to avoid iron overload.[33] A fasting morning percent saturation is preferred because a value

greater than 45% is 1 of the best indicators of possible hemochromatosis.[22]

Pharmacologic therapy Dopamine agonists, antiepileptic drugs (AEDs), opioids, and benzodiazepines are the recommended medication classes of choice when treating RLS.[31]

Dopaminergic agents Dopaminergic agents (DA) are considered to be the gold standard and 2 of the medications (ropinirole and pramipexole) are the only medications approved by the US Food and Drug Administration for the treatment of RLS. Levodopa is recommended for occasional sedentary activities (such as flights or long meetings) or for intermittent symptoms at bedtime.[33] Levodopa use more than twice a week is not recommended because of the high potential for augmentation (see later discussion). Dopamine agonists, therefore, are the medications of choice for patients with persistent daily RLS symptoms. Dopamine agonists have a longer half-life than levodopa and have a reduced risk of developing augmentation (see later discussion) compared with levodopa, making them the ideal choice for idiopathic RLS.[33] The rotigotine transdermal patch may be another consideration for patients in the future after RLS.[28] Rotigotine is associated with less augmentation and fewer side effects than other DA. Rotigotine was withdrawn in the United States

Table 1
Medication aggravators of RLS, PLMS, and PLMD

Type of Drug	Common or Trade Name	Generic
Antidepressants	Elavil Prozac Paxil	Amitriptyline Fluoxetine Paroxetine
Antihistamines	Allegra Benadryl Chlor-Trimeton Claritin	Fexofenadine Diphenhydramine Chlorpheniramine Loratadine
Antiemetics	Compazine Reglan	Prochlorperazine Metoclopramide
Lithium	Eskalith Lithobid Lithonate Lithotabs	Lithium carbonate
Calcium channel blockers	Calan Cardizen Norvasc Procardia	Verapamil Diltazem Amlodipine Nifedipine
Major tranquilizers	Haldol Phenothiazines Trilafon Thorazine	Haloperidol Phenothiazines Perphenazine Chlorpromazine

because of crystallization of the drug within the transdermal patch, leading to unpredictable delivery of the drug. However, it is expected to be available in the United States again soon. Side effects of DA include excessive daytime sleepiness, nausea, vomiting, nasal congestion, edema, hallucinations, chest pain, and insomnia.[33,34] Augmentation and dopamine dysregulation syndrome (DDS) are 2 commonly encountered side effects related to DA treatment and therefore require specific discussion.

Differentiating DA-related augmentation from other RLS treatment-related patterns Augmentation is the worsening of RLS symptoms while the patient is on a DA.[35] Augmentation occurs in approximately 80% of patients with RLS treated with levodopa.[36] Dopamine agonists (pramipexole and ropinirole) have a longer half-life than levodopa and therefore are less likely to result in more rapid augmentation.[36,37] However, it is believed that most patients on DA experience augmentation at some point in their therapy. There are 4 main features of augmentation related to changes in the duration, severity, frequency and location of RLS symptoms. Symptoms that may have once been intermittent begin to occur daily; this is the most prevailing feature. Initially, most patients with RLS report onset of symptoms at bedtime as a result of the circadian nature of RLS. However, in those with augmentation, the symptoms begin to present earlier in the day. Those patients who once had symptoms in the evening now report problems in the early afternoon, with greater symptom intensity. At initial presentation, sensations typically affect specific and localized areas of the body such as the legs. Once a patient has become augmented, affected areas begin to expand beyond the initial area to include in some patients the arms and trunk and in some patients, the face. Augmentation, RLS exacerbation, and RLS disease progression need to be differentiated as therapy may be different.[38] The previously met RLS diagnostic criteria by the patient before initiation of treatment may no longer be apparent, which may make one question the RLS diagnosis. Therefore it is imperative that the health care provider perform a thorough history to make sure the RLS diagnostic criteria were initially met. If so, progression and intensity of the symptoms while on DA are highly suggestive of augmentation; this is especially true in the absence of iron deficiency or other RLS aggravators. Once a patient is tapered from the DA, symptoms usually improve (after a withdrawal period) back to baseline. If symptoms do not improve, it is most likely progression of the RLS itself and not augmentation.

It is also important to differentiate augmentation from medication rebound and early morning rebound (EMR). Medication rebound is considered a pharmacokinetic end-of-the-dose rebound of symptoms. EMR is another complication of DA that is characterized by recurrence of RLS symptoms in the early morning, often awakening patients from sleep. EMR is primarily observed in 20% to 35% of patients taking levodopa as a result of its short half-life and is usually of lesser clinical significance for the patient than augmentation.[38] EMR presentation does not show the dramatic evolution of symptoms from baseline compared with augmentation. For instance, individuals with EMR do not report an increase in symptom intensity or radiation of symptoms to other parts of the body. In EMR, RLS symptoms worsen at the end of effective medication treatment each day (usually morning) as opposed to augmentation, in which RLS symptoms are worse usually in the afternoon. Switching to a long-acting dopamine agonist or changing the timing of the dopamine agonist usually improves symptoms of EMR. A health care provider may also consider a dose of levodopa to treat middle-of-the-night symptoms if these occur no more than twice a week.

Augmented patients with RLS most likely experience withdrawal effects while tapering off the DA. Withdrawal symptoms can be severe and patients must be educated on this occurrence. Patients usually experience severe restlessness and discomfort and may report excruciating RLS symptoms. This withdrawal phenomenon is common, especially with higher doses of DA. Health care providers should manage patients on a case-by-case basis when tapering off the DA. It remains controversial whether levodopa or the DA should be stopped immediately or tapered slowly.[39,40]

DDS: a newly observed DA-related presentation in RLS Punding, excessive gambling, shopping, and hypersexuality are types of compulsive behaviors defining DDS.[41] DDS is a neuropsychological behavioral disorder associated with substance misuse and addiction that was initially recognized in individuals treated for PD on dopamine replacement therapy.[41] DDS has also been linked to RLS in several published case reports.[38,42,43] DDS has been associated with impaired cognition and executive function in PD, but not in RLS. The cognitive deficits experienced by patients with RLS are most likely associated with sleep loss, not with the underlying disease as seen in PD.[44,45] Withdrawal of the DA usually results in almost immediate resolution of DDS symptoms. Important features noted in patients with RLS with DDS is that there is little insight of the compulsive behaviors until after being tapered off the DA and that these behaviors usually do not result in significant social consequences as typically seen in PD patients, perhaps because of the smaller medication doses used in patients with RLS compared with patients with PD.[42] However, this raises some potential concerns for patients with RLS as they may not be aware of the subtle behavioral changes during the duration of therapy, which can last for years.

AEDs AEDs commonly used in the treatment of RLS include carbamazepine, gabapentin, pregabalin, and lamotrigine. AEDs may be considered first-line therapy for patients with RLS with concomitant neuropathy or painful dysthesias. Typical side effects of gabapentin, pregabalin, and lamotrigine include sleepiness, dizziness, fluid retention, and increased appetite.[33] There is a higher risk of allergic skin reactions, including the rare Stevens-Johnson syndrome, when using lamotrigine. Therefore lamotrigine should be titrated slowly (no more than 25 mg/wk).[33]

Opioids Opioids have been shown to be effective in the treatment of RLS and may be considered as therapy for patients with RLS presenting with neuropathy or painful dysthesias.[33,44] Short-acting agents such as hydrocodone, oxycodone, and codeine may be used for intermittent symptoms or symptoms occurring only at night.[33] For more severe disease, long-acting opioids (oxycodone, methadone, or the fentanyl patch) can also be used.[33] Side effects of long-term opioid use include development or exacerbation of sleep apnea.[46] Of patients on chronic opioids, 75% have either obstructive or central sleep apnea.[47] Opioids may also decrease rapid eye movement (REM) and slow wave sleep.[47] Sedation, fatigue, and constipation are also common side effects. The risk of addiction is no different in patients with RLS than in the general population. Augmentation or tolerance does not seem to develop with long-term use of the opioids, which makes this class an alternative for augmented patients.[33,34] However, Q-T interval prolongation and torsades de pointes have been associated with the use of methadone and are potentially fatal adverse effects; for this reason a thorough patient history and electrocardiogram monitoring are encouraged for patients treated with methadone.[48]

Benzodiazepine receptor agonists Although not usually the first-line choice, benzodiazepine receptor agonists (BRAs) may be useful in particular situations in which symptoms are primarily related to initiation of sleep.[49] Side effects of the BRAs include sedation and the development of

tolerance,[34] although this is less of an issue for the longer-acting BRAs.

General updates on underlying RLS pathophysiology and genetic associations

Idiopathic RLS tends to occur at a greater rate among family members.[50,51] A positive family history is particularly common in patients with RLS with onset of symptoms before 40 years of age.[52] Patients with RLS with onset of symptoms after 50 years of age generally have peripheral neuropathy and/or an increased rate of disease progression[33,52,53] Genetic studies have linked chromosomal loci (12q, 14q, and 9p) to RLS.[33,45,54,55] Another study reported a genome-wide significant association with a common variant in an intron (*BTBD9*) on chromosome 6p; this specific variant showed that the population attributable risk of RLS with PLMS was 50%.[56]

Because levodopa and iron can be used to treat RLS, the dopamine and iron system have been the main focus of RLS research.[57,58] Differences in dopamine- and iron-related markers have also been shown in the cerebrospinal fluid of individuals with RLS.[59] A connection between these 2 systems is shown by the finding of low iron levels in the substantia nigra of patients with RLS, although other areas may also be involved.[2]

PLMS

Diagnosing PLMS: supportive features and diagnostic tools

As discussed in the opening section of this article, PLMS represent polysomnographic findings based on specific scoring criteria as defined by the AASM scoring manual.[2] PLMS, similar to RLS, may be associated with some medical conditions, including uremia, anemia, chronic lung disease, myelopathies, and peripheral neuropathies. Use of certain medications, such as tricyclic antidepressants and lithium carbonate, and withdrawal from benzodiazepines and anticonvulsants can also cause or exacerbate PLMS. PLMS should not be confused with other limb movements or EMG bursts encountered on the PSG: REM twitches, hypnagogic foot tremors, myoclonus, or alternating leg muscle activation (ALMA). REM twitches occur in REM sleep as a normal physiologic component of phasic REM, whereas PLMS primarily occur during non-REM sleep. Foot tremors, myoclonus, and ALMA are usually of shorter duration than PLMS, are less likely to occur in a repetitive periodic pattern, and are generally considered to be of little or at least unknown clinical relevance.

PLMS are not limited to the legs and can occur in the arms. However, only the lower extremities are routinely included in the PSG and therefore have diagnostic value. As the name implies, the movements occur at regular, periodic intervals, usually every 30 seconds. They typically consist of an extension of the big toe, with an upward bending of the ankle, knee, or hip. These movements may be similar to jerking or kicking. PLMS usually do not occur continuously throughout the night, but instead cluster in the first half of the night. If an individual experiences periodic leg movements 5 or more times during each hour of sleep, sleep may be disrupted. The sleep disruption caused by repeated and brief awakenings secondary to PLMS may result in excessive daytime sleepiness. PLMS may also cause several other problems, some of which may affect the bed-partner. The bed-partner may report being kicked at night, that the bedding becomes disheveled, or that limb movements shake the bed.[2]

Individuals not meeting the diagnostic criteria for other sleep disorders such as RLS or sleep apnea or who deny daytime symptoms such as hypersomnolence can be diagnosed with idiopathic PLMS. Individuals reporting hypersomnolence in the context of PLMS not attributed to any other disorder (including RLS) can be diagnosed with PLMD.

How common are PLMS?

PLMS affect a small percentage of people aged 30 to 50 years, one-third of people age 50 to 65 years, and almost half of people more than age 65 years. Therefore, PLMS become more common with age and are rarely seen in individuals younger than 30 years of age.[60] Men and women are equally likely to be affected. As mentioned earlier, PLMS occurring in the context of symptoms resulting in PLMD are rare.

PLMS and associated comorbid sleep and medical conditions

PLMS are a nonspecific PSG finding that are associated with several medical, neurologic, and sleep conditions (**Box 3**).

PLMS and cardiovascular disease

Whereas Winkelman and colleagues[15] noted only a weak association between RLS and hypertension, Siddiqui and colleagues[61] reported a significant sleep-time increase of heart rate and systolic blood pressure (SBP) during PLMS associated with RLS, possibly caused by increases in autonomic activation during PLM episodes. Such patients present with decreased nocturnal sleep-time dipping in BP (<10%), which has been associated with severe organ damage, such as left ventricular hypertrophy. Unruh and colleagues[62] also reported that RLS and PLMS play a factor in

---

Box 3
Conditions associated with periodic limb movements of sleep (PLMS)

Aging

Attention deficit hyperactivity disorder

Chronic obstructive pulmonary disease

Chronic renal failure

Drugs (ie, neuroleptics and antidepressants)

Iron deficiency anemia

Narcolepsy

Neuropathy

Parkinson's disease

Posttraumatic stress disorder

Pregnancy

REM behavioral sleep disorder

Restless legs syndrome

Rheumatic diseases

Sleep apnea

Sleep-disordered breathing events

Spinal cord injury

Spinal cord lesion

---

nondipping nocturnal BP and sleep-time hypertension seen in renal failure patients. Portaluppi and colleagues[63] hypothesized that RLS may provide a causal role in increasing night-time SBP, leading to increased risk for CVD and morbidity in renal patients.

PLMS and medications

Medications can affect PLMS, and health care providers should be aware of them. Some antidepressant medications can increase the frequency of PLMS. Selective serotonin reuptake inhibitors (SSRIs), for example, have been reported to worsen RLS symptoms. However, a review of the literature indicates that SSRIs worsen PLMS and are not necessarily associated with the worsening of RLS symptoms. Moreover, some studies have suggested that some of the same factors associated with RLS (eg, hereditary, iron deficiency) may be associated with the development of PLMS as well as the presence of PLMS in the context of PLMD.

PLMS treatment and management considerations

PLMS should be reported when noted on a PSG as they may reflect a greater degree of disrupted sleep at night, which can affect daytime functioning.[64]

Identification of PLMS is also important because treatment with medications such as DA may improve sleep quality in patients with PLMS associated with other sleep disorders. However, a decision on whether or not to treat PLMS should be considered only once other medical disorders, including sleep disorders, have been thoroughly investigated and treated. Treatment of PLMS in the context of other disorders may improve nocturnal sleep but may exacerbate other symptoms such as daytime sleepiness.[65]

PLMD

Diagnosing PLMD: a diagnosis of exclusion

PLMD is another sleep-related movement disorder associated with night-time limb movement complaints that results in disruption in sleep quality and daytime functioning. Individuals with PLMD, however, do not complain about the sensory creepy-crawly symptoms or the overwhelming urge to move experienced by those with RLS. Instead, individuals with PLMD are observed to have involuntary leg kicks by their bed-partner or on a sleep study. Evidence of PLMS along with complaints of sleep disturbance or disruption in daytime functioning are required for an individual to have the diagnosis of PLMD. Although individuals with RLS often display increased PLMS, PLMS are not required for the diagnosis of RLS but are required for the diagnosis of PLMD. For this reason, unlike RLS, which is a clinical diagnosis based on 4 diagnostic clinical features and therefore does not require a PSG, diagnosing PLMD does require a sleep study to establish the presence of PLMS. Other conditions to consider in the differential diagnosis for PLMD include such conditions as hypnic myoclonus, sleep-related leg cramps, and akathesias as well as other conditions often considered in the differential for RLS. Thus, after all other sleep disorders known to cause leg kicks and sleep disruption leading to excessive daytime sleepiness have been excluded (eg, RLS, sleep apnea, medications), then an individual can be given the PLMD diagnosis.

How common is PLMD?

Although the specific prevalence of PLMD is unknown, the diagnosis is considered to be uncommon to rare amongst the experts in the field.[1]

PLMD treatment and management considerations

The pharmacologic treatment options for PLMD are similar to RLS and therefore readers are referred to that section for complete discussion of the different medical therapies. Treatment of PLMS and PLMD is usually recommended in patients reporting daytime sleepiness that is not attributed to any other disorder.

SUMMARY

RLS, PLMS, and PLMD, which are listed in the ICSD-2 as sleep-related movement disorders, are a group of conditions that merit awareness from the medical community. These disorders are commonly encountered yet often confused and misdiagnosed by health care professionals. Therefore it is imperative that health care providers are able to recognize, diagnose and proficiently manage or properly refer patients with these conditions.

REFERENCES

1. American Academy of Sleep Medicine. International classification of sleep disorders. 2nd edition. Diagnostic and Coding Manual. Westchester (IL): American Academy of Sleep Medicine; 2005.
2. Iber C, Ancoli-Israel S, Chesson AL, et al. The AASM manual for the scoring of sleep and associated events: rules, terminology specifications. Westchester (IL): American Academy of Sleep Medicine; 2007.
3. Montplaisir J, Boucher S, Nicolas A, et al. Immobilization tests and periodic leg movements in sleep for the diagnosis of restless leg syndrome. Mov Disord 1998;13(2):324–9.
4. Michaud M, Poirier G, Lavigne G, et al. Restless legs syndrome: scoring criteria for leg movements recorded during the suggested immobilization test. Sleep Med 2001;2(4):317–21.
5. Michaud M, Paquet J, Lavigne G, et al. Sleep laboratory diagnosis of restless legs syndrome. Eur Neurol 2002;48(2):108–13.
6. Winkelman JW, Redline S, Baldwin CM, et al. Polysomnographic and health-related quality of life correlates of restless legs syndrome in the Sleep Heart Health Study. Sleep 2009;32(6):772–8.
7. Salas RE, Gamaldo CE, Allen RP, et al. Quiescegenic nocturnal dyskinesia: a restless legs syndrome (RLS) variant or a new syndrome? Sleep Med 2009;10(3):396–7.
8. Rajaram SS, Walters AS, England SJ, et al. Some children with growing pains may actually have restless legs syndrome. Sleep 2004;27(4):767–73.
9. Gamaldo CE, Benbrook AR, Allen RP, et al. Childhood and adult factors associated with restless legs syndrome (RLS) diagnosis. Sleep Med 2007; 8(7–8):716–22.
10. Sharifian A, Firoozeh M, Pouryaghoub G, et al. Restless legs syndrome in shift workers: a cross sectional study on male assembly workers. J Circadian Rhythms 2009;7:12.

11. Ohayon MM, Roth T. Prevalence of restless legs syndrome and periodic limb movement disorder in the general population. J Psychosom Res 2002; 53(1):547–54.
12. Schonbrunn E, Riemann D, Hohagen F, et al. [Restless legs and sleep apnea syndrome–random coincidence or causal relation?] Nervenarzt 1990;61(5): 306–11 [in German].
13. Rodrigues RN, Abreu e Silva Rodrigues AA, Pratesi R, et al. Outcome of sleepiness and fatigue scores in obstructive sleep apnea syndrome patients with and without restless legs syndrome after nasal CPAP. Arq Neuropsiquiatr 2007;65(1):54–8.
14. Ahlberg K, Ahlberg J, Könönen M, et al. Reported bruxism and restless legs syndrome in media personnel with or without irregular shift work. Acta Odontol Scand 2005;63(2):94–8.
15. Winkelman JW, Shahar E, Sharief I, et al. Association of restless legs syndrome and cardiovascular disease in the Sleep Heart Health Study. Neurology 2008;70(1):35–42.
16. Weinstock LB, Walters AS, Mullin GE, et al. Celiac disease is associated with restless legs syndrome. Dig Dis Sci 2009, September 3.
17. Abetz L, Allen R, Follet A, et al. Evaluating the quality of life of patients with restless legs syndrome. Clin Ther 2004;26(6):925–35.
18. Allen RP, Walters AS, Montplaisir J, et al. Restless legs syndrome prevalence and impact: REST general population study. Arch Intern Med 2005; 165(11):1286–92.
19. Freye E, Levy JV, Partecke L. Use of gabapentin for attenuation of symptoms following rapid opiate detoxification (ROD)–correlation with neurophysiological parameters. Neurophysiol Clin 2004;34(2):81–9.
20. Dinges DF, Pack F, Williams K, et al. Cumulative sleepiness, mood disturbance, and psychomotor vigilance performance decrements during a week of sleep restricted to 4-5 hours per night. Sleep 1997;20(4):267–77.
21. Van Dongen HP, Maislin G, Mullington JM, et al. The cumulative cost of additional wakefulness: dose-response effects on neurobehavioral functions and sleep physiology from chronic sleep restriction and total sleep deprivation. Sleep 2003;26(2):117–26.
22. Allen RP. Restless legs syndrome (RLS) and periodic limb movement disorder (PLMD). In: Carney P, Berry R, Geyer J, editors. Clinical sleep disorders. Philadelphia: Lippincott: Williams & Wilkins; 2005. p. 209–23.
23. Bassetti CL, Mauerhofer D, Gugger M, et al. Restless legs syndrome: a clinical study of 55 patients. Eur Neurol 2001;45(2):67–74.
24. Pearson VE, Allen RP, Dean T, et al. Cognitive deficits associated with restless legs syndrome (RLS). Sleep Med 2006;7(1):25–30.
25. Saletu M, Anderer P, Saletu B, et al. EEG mapping in patients with restless legs syndrome as compared with normal controls. Psychiatry Res 2002;115(1–2): 49–61.
26. Gamaldo C, Benbrook AR, Allen RP, et al. Evaluating daytime alertness in individuals with Restless Legs Syndrome (RLS) compared to sleep restricted controls. Sleep Med 2009;10(1):134–8.
27. Gamaldo CE, Benbrook AR, Allen RP, et al. A further evaluation of the cognitive deficits associated with restless legs syndrome (RLS). Sleep Med 2008;9(5): 500–5.
28. Edinger JD. Cognitive and behavioral anomalies among insomnia patients with mixed restless legs and periodic limb movement disorder. Behav Sleep Med 2003;1(1):37–53.
29. Cortese S, Konofal E, Lecendreux M, et al. Restless legs syndrome and attention-deficit/hyperactivity disorder: a review of the literature. Sleep 2005;28(8):1007–13.
30. Zak R, Fisher B, Couvadelli BV, et al. Preliminary study of the prevalence of restless legs syndrome in adults with attention deficit hyperactivity disorder. Percept Mot Skills 2009;108(3):759–63.
31. Daviss WB, Perel JM, Birmaher B, et al. Steady-state clinical pharmacokinetics of bupropion extended-release in youths. J Am Acad Child Adolesc Psychiatry 2006;45(12):1503–9.
32. Monuteaux MC, Spencer TJ, Faraone SV, et al. A randomized, placebo-controlled clinical trial of bupropion for the prevention of smoking in children and adolescents with attention-deficit/hyperactivity disorder. J Clin Psychiatry 2007;68(7):1094–101.
33. Gamaldo CE, Earley CJ. Restless legs syndrome: a clinical update. Chest 2006;130(5):1596–604.
34. Earley CJ. Restless legs syndrome. N Engl J Med 2003;348(21):2103–9.
35. Oner P, Dirik EB, Taner Y, et al. Association between low serum ferritin and restless legs syndrome in patients with attention deficit hyperactivity disorder. Tohoku J Exp Med 2007;213(3):269–76.
36. Evans AH, Strafella AP, Weintraub D, et al. Impulsive and compulsive behaviors in Parkinson's disease. Mov Disord 2009;24(11):1561–70.
37. Benbir G, Guilleminault C. Pramipexole: new use for an old drug - the potential use of pramipexole in the treatment of restless legs syndrome. Neuropsychiatr Dis Treat 2006;2(4):393–405.
38. Berger K, Luedemann J, Trenkwalder C, et al. Sex and the risk of restless legs syndrome in the general population. Arch Intern Med 2004;164(2):196–202.
39. Earley CJ. Clinical practice. Restless legs syndrome. N Engl J Med 2003;348(21):2103–9.
40. Garcia-Borreguero D, Allen RP, Benes H, et al. Augmentation as a treatment complication of restless legs syndrome: concept and management. Mov Disord 2007;22(Suppl 18):S476–84.
41. Hening WA, Allen RP, Washburn M, et al. Validation of the Hopkins telephone diagnostic interview for restless legs syndrome. Sleep Med 2008;9(3):283–9.

42. Wang J, O'Reilly B, Venkataraman R, et al. Efficacy of oral iron in patients with restless legs syndrome and a low-normal ferritin: a randomized, double-blind, placebo-controlled study. Sleep Med 2009; 10(9):973–5.

43. Ferri R, Manconi M, Lanuzza B, et al. Age-related changes in periodic leg movements during sleep in patients with restless legs syndrome. Sleep Med 2008;9(7):790–8.

44. Walters AS. Review of receptor agonist and antagonist studies relevant to the opiate system in restless legs syndrome. Sleep Med 2002;3(4):301–4.

45. Winkelmann J, Lichtner P, Putz B, et al. Evidence for further genetic locus heterogeneity and confirmation of RLS-1 in restless legs syndrome. Mov Disord 2006;21(1):28–33.

46. Walters AS, Winkelmann J, Trenkwalder C, et al. Long-term follow-up on restless legs syndrome patients treated with opioids. Mov Disord 2001; 16(6):1105–9.

47. Salas R. Long-term treatment of RLS: augmentation, compulsive behaviors, and sleep-disordered breathing. 23rd Annual Meeting of Associated Professional Sleep Societies. Seattle, Washington, June 8–10, 2009.

48. Stringer J, Welsh C, Tommasello A. Methadone-associated Q-T interval prolongation and torsades de pointes. Am J Health Syst Pharm 2009;66(9):825–33.

49. Hening W, Allen R, Earley C, et al. The treatment of restless legs syndrome and periodic limb movement disorder. Sleep 1999;22(7):970–99.

50. Montplaisir J, Boucher S, Poirier G, et al. Clinical, polysomnographic, and genetic characteristics of restless legs syndrome: a study of 133 patients diagnosed with new standard criteria. Mov Disord 1997;12(1):61–5.

51. Ondo W, Jankovic J. Restless legs syndrome: clinicoetiologic correlates. Neurology 1996;47(6):1435–41.

52. Allen RP, Earley CJ. Defining the phenotype of the restless legs syndrome (RLS) using age-of-symptom-onset. Sleep Med 2000;1(1):11–9.

53. Polydefkis M, Allen RP, Hauer P, et al. Subclinical sensory neuropathy in late-onset restless legs syndrome. Neurology 2000;55(8):1115–21.

54. Bonati MT, Ferini-Strambi L, Aridon P, et al. Autosomal dominant restless legs syndrome maps on chromosome 14q. Brain 2003;126(Pt 6):1485–92.

55. Chen S, Ondo WG, Rao S, et al. Genomewide linkage scan identifies a novel susceptibility locus for restless legs syndrome on chromosome 9p. Am J Hum Genet 2004;74(5):876–85.

56. Stefansson H, Rye DB, Hicks A, et al. A genetic risk factor for periodic limb movements in sleep. N Engl J Med 2007;357(7):639–47.

57. Allen R. Dopamine and iron in the pathophysiology of restless legs syndrome (RLS). Sleep Med 2004; 5(4):385–91.

58. Clemens S, Rye D, Hochman S. Restless legs syndrome: revisiting the dopamine hypothesis from the spinal cord perspective. Neurology 2006;67(1): 125–30.

59. Allen RP, Connor JR, Hyland K, et al. Abnormally increased CSF 3-Ortho-methyldopa (3-OMD) in untreated restless legs syndrome (RLS) patients indicates more severe disease and possibly abnormally increased dopamine synthesis. Sleep Med 2009;10(1):123–8.

60. Avidan AY. Sleep disorders in the older patient. Prim Care 2005;32(2):563–86.

61. Siddiqui F, Strus J, Ming X, et al. Rise of blood pressure with periodic limb movements in sleep and wakefulness. Clin Neurophysiol 2007;118(9):1923–30.

62. Unruh ML, Levey AS, D'Ambrosio C, et al. Restless legs symptoms among incident dialysis patients: association with lower quality of life and shorter survival. Am J Kidney Dis 2004;43(5):900–9.

63. Portaluppi F, Cortelli P, Buonaura GC, et al. Do restless legs syndrome (RLS) and periodic limb movements of sleep (PLMS) play a role in nocturnal hypertension and increased cardiovascular risk of renally impaired patients? Chronobiol Int 2009; 26(6):1206–21.

64. Connor JR, Wang XS, Patton SM, et al. Decreased transferrin receptor expression by neuromelanin cells in restless legs syndrome. Neurology 2004; 62(9):1563–7.

65. Norlander N. Therapy in restless legs. Acta Med Scand 1953;145:453–7.

Medication Effects on Sleep

Francoise J. Roux, MD, PhD[a,b,*], Meir H. Kryger, MD[c,d]

KEYWORDS

- Medications • Sleep architecture • Insomnia
- Excessive daytime somnolence

Sleep and wake states encompass a complex interaction of neuronal networks, involving multiple neurotransmitters with a delicate balance governing the transition from one state to the other. Medications can directly alter this delicate balance depending on their effects on specific neurotransmitters. As a result, medications can promote insomnia or hypersomnia or even act indirectly to disturb sleep. The mechanisms and functions of sleep are still not entirely elucidated, but there is now mounting evidence that good quality of sleep is essential to maintain general good health and adequate daily functioning. In this article, the different neurologic networks and neurotransmitters involved in the wake and sleep states, and how commonly used medications can directly or indirectly affect wakefulness or sleep, are reviewed.

NEUROPHARMACOLOGY OF WAKEFULNESS AND SLEEP
Wakefulness

The mesopontine ascending reticular activating system in the brainstem is a major contributor to wakefulness. The main wake-promoting nuclei in the brainstem are the pedunculopontine and the laterodorsal tegmental nuclei, which project through cholinergic neurons to the reticular thalamic nuclei toward the cortex to produce arousal signals. The ascending arousal system also sends signals from the noradrenergic locus coeruleus nucleus, the serotoninergic dorsal and median raphe nuclei, and the histaminergic tuberomamillary nucleus of the brainstem and posterior hypothalamus, respectively, through the lateral hypothalamus to the cortex. These neurons are also joined in the hypothalamic area by the hypocretinergic neurons, which help maintain and stabilize wakefulness by increasing the activity of the aminergic neurons in the ascending arousal system. These hypocretinergic neurons also send projections to the cortex to contribute to wakefulness. The ascending arousal system projects from the brainstem to the hypothalamus and thalamus, which in turn lead to diffuse cortical activation, with wakefulness as an end result. More recent studies in animals point also toward a role for dopamine (D) as a contributor to arousal through the activation of D_1 and D_2 receptors.[1] The locus coeruleus can also promote wakefulness by inhibiting the sleep-promoting areas such as the ventrolateral preoptic (VLPO). Acetylcholine, noradrenaline, and serotonin can all inhibit the neuronal activity of the VLPO, promoting arousal.

Sleep

The complex arousal system needs to be turned off to allow sleep induction. The role of sleep is still not completely understood. However, sleep seems to play an essential restorative function and promote memory consolidation. Sleep is divided into non–rapid eye movement (NREM)

[a] Section of Pulmonary and Critical Care Medicine, Yale University School of Medicine, 333 Cedar Street, Post Office Box 208057, New Haven, CT 06520-8057, USA
[b] Yale Center for Sleep Medicine, Yale University School of Medicine, 40 Temple Street, Suite 3C, New Haven, CT 06520, USA
[c] University of Connecticut School of Medicine, CT, USA
[d] Gaylord Sleep Medicine, 400 Gaylord Farm Road, Wallingford, CT 06492, USA
* Corresponding author. Section of Pulmonary and Critical Care Medicine, Yale University School of Medicine, 333 Cedar Street, Post Office Box 208057, New Haven, CT 06520-8057.
E-mail address: francoise.roux@yale.edu

Clin Chest Med 31 (2010) 397–405
doi:10.1016/j.ccm.2010.02.008

and rapid eye movement (REM) sleep. NREM sleep is further subdivided into stages N1, N2, and N3. Stages N1 and N2 (formerly called stages 1 and 2) are light sleep, whereas stage N3 (formerly called stages 3 and 4) is considered deep sleep or delta sleep. REM sleep is the stage of sleep where the muscle tone is the lowest and the most dreaming occurs. During the night, there are 3 to 4 cycles of NREM sleep, with episodes of REM sleep about every 90 minutes between the cycles. The anterior hypothalamus is the main area responsible for the induction of sleep. The VLPO area in the anterior hypothalamus contains γ-aminobutyric acid (GABA) and galanin neurons, which project to and inhibit the wake-promoting areas, including the monoaminergic systems and the tuberomamillary nucleus. The cholinergic neurons of the pedunculopontine and the latero-dorsal tegmental nuclei promote REM sleep. The ablation of the VLPO area results in a state of prolonged wakefulness. During wakefulness, there is also a progressive increase in adenosine, which accumulates in the forebrain and promotes NREM sleep. Adenosine binds to the adenosine A_1 receptors, which inhibit the cholinergic centers in the brainstem and decrease the cortical arousal. Another nucleus in the brain has been implicated in the regulation of the sleep-wake cycle by playing a role in the control of circadian rhythms. The circadian clock of the brain is the suprachiasmatic nucleus (SCN) of the hypothalamus. The SCN has a significant impact on the timing of the sleep-wake cycle.[2] The SCN regulates the production of melatonin in a circadian pattern, with high levels secreted at night. As the day progresses, the onset of melatonin production favors sleep initiation.

The sleep-wake interaction is made of mutual inhibitory groups of neurons, one promoting arousal and inhibiting sleep and the other inhibiting arousal and promoting sleep, creating a delicate reciprocal relationship. Medications can exert their effects in a regionally specific manner, which would tip the balance from one side to the other, leading to symptoms of either hypersomnolence or insomnia.

DRUGS INDUCING EXCESSIVE DAYTIME SOMNOLENCE
Hypnotics

Benzodiazepines
Benzodiazepines are among the most widely prescribed hypnotics. Benzodiazepines replaced the barbiturates, which had potential for abuse and significant side effects. The benzodiazepines bind nonselectively to the various subunits of the $GABA_A$ receptor in the brain. $GABA_A$ is the predominant central nervous system inhibitory neurotransmitter. $GABA_A$ allows the entrance of negative chloride ions into the cells, creating increased membrane polarization and an inhibitory effect. A meta-analysis was done on the effects of about 2 weeks of benzodiazepines for the treatment of insomnia. The investigators concluded that benzodiazepines can effectively reduce sleep latency, increase sleep time, reduce the number of awakenings after sleep onset, and improve overall sleep quality.[3] However, benzodiazepines can alter sleep architecture. Benzodiazepines effectively suppress delta sleep and, to some extent, slightly decrease REM sleep. The latency of REM sleep is prolonged, stage 2 is increased, and so are all fast activities, especially spindles, which are called pseudospindles and are electroencephalographic markers of benzodiazepine use.

This nonselective binding to the $GABA_A$ receptor is responsible not only for the hypnotic effect of the benzodiazepines but also for their various side effects, such as daytime sedation, cognitive impairment, anterograde amnesia, ataxia, muscle relaxation, and dependency. Hypnotic benzodiazepine medications include temazepam, estazolam, flurazepam, quazepam, and triazolam. These agents differ from each other in terms of onset and duration of action, which are summarized in **Table 1**. Triazolam has the shortest duration of action and is cleared rapidly, leading to less daytime sedation. However, because of its short duration of action, it might lead to withdrawal and sleep fragmentation at the end of the night. In contrast, flurazepam and quazepam have the longest duration of action, with active metabolites causing more daytime sedation and cognitive effects. Short-acting benzodiazepines are more likely to cause anterograde amnesia and rebound insomnia. Rebound insomnia is characterized by sudden exacerbation of insomnia compared with baseline levels after discontinuation of benzodiazepine use. Benzodiazepine withdrawal results in worsening insomnia with anxiety, tremor, irritability and, in rare instances, seizures. These symptoms are also more common with short-acting benzodiazepines. A rebound in REM sleep can also occur, with resultant nightmares. Benzodiazepines should be tapered slowly to allow a gradual decline in plasma concentration, avoiding rebound insomnia or withdrawal symptoms. Because benzodiazepines are sedatives and muscle relaxants, they can also affect nighttime breathing in susceptible hosts.[4] Benzodiazepines have been shown to worsen sleep-disordered breathing and cause hypoventilation in patients with underlying lung impairment, with resulting nocturnal sleep disruption.[5]

Table 1
Profiles of various benzodiazepines

Medication	Half-life (h)	Duration of Action	Characteristics
Temazepam	3.5–20	Intermediate	Delayed-onset Intermediate-acting
Estazolam	8–24	Intermediate	Delayed-onset Intermediate-acting
Quazepam	39–73	Long	Rapid-onset Long-acting
Triazolam	1.5–5.5	Short	Rapid-onset Short-acting

Nonbenzodiazepines

The side effects observed with the classic benzodiazepines prompted the discovery of more selective agents such as the nonbenzodiazepines (eg, zolpidem, zopiclone, zaleplon, eszopiclone). The nonbenzodiazepines are structurally different from the benzodiazepines and bind selectively to the α_1 subunit of the $GABA_A$ receptor, leading to sedation but fewer side effects. The hypnotic effect is comparable to the benzodiazepines, but they exhibit a lower risk of dependency, abuse, and rebound insomnia. Because of their selectivity they have no antianxiety, myorelaxant, or anticonvulsant properties. The duration of action varies from ultrashort to short to intermediate for zaleplon, zolpidem, and eszopiclone, respectively (**Table 2**). As a result, zaleplon is better suited for the treatment of initiation rather than maintenance of insomnia. Zolpidem is the most commonly prescribed agent among the nonbenzodiazepine group. Polysomnographic data in patients with chronic insomnia showed that zolpidem decreased sleep latency and increased total sleep time and sleep efficiency, like other nonbenzodiazepine agents.[6] In contrast to the benzodiazepines, zolpidem preserves the sleep architecture, including delta sleep.[7] Some reports indicate that it might even increase delta sleep.[8] The repeated administration of zolpidem for 8 days did not alter nocturnal ventilation and oxygenation in patients with chronic obstructive lung disease.[7] The study by Krystal and colleagues[9] showed a sustained efficacy of eszopiclone over 6 months of nightly treatment, with improved sleep latency and quality, increased total sleep time, and decreased number of awakenings. An absence of tolerance has been shown for nonbenzodiazepines for up to 12 months of treatment duration, as well as an absence of rebound insomnia on discontinuation.[10] Fewer clinically significant interactions with other medications have been reported with the nonbenzodiazepines compared with the benzodiazepines, which is likely because of the difference in cytochrome P-450 metabolism.[11]

Antidepressants

Since the late 1980s, the number of antidepressants prescribed for the treatment of insomnia has increased steadily. The usage of antidepressants in this setting has not been as well studied as the usage of benzodiazepines, especially in patients without depression. Most depressive patients experience prolonged sleep latency, decreased sleep efficiency, early morning awakenings, and reduced total sleep time.

Tricyclic antidepressants

The tricyclic antidepressants (TCAs) have multiple mechanisms of action; they inhibit the reuptake of serotonin and noradrenaline and block histamine (H) H_1 and muscarinic cholinergic receptors, and most of them also block α_1-adrenoceptors. TCAs are associated with daytime somnolence, especially those with greater effect on serotonin than noradrenaline reuptake, such as clomipramine, amitriptyline, and doxepin.[12] Tricyclics in general reduce REM sleep and prolong REM latency. Clomipramine especially is a very potent REM suppressor. The REM suppressant's effects tend to lessen over time but do not return to baseline values. In contrast, trimipramine does not have the same effect on REM sleep as other TCAs; it is not a serotonin reuptake inhibitor. Sedating

Table 2
Profiles of nonbenzodiazepines

Medication	Half-life (h)	Duration of Action
Eszopiclone	5–7	Intermediate
Zolpidem	1.5–4	Short
Zaleplon	1	Very short

TCAs, such as amitriptyline, nortriptyline, doxepin, and clomipramine, reduce sleep-onset latency and improve total sleep time and sleep efficiency. Trimipramine, desipramine, and protriptyline are less sedating and can decrease total sleep time. TCAs can exacerbate the frequency of periodic leg movements during sleep and worsen REM-sleep behavior disorder.

Selective serotonin reuptake inhibitors

Selective serotonin reuptake inhibitors (SSRIs) are perhaps the most commonly prescribed medications to treat depression because they exhibit significantly fewer side effects than the TCAs. SSRIs are also indicated for generalized anxiety disorder, social phobia, and obsessive-compulsive disorder. SSRIs primarily block the reuptake of serotonin but can also affect different receptors. SSRIs may be associated with daytime sedation or insomnia, which may be because of the effects on different serotonin (5-hydroxytryptamine [5-HT]) receptor subtypes based on the individual SSRI.[12] Paroxetine and fluvoxamine are among the most sedating SSRIs, whereas fluoxetine is more alerting. In patients with primary insomnia, paroxetine resulted in subjective improvements in sleep quality, although polysomnographic data demonstrated worsening sleep-onset latency but improved total sleep time. Electroencephalographic studies reveal that SSRIs induce sleep fragmentation. Polysomnographic data of normal patients and patients with depression showed that SSRIs increased sleep and REM sleep latency, and decreased REM sleep and sleep efficiency.[13] Feige and colleagues[14] examined the effect of a 3-week administration of fluoxetine on sleep parameters in healthy subjects. These investigators found that fluoxetine worsened total sleep time and sleep efficiency and decreased REM sleep. However, discontinuation of fluoxetine restored these indexes within 2 to 4 days and led to a rebound in REM sleep. SSRIs can also induce prominent eye movement during NREM sleep, which was present in 36% of patients chronically on SSRIs in one study.[15] Serotonergic antidepressants can also induce REM-sleep behavior disorder[16] and increase the number of periodic leg movements during sleep.[17]

Atypical Antidepressants

Trazodone is commonly prescribed for insomnia, even for patients without depression; unfortunately, few studies look at the effect of trazodone in this patient population. Trazodone and nefazodone are weak serotonin reuptake inhibitors. These agents are also 5-HT$_2$ receptor antagonists and block α_1-adrenoceptor activity. Trazodone also blocks histamine H$_1$ receptor. Very few studies have examined the objective effect of trazodone on polysomnographic parameters, and most of these were done in patients with depression. A review of these studies showed that trazodone decreased the number of awakenings during the night, but evidence for its efficacy is overall limited.[18] Trazodone has been noted to increase deep sleep; it causes drowsiness and next-day sedation even at low doses. Further, the optimal dose for the treatment of insomnia in patients without depression has not yet been established. Trazodone is not approved by the Food and Drug Administration (FDA) for the treatment of insomnia. Further, trazodone induced significant side effects such as syncope, ventricular arrhythmias, QTc prolongation, exacerbation of ischemic attacks, and orthostatic hypotension, which should raise concern, especially in the elderly. In contrast to most other antidepressants, nefazodone has been shown to either have no effect on REM sleep[19] or increase it in healthy and depressed subjects. Nefazodone can cause drowsiness but, according to some studies, does not improve sleep continuity in healthy subjects.[20] Mirtazapine blocks α_2-adrenergic, histamine H$_1$, and 5-HT$_2$ and 5-HT$_3$ serotonergic receptors, and is an effective antidepressant. Mirtazapine is associated with daytime somnolence and significant weight gain. Aslan and colleagues[21] found that mirtazapine improved sleep efficiency, increased deep sleep, and decreased the number of awakenings but, in contrast to other antidepressants, did not decrease REM sleep in healthy subjects. Another recent study in patients with depression confirmed its sedative properties, with improvement in sleep continuity and total sleep time with increased delta sleep, which were maintained even after 28 days of treatment.[22]

Antipsychotics

Most schizophrenic patients suffer from sleep disturbances[23] such as insomnia and circadian rhythm shift. Polysomnographic studies in schizophrenics reveal a reduced sleep efficiency and short REM sleep latency, which seem to correlate with greater severity of the disease. Both the traditional and newest antipsychotics exhibit sedative properties, most likely because of their antagonism of histaminergic, serotonergic, and α_1-adrenergic receptors. However, these medications will also improve sleep quality by decreasing psychotic symptoms. A review of polysomnographic studies in schizophrenic and healthy patients[24] showed that antipsychotics improve total sleep time, decreased awakenings, and shortened sleep latency, especially quetiapine, thiothixene, and haloperidol. Ziprasidone, olanzapine, and risperidone have been shown to increase delta sleep. Risperidone and ziprasidone are the strongest REM suppressant agents among antipsychotics. Clozapine, olanzapine, thioridazine, and chlorpromazine are the most sedating antipsychotics and can impair daytime functioning. Conversely, aripiprazole is the least sedating agent. Antipsychotics can also elicit akathisia due to their extrapyramidal side effects. An increased number of periodic leg movements and the onset of restless legs syndrome caused by their dopamine antagonism can also be induced by these medications. Weight gain induced by these antipsychotic medications can also eventually promote sleep-disordered breathing.

Lithium

Lithium is used mainly to treat manic-depressive disease and is associated with excessive daytime somnolence; it has been shown to decrease REM sleep in depressed and normal subjects. Lithium was also shown to increase delta sleep in healthy subjects, likely through a decrease in $5\text{-}HT_2$ receptor function.[25] Lithium can also worsen restless legs syndrome, affecting sleep quality.

Antiepileptic Drugs

Poorly controlled epilepsy can directly disrupt sleep with decreased REM sleep. Poor sleep quality can further worsen epilepsy, with impaired daytime alertness as a consequence. Patients with epilepsy complain of excessive daytime somnolence, which can be multifactorial, including adverse effects of antiepileptic drugs (AEDs). Most AEDs lead to daytime sedation, and some patients may need multiple medications to adequately control seizures, further affecting daytime alertness. Daytime somnolence is a common side effect of barbiturates and benzodiazepines (see earlier discussion). Barbiturates such as phenobarbital decrease sleep latency, increase sleep continuity, and decrease arousals and REM sleep. Benzodiazepines such as diazepam decrease sleep latency as well as delta and REM sleep. Barbiturates and benzodiazepines can also promote sleep-disordered breathing, which could further worsen seizure control. Phenytoin, valproate, and carbamazepine have been shown to increase daytime drowsiness by objective measures. The classic antiepileptic medications such as carbamazepine and phenytoin decrease REM sleep. Newer AEDs

include gabapentin, lamotrigine, tiagabine, felbamate, topiramate, and levetiracetam. Gabapentin and tiagabine increase GABA concentrations[12] and delta sleep. Gabapentin and lamotrigine seem to increase REM sleep when added to other AEDs. Gabapentin is effective for the treatment of restless legs syndrome and periodic leg movements, which can improve sleep quality. Cicolin and colleagues[26] examined the effect of levetiracetam for 3 weeks on sleep architecture and daytime alertness, using polysomnography and a multiple sleep latency test (MSLT) in healthy subjects. Levetiracetam increased sleep efficiency, total sleep time, and delta sleep, but daytime sleep latencies were normal. Bonanni and colleagues[27] evaluated daytime sleep latencies using MSLT in drug-naïve epileptic patients receiving topiramate for 2 months. The investigators found that topiramate did not impair daytime alertness in epileptic patients. Felbamate, lamotrigine, and zonisamide can have an alerting effect and should be administered early in the day.[28] The time of administration of an AED should be individualized to optimize daytime function.

Antiparkinsonian Drugs

Excessive daytime somnolence and sleep disruption are inherent to Parkinson disease, occurring in 50% to 80% of patients compared with controls. Sleep disruption is multifactorial in this patient population and can result from periodic leg movement disorder, REM sleep behavior disorder, sleep-disordered breathing, depression, or even dementia in the late stages of the disease. The antiparkinsonian drugs include the dopamine precursors such as levodopa, the ergot derivative dopamine agonists such as pergolide, and the nonergot dopamine agonists such as pramipexole and ropinirole acting at the $D_2\text{-}D_3$ receptors. Hypersomnia has been reported with most antiparkinsonian medications, but sudden sleep attacks have been linked to the new dopaminergic agonists. A randomized placebo-controlled study in healthy subjects showed that ropinirole significantly decreased the sleep latency measured by MSLT compared with placebo.[29] Decreased sleep latencies were also demonstrated in patients with Parkinson disease who were treated with pramipexole, which normalized after its withdrawal. Kaynak and colleagues[30] examined sleep and sleepiness in patients with mild to moderate Parkinson disease before any treatment and after 10 months of dopaminergic treatment, using polysomnography, the Epworth sleepiness scale, and MSLT. These investigators found that the sleep architecture was not significantly altered by the treatment, although there was a trend toward an increase in total sleep time and sleep efficiency with treatment. In contrast, the dopaminergic treatment elicited a significant increase in subjective and objective daytime sleepiness in patients with Parkinson disease, especially when a higher dose of L-dopa was given, compared with before treatment. Anticholinergic drugs such as benztropine are also sedative.

Opiates

Pain is a major contributor to sleep disruption. Opioid use, whether acute or chronic, has dramatically increased in the last decade. Opioid receptors are present in the brain and the peripheral nervous system. Opioid medications, morphine and methadone for example, activate the opioid μ receptors present in the brainstem respiratory centers and on pain neurons. Acute administration of morphine disrupts sleep with increased arousals and wakefulness after sleep onset,[31] and reduces delta and REM sleep[32] in healthy subjects. With chronic morphine use, REM sleep is still decreased, and there are increased wake episodes during the night. In contrast, chronic methadone use does not affect the sleep architecture much; a decrease in waking state was the only abnormality noted.[33] Fatigue and excessive daytime somnolence are observed during chronic opioid use. Acute opioid administration decreases respiratory rate and tidal volume but could lead to respiratory depression in the case of overdose or in patients with underlying pulmonary compromise. A retrospective cohort study[34] assessed the effect of chronic opiate use for at least 6 months on respiration compared with patients not on opiates. Chronic opioid use was associated with the development of central apneas with a significant dose response effect. These central apneas (**Fig. 1**) are distinct from Cheyne-Stokes respiration, and are characterized by an irregular pattern of breathing during NREM sleep termed as Biot respiration or ataxic breathing. Other studies have confirmed these findings; one of them even showed a correlation between the occurrence of the central apneas and the blood level of methadone.[31] However, opiates can be useful in improving restless legs syndrome.

Antihistamines

Histamine (H) is one of the major wake-promoting neurotransmitters. Antihistamines will block the postsynaptic H_1 receptor. However, antihistamines are multifunctional drugs that can also block muscarinic cholinergic and adrenergic receptors. The first generation of antihistamines readily penetrates the blood-brain barrier because of its high lipophilic properties, with daytime sedation as a consequence. These antihistamines tend to decrease sleep latency and improve sleep continuity; they include hydroxyzine, diphenhydramine, doxylamine, chlorpheniramine, clemastine, and promethazine. These agents are mainly useful to treat symptoms of allergy, but diphenhydramine is often self-prescribed as an over-the-counter hypnotic medication because of its sedative properties. Hydroxyzine is, however, the most sedating antihistamine. Considering these undesirable side effects, a second generation of antihistamines has emerged. This generation includes cetirizine and loratadine, which are hydrophilic and penetrate the blood-brain barrier less but can still be sedative at high dose. The most recently developed antihistamines are levocetirizine, fexofenadine, and desloratadine, which have no anticholinergic properties and are not sedative.[35]

Cardiovascular Medications

$α_2$-AGONISTS

Clonidine is a common antihypertensive agent. In healthy subjects, morning administration of clonidine resulted in significant sleepiness compared with controls who persisted without sleep throughout the day, as well as a decrease in REM sleep compared with controls.[36] Clonidine was also shown to reduce sleep latency and significantly decrease REM sleep among hypertensive subjects.[37] Methyldopa has also been associated with sedation.

$α_1$-ANTAGONISTS

Prazosin and terazosin can be sedating. In patients with posttraumatic stress disorder, prazosin was found to significantly increase total sleep time and REM sleep compared with placebo.[38]

DRUGS INDUCING ALERTNESS OR INSOMNIA

Multiple neurotransmitters, such as acetylcholine, serotonin, noradrenaline, histamine, hypocretin, dopamine, and glutamate, are involved in the promotion of wakefulness.

Amphetamines

Stimulants are mostly prescribed for attention-deficit hyperactivity disorders and narcolepsy. Stimulants include amphetamines, methylphenidate, and dextroamphetamine. These agents promote wakefulness by blocking the reuptake and increasing the release of dopamine, norepinephrine, and serotonin in the central nervous system. Dopamines seem to play a major role in this process.[39] Dopamines increase sleep latency,

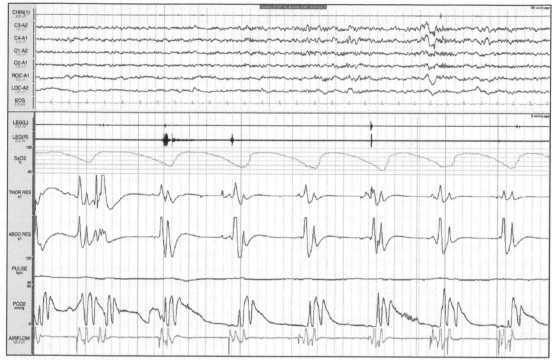

Fig. 1. Central apnea related to opiate. These data are from a 44-year-old soldier treated for severe nerve pain related to an ankle injury. He suffered from snoring and severe sleepiness, and witnessed apnea for 2 to 3 years. He was treated with morphine for pain. He had a breathing frequency of only 4 or 5 breaths per minute and repetitive cycles of 2 to 3 breaths followed by central apneic episodes. The bottom window is 5 minutes. It is likely that this pattern is related to the morphine. The patient also had central apneas during wakefulness. (*Adapted from* Kryger MH. Atlas of clinical sleep medicine. Philadelphia: Elsevier; 2010; with permission.)

reduce total sleep time, and decrease delta and REM sleep. Unfortunately, this increased wakefulness comes at the expense of significant cardiovascular side effects, including increases in blood pressure and heart rate. Insomnia and, more rarely, hallucinations and paranoid ideation have been reported. It is of concern that abuse, tolerance, and dependence are more likely with these medications.

Modafinil and Armodafinil

Modafinil and armodafinil, under a new class of medications, have been approved by the FDA as a first-line treatment for narcolepsy as well as for patients suffering from shift work sleep disorder and sleep-disordered breathing with residual hypersomnia. The increased use of these medications is due to their minor side effects and low potential for abuse in comparison with the amphetamines. The exact mechanisms of action of modafinil or armodafinil have still not been totally elucidated but might involve some effect at the dopamine and noradrenergic transporters in the central nervous system. A study in animals

suggests that the dopaminergic D_1 and D_2 receptors are essential for the wakefulness effect of modafinil.[40] Armodafinil is the R-enantiomer of modafinil and has a much longer half-life. Maintenance wakefulness tests have shown that modafinil and armodafinil promote wakefulness compared with placebo in narcoleptic patients.[41] Both are well tolerated, headache is the most common side effect, and insomnia is a rare occurrence, affecting only about 5% of patients.

Theophylline

Adenosine concentration increases during the day and seems to contribute to the pressure to sleep at the end of the day. Antagonism of adenosine receptors by theophylline can induce alertness. Theophylline is a bronchodilator mainly used in patients with chronic obstructive lung disease. The effect of theophylline on sleep and wakefulness was assessed in healthy subjects using MSLT and polysomnography.[42] Nighttime administration of theophylline, at a therapeutic level, delayed nocturnal sleep latency, increased the number of arousals and wake time, and decreased the total sleep time by 1 hour. Theophylline also increased alertness during the daytime with prolonged latency during the MSLT compared with placebo. Sleep quality among asthmatics was shown to improve with salmeterol treatment but not with theophylline.

Cardiovascular Drugs

β-BLOCKERS

β-Blockers can vary significantly from each other depending on their degree of lipophilicity versus hydrophilicity. A higher lipophilicity index allows for a better penetration into the central nervous system and might lead to more central nervous system side effects. β-Blockers have been associated with increased rates of nightmares, hallucinations, and insomnia, especially with lipophilic agents such as propranolol and pindolol, although other pharmacologic properties may also be at play. Switching to a more hydrophilic β-blocker would be beneficial. β-Blockers can also decrease melatonin release, which could contribute to sleep disruption.

Corticosteroids

Corticosteroids have a wide range of effects on multiple organs and can also affect sleep. Insomnia has been reported in patients on steroids. In healthy volunteers, dexamethasone increased the wake time after sleep onset and reduced REM sleep compared with placebo.[43] Dexamethasone can increase daytime alertness after nocturnal administration. Endogenous glucocorticoid secretion is inhibited during early nocturnal sleep, and delta sleep is believed to play a significant role for declarative memory formation. In some studies, dexamethasone has been shown to decrease delta sleep. Administration of dexamethasone resulted in impaired sleep-facilitating declarative memory in healthy subjects.[44]

SUMMARY

Numerous drugs have been developed that can affect multiple neurotransmitters and/or receptors and thereby directly or indirectly affect sleep and the waking state. Molecular studies have shown that hypnotics still cannot reproduce a good night of natural sleep, based on transcription factors analysis.[45] An understanding of pharmacokinetics and receptor targets of these various complex medications is important to decrease possible side effects in more susceptible patient populations. The future resides in designing extremely selective medications with fewer side effects and, hopefully, with minimal impact on the sleep-wake cycle to prevent detrimental health consequences.

REFERENCES

1. Isaac SO, Berridge CW. Wake-promoting actions of dopamine D1 and D2 receptor stimulation. J Pharmacol Exp Ther 2003;307(1):386–94.
2. Moore RY. Suprachiasmatic nucleus in sleep-wake regulation. Sleep Med 2007;8(Suppl 3):27–33.
3. Nowell PD, Mazumdar S, Buysse DJ, et al. Benzodiazepines and zolpidem for chronic insomnia: a meta-analysis of treatment efficacy. JAMA 1997; 278(24):2170–7.
4. Roth T. Hypnotic use for insomnia management in chronic obstructive pulmonary disease. Sleep Med 2009;10(1):19–25.
5. Guilleminault C. Benzodiazepines, breathing, and sleep. Am J Med 1990;88(3A):25S–8S.
6. Monti JM. Effect of zolpidem on sleep in insomniac patients. Eur J Clin Pharmacol 1989;36(5):461–6.
7. Girault C, Muir JF, Mihaltan F, et al. Effects of repeated administration of zolpidem on sleep, diurnal and nocturnal respiratory function, vigilance, and physical performance in patients with copd. Chest 1996;110(5):1203–11.
8. Besset A, Tafti M, Villemin E, et al. Effects of zolpidem on the architecture and cyclical structure of sleep in poor sleepers. Drugs Exp Clin Res 1995; 21(4):161–9.
9. Krystal AD, Walsh JK, Laska E, et al. Sustained efficacy of eszopiclone over 6 months of nightly treatment: results of a randomized, double-blind, placebo-controlled study in adults with chronic insomnia. Sleep 2003;26(7):793–9.
10. Fry J, Scharf M, Mangano R, et al. Zaleplon improves sleep without producing rebound effects in outpatients with insomnia. Zaleplon clinical study group. Int Clin Psychopharmacol 2000; 15(3):141–52.
11. Hesse LM, von Moltke LL, Greenblatt DJ. Clinically important drug interactions with zopiclone, zolpidem and zaleplon. CNS Drugs 2003;17(7): 513–32.
12. DeMartinis NA, Winokur A. Effects of psychiatric medications on sleep and sleep disorders. CNS Neurol Disord Drug Targets 2007;6(1):17–29.
13. Oberndorfer S, Saletu-Zyhlarz G, Saletu B. Effects of selective serotonin reuptake inhibitors on objective and subjective sleep quality. Neuropsychobiology 2000;42(2):69–81.
14. Feige B, Voderholzer U, Riemann D, et al. Fluoxetine and sleep EEG: effects of a single dose, subchronic treatment, and discontinuation in healthy subjects. Neuropsychopharmacology 2002;26(2): 246–58.

15. Geyer JD, Carney PR, Dillard SC, et al. Antidepressant medications, neuroleptics, and prominent eye movements during NREM sleep. J Clin Neurophysiol 2009;26(1):39–44.

16. Schenck CH, Mahowald MW, Kim SW, et al. Prominent eye movements during NREM sleep and REM sleep behavior disorder associated with fluoxetine treatment of depression and obsessive-compulsive disorder. Sleep 1992;15(3):226–35.

17. Yang C, White DP, Winkelman JW. Antidepressants and periodic leg movements of sleep. Biol Psychiatry 2005;58(6):510–4.

18. Mendelson WB. A review of the evidence for the efficacy and safety of trazodone in insomnia. J Clin Psychiatry 2005;66(4):469–76.

19. Vogel G, Cohen J, Mullis D, et al. Nefazodone and REM sleep: how do antidepressant drugs decrease REM sleep? Sleep 1998;21(1):70–7.

20. Sharpley AL, Williamson DJ, Attenburrow ME, et al. The effects of paroxetine and nefazodone on sleep: a placebo controlled trial. Psychopharmacology (Berl) 1996;126(1):50–4.

21. Aslan S, Isik E, Cosar B. The effects of mirtazapine on sleep: a placebo controlled, double-blind study in young healthy volunteers. Sleep 2002;25(6):677–9.

22. Schmid DA, Wichniak A, Uhr M, et al. Changes of sleep architecture, spectral composition of sleep EEG, the nocturnal secretion of cortisol, ACTH, GH, prolactin, melatonin, ghrelin, and leptin, and the DEX-CRH test in depressed patients during treatment with mirtazapine. Neuropsychopharmacology 2006;31(4):832–44.

23. Cohrs S. Sleep disturbances in patients with schizophrenia: impact and effect of antipsychotics. CNS Drugs 2008;22(11):939–62.

24. Krystal AD, Goforth HW, Roth T. Effects of antipsychotic medications on sleep in schizophrenia. Int Clin Psychopharmacol 2008;23(3):150–60.

25. Friston KJ, Sharpley AL, Solomon RA, et al. Lithium increases slow wave sleep: possible mediation by brain 5-HT2 receptors? Psychopharmacology (Berl) 1989;98(1):139–40.

26. Cicolin A, Magliola U, Giordano A, et al. Effects of levetiracetam on nocturnal sleep and daytime vigilance in healthy volunteers. Epilepsia 2006;47(1):82–5.

27. Bonanni E, Galli R, Maestri M, et al. Daytime sleepiness in epilepsy patients receiving topiramate monotherapy. Epilepsia 2004;45(4):333–7.

28. Bazil CW. Effects of antiepileptic drugs on sleep structure: are all drugs equal? CNS Drugs 2003;17(10):719–28.

29. Ferreira JJ, Galitzky M, Thalamas C, et al. Effect of ropinirole on sleep onset: a randomized, placebo-controlled study in healthy volunteers. Neurology 2002;58(3):460–2.

30. Kaynak D, Kiziltan G, Kaynak H, et al. Sleep and sleepiness in patients with Parkinson's disease before and after dopaminergic treatment. Eur J Neurol 2005;12(3):199–207.

31. Wang D, Teichtahl H. Opioids, sleep architecture and sleep-disordered breathing. Sleep Med Rev 2007;11(1):35–46.

32. Shaw IR, Lavigne G, Mayer P, et al. Acute intravenous administration of morphine perturbs sleep architecture in healthy pain-free young adults: a preliminary study. Sleep 2005;28(6):677–82.

33. Kay DC. Human sleep during chronic morphine intoxication. Psychopharmacologia 1975;44(2):117–24.

34. Walker JM, Farney RJ, Rhondeau SM, et al. Chronic opioid use is a risk factor for the development of central sleep apnea and ataxic breathing. J Clin Sleep Med 2007;3(5):455–61.

35. McDonald K, Trick L, Boyle J. Sedation and antihistamines: an update. Review of inter-drug differences using proportional impairment ratios. Hum Psychopharmacol 2008;23(7):555–70.

36. Carskadon MA, Cavallo A, Rosekind MR. Sleepiness and nap sleep following a morning dose of clonidine. Sleep 1989;12(4):338–44.

37. Danchin N, Genton P, Atlas P, et al. Comparative effects of atenolol and clonidine on polygraphically recorded sleep in hypertensive men: a randomized, double-blind, crossover study. Int J Clin Pharmacol Ther 1995;33(1):52–5.

38. Taylor FB, Martin P, Thompson C, et al. Prazosin effects on objective sleep measures and clinical symptoms in civilian trauma posttraumatic stress disorder: a placebo-controlled study. Biol Psychiatry 2008;63(6):629–32.

39. Boutrel B, Koob GF. What keeps us awake: the neuropharmacology of stimulants and wakefulness-promoting medications. Sleep 2004;27(6):1181–94.

40. Qu WM, Huang ZL, Xu XH, et al. Dopaminergic D1 and D2 receptors are essential for the arousal effect of modafinil. J Neurosci 2008;28(34):8462–9.

41. Lankford DA. Armodafinil: a new treatment for excessive sleepiness. Expert Opin Investig Drugs 2008;17(4):565–73.

42. Roehrs T, Merlotti L, Halpin D, et al. Effects of theophylline on nocturnal sleep and daytime sleepiness/alertness. Chest 1995;108(2):382–7.

43. Moser NJ, Phillips BA, Guthrie G, et al. Effects of dexamethasone on sleep. Pharmacol Toxicol 1996;79(2):100–2.

44. Plihal W, Pietrowsky R, Born J. Dexamethasone blocks sleep induced improvement of declarative memory. Psychoneuroendocrinology 1999;24(3):313–31.

45. Wisor JP, Morairty SR, Huynh NT, et al. Gene expression in the rat cerebral cortex: comparison of recovery sleep and hypnotic-induced sleep. Neuroscience 2006;141(1):371–8.

Index

Note: Page numbers of article titles are in **boldface** type.

A

Acromegaly, CSA in, 242

Actigraphy, in excessive sleepiness assessment, 346

Advanced sleep phase syndrome, 320
  excessive sleepiness due to, 344

AEDs. See *Antiepileptic drugs (AEDs)*.

Age, as factor in OSAHS, 181–182

α_2-Agonists, excessive daytime somnolence due to, 402

Air flow measurement, in sleep studies, 289

Airway(s), upper, surgery of, in OSAS management, 195–196

Alertness, drugs inducing, 402–404

Altitude, high, eucapnic-hypocanic CSA and, 239–240

Alveolar hypoventilation syndromes, with normal pulmonary function, CSA due to, 240

Amphetamines, alertness or insomnia due to, 402–403

α_1-Antagonists, excessive daytime somnolence due to, 402

Antidepressants, excessive daytime somnolence due to, 399–400

Antiepileptic drugs (AEDs)
  excessive daytime somnolence due to, 401
  for RLS, 391

Antihistamines, excessive daytime somnolence due to, 402

Antiparkinsonian drugs, excessive daytime somnolence due to, 401–402

Antipsychotics, excessive daytime somnolence due to, 400–401

Anxiety disorders, insomnia associated with, 331

APAP devices
  in ambulatory management of sleep apnea, 303
  in OSAS management, 192–194
    described, 192–193
    titrations of, in determination of therapeutic pressure setting for conventional fixed CPAP devices, 194
    types of, 193–194
    unattended home APAP, 194
    vs. CPAP, 193
  unattended home, in OSAS management, 194

Apnea(s)
  defined, 179
  RLS and, 387

sleep. See Obstructive sleep apnea syndrome (OSAS); Sleep apnea; *specific types, e.g.,* Obstructive sleep apnea (OSA).

Apneic threshold, in CSA, 235–236

Armodafinil, alertness or insomnia due to, 403

Arousal(s), confusional, 354–356

Arrhythmia(s)
  atrial, CPAP for, 211–212
  in OSA, 210–212. See also *Obstructive sleep apnea (OSA), arrhythmias in.*
  OSA in cardiovascular disease and, 206
  sinus, 211
  ventricular, 211

Asthma, bronchial, hypoventilation due to, 258–259

Atrial arrhythmias, CPAP for, 211–212

Atrial fibrillation, 211

Atrial overdrive, 212

Autonomic system, alterations of, OSA and, 281

B

Bariatric surgery, in OSAS management, 196

Benzodiazepine(s), excessive daytime somnolence due to, 398

Benzodiazepine receptor agonists, for RLS, 391

Bilevel positive pressure therapy, in OSAS management, 191–192

ß-Blockers, alertness or insomnia due to, 404

Brainstem disorders, CSA due to, 241

Breathing disorders, sleep-related
  categories of, 179
  glucose metabolism disorders in, **271–285.** See also *Obstructive sleep apnea (OSA), glucose metabolism disorders in.*

Bronchial asthma, hypoventilation due to, 258–259

Bruxism, RLS and, 387

C

Cardiovascular disease
  CPAP and, 189–190
  OSA in, pathophysiologic influence of, 204–207
    abnormal coagulation, 206–207
    arrhythmias, 206
    heart failure, 205
    heart rate variability, 206
    inflammation, 204–205

Clin Chest Med 31 (2010) 407–414
doi:10.1016/S0272-5231(10)00049-3
0272-5231/10/$ – see front matter

chestmed.theclinics.com

Moving?

Make sure your subscription moves with you!

To notify us of your new address, find your **Clinics Account Number** (located on your mailing label above your name), and contact customer service at:

Email: journalscustomerservice-usa@elsevier.com

800-654-2452 (subscribers in the U.S. & Canada)
314-447-8871 (subscribers outside of the U.S. & Canada)

Fax number: 314-447-8029

Elsevier Health Sciences Division
Subscription Customer Service
3251 Riverport Lane
Maryland Heights, MO 63043

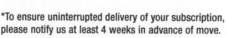
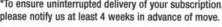

*To ensure uninterrupted delivery of your subscription, please notify us at least 4 weeks in advance of move.

Printed and bound by CPI Group (UK) Ltd, Croydon, CR0 4YY

03/10/2024

01040354-0009